CANCER IMMUNOTHERAPY
AND ITS IMMUNOLOGICAL BASIS

GANN Monograph on Cancer Research

The series of GANN Monograph on Cancer Research was initiated in 1966 by the late Dr. Tomizo Yoshida (1903–73) for the purpose of publishing proceedings of international conferences and symposia on cancer and allied research fields, and papers on specific subjects of importance in cancer research.

The decision to publish a monograph is made by the Editorial Board of the Japanese Cancer Association, with the final approval of the Board of Directors. It is hoped that the series will serve as an important source of information in cancer research.

Japanese Cancer Association

The publication of this monograph owes much to the financial support given by the late Professor Kazushige Higuchi of Jikei University.

JAPANESE CANCER ASSOCIATION

GANN Monograph on Cancer Research No.21

CANCER IMMUNOTHERAPY AND ITS IMMUNOLOGICAL BASIS

YUICHI YAMAMURA
Edited by MASAYASU KITAGAWA[†]
ICHIRO AZUMA

JAPAN SCIENTIFIC SOCIETIES PRESS, Tokyo
UNIVERSITY PARK PRESS, Baltimore

Published jointly by
JAPAN SCIENTIFIC SOCIETIES PRESS
Tokyo
and
UNIVERSITY PARK PRESS
Baltimore

Library of Congress Cataloging in Publication Data
Symposium on Cancer Immunotherapy and Its Immunological Basis, Osaka, 1977.
Cancer immunotherapy and its immunological basis.

(Gann monograph on cancer research; 21)
At head of title: Japanese Cancer Association.
Bibliography: p.
Includes index.
1. Cancer—Chemotherapy—Congresses. 2. Immunotherapy—Congresses. 3. BCG—Therapeutic use—Congresses. I. Yamamura, Yūichi, 1918–
II. Kitagawa, Masayasu. III. Azuma, Ichirō.
IV. Nippon Gan Gakkai. V. Title. VI. Series.
RC271. 145S88 1977 616.9′94′061 78-15589
ISBN 0-8391-1313-7

PREFACE

Recent progress in cancer immunotherapy has been promoted by rapidly advancing modern immunology. Tumor-specific antigens of various kinds of malignant cells were demonstrated by specified immunological techniques. The mechanisms of immune responses to tumor cells with special reference to cell-mediated cytotoxicity against cancer cells has also been clarified by many investigators.

The Symposium on "Cancer Immunotherapy and Its Immunological Basis," sponsored by the Japanese Cancer Association, was held in Osaka on May 28th and 29th, 1977. Twenty-three papers, including three papers by guest speakers from the United States, were presented.

The immunological basis of tumor immunotherapy has been summarized in the first part of this monograph.

The relationships of the antigenicity of tumor cells and tumor immunotherapy, the regulatory mechanism of the immune response to tumor cells, and the role of T cells as well as macrophages in the immune response to tumor cells were discussed; further, the trial to elevate tumor cell antigenicity by xenogenization or various kinds of adjuvant active substances, such as BCG and its cell-wall skeleton or *Propionibacterium acnes* were described and discussed.

BCG and other immunopotentiating substances are being used widely in order to enhance antitumor activities on an immunological basis both in experimental tumor systems and in human cancer patients. Some adjuvant active agents have been reported to induce antitumor immunity and have been used successfully in the treatment of cancer, however, many important problems remain unsolved.

Although BCG shows potent adjuvant activities in enhancing T cell functions such as induction of delayed-type hypersensitivity and cell-mediated cytotoxicity to tumor cells, BCG has many hazardous side-effects. Cancer patients are usually treated by radiotherapy and chemotherapy, which are mostly active in the sense of immunosuppression. Further, cancer patients are forced into an immunosuppressive state by some mechanisms due to the tumor-bearing state. For these reasons, BCG often exhibits unexpected side-effects in cancer patients. Consequently, in order to eliminate the side-effects of BCG, attempts have been made to isolate its active principle for tumor immunotherapy and to eliminate side-effects induced by these substances. For this purpose, BCG cell-wall skeleton (BCG-CWS), methanol-extraction residue (MER), cord factor, wax D, and water-soluble adjuvant substances were purified. Among these immunopotentiators, BCG-CWS and MER are being used clinically in the treatment of lung cancer, leukemia, melanoma, gastrointestinal cancer, and other malignant tumors. In this monograph, a comparison was made on the mechanism and clinical efficacy of BCG, BCG-CWS, MER, and *P. acnes*.

The term "Cancer Immunotherapy" is often widely used now, but this term should be defined clearly and scientifically to promote this new approach to cancer therapy.

"Cancer Immunotherapy" should be defined as follows:

1) Antitumor activities on the immunological mechanisms should be proved on an syngeneic or autochthonous tumor system of experimental animals.

2) Statistically evaluated efficacy should be confirmed by clinical application to cancer patients.

The following problems relating to "Cancer Immunotherapy" were emphasized in this monograph.

1) Elucidation of the mechanism of the immune response to tumor cells, which is related to the immunotherapy of tumor.

2) Development of the most effective way to enhance the immune response to tumor cells by the use of adjuvant active agents.

3) Evaluation of clinical efficacy of adjuvant active agents in the treatment of various kinds of cancer patients.

Dr. Masayasu Kitagawa, a member of an Organizing Committee of this Cancer Symposium and co-editor of this GANN Monograph on Cancer Research, passed away suddenly owing to subarachnoid bleeding on November 7th, 1977 at the age of 50 years. Dr. Kitagawa graduated from Kyushu University Medical School in 1953. From 1953 to 1963, he was a research associate and instructor at the Department of Medical Chemistry, Kyushu University Medical School. In 1963, he moved to the Institute for Cancer Research, Osaka University Medical School as Associate Professor and continued his work in the Rosewell Park Memorial Institute, U.S.A. from 1963 to 1965. In 1966, he was appointed as Professor and Chairman of the Department of Oncogenesis in the Institute for Cancer Research, Osaka University Medical School, and accomplished a tremendous amount of brilliant work in cellular immunology and tumor immunology before his tragic death.

The major works of Dr. Kitagawa in the field of tumor immunology consisted mainly of three parts: (a) Based on his deep knowledge of basic cellular immunology and immunochemistry, he clarified the selective suppression of T cell activity in a tumor-bearing host and in the process of chemical carcinogenesis; (b) with reference to the importance of T cell activity in tumor immunology, he attempted experimentally to improve the impaired T cell activity against the tumor (tumor-associated transplantation antigens), and established his concept oriented to tumor immunotherapy; (c) besides these experimental approaches for immunotherapy, he also clarified many intriguing cellular mechanisms associated with tumor immunology.

Dr. Kitagawa had always shown heart-warming sincerity to his friends, but was strict with himself. Anyone who had any contact with Dr. Kitagawa will keep a respectful memory of him. All the participants of the Cancer Symposium in Osaka pay their deepest respects to Dr. Kitagawa for his outstanding work on tumor immunology and for his cooperation.

August 1978

Yuichi Yamamura
Ichiro Azuma

CONTENTS

CLINICAL TRIALS. IV.
IMMUNOTHERAPY OF MALIGNANT MELANOMA

SUMMARY REMARKS

EXPERIMENTAL STUDY. I. CELLULAR MECHANISMS OF IMMUNE RESPONSES TO TUMOR ANTIGENS

GANN Monograph on Cancer Research 21, 1978

CHARACTERISTICS OF TUMOR-ASSOCIATED ANTIGEN IN CHEMICALLY INDUCED URINARY BLADDER CANCERS OF RATS

Yoshiyuki HASHIMOTO

*Department of Hygienic Chemistry, Pharmaceutical Institute, Tohoku University**

Antigen characteristics of urinary bladder cancers induced by N-butyl-N-(4-hydroxybutyl)nitrosamine in ACI/N rats were studied by several immunological methods. 1) Tumor-associated cell surface antigen was detected by a membrane immunofluorescence test with serum which was induced in allogeneic rats by a bladder cancer and absorbed with normal ACI rat cells. The serum showed positive immunofluorescence against 3 out of 7 bladder cancer lines, suggesting the presence of a common antigen among the cancers. 2) By transplantation immunity in syngeneic rats, 2 out of 6 cancer lines were found to have high antigenicity but antigenicities of the other 4 cancer lines were low or undetectable level. Cross transplantation resistance was observed in the 2 high antigenic cancer lines. 3) *In vitro* cytotoxicity of lymphoid cells from rats immunized with a high antigenic cancer was demonstrated specifically to cancer cells of the immunizing line but not to cancer cells of the other lines.

The difference between the antigens detected was summarized and discussed.

Tumor-associated antigen (TAA) is a general term for antigens which are present in tumors but not in normal cells. When an antigen is immunogenic against histocompatible (syngeneic or autochthonous) host and unless it is present in cells of any normal state, it can be defined as a tumor-specific antigen. If a tumor-associated or tumor-specific antigen is capable of inducing transplant rejection of a tumor, it is called tumor-associated transplantation antigen (TATA) or tumor-specific transplantation antigen (TSTA). It has been widely accepted that virus-induced tumors are characterized by the sharing of common antigens between different tumors induced by the same virus (2, 7, 10), whereas a majority of chemically induced murine tumors have TSTA characteristic to each individual tumor, although several reports (6, 8, 12, 22) have suggested the existence of a common TAA among certain types of tumors. The common antigen of chemically induced tumors was frequently identified as fetal antigen, as shown in aminoazo dye-induced hepatomas (1) and 3-methylcholanthrene (MCA)-induced fibrosarcomas in rats (20).

In urinary bladder tumors induced in mice and rats by MCA, Taranger *et al.* (19) demonstrated a wide distribution of a common TAA utilizing an *in vitro* cytotoxicity test, and they referred to such TAA as tissue type-specific antigen. Tissue type-specific

---

* Aobayama, Aramaki, Sendai 980, Japan (橋本嘉幸).

TAA has also been demonstrated by an *in vitro* cell-mediated cytotoxicity test in human urinary bladder tumors by several authors (*3–5, 15, 16*). In contrast, Wahl *et al.* (*21*) failed to detect a common antigen in MCA-induced mouse bladder tumors by transplantation immunity. Whether this discrepancy is derived from different analytical methods or different etiology of the tumors is not known.

We induced bladder cancers in ACI/N rats of an inbred strain by a nitrosamine derivative, N-butyl-N-(4-hydroxybutyl)nitrosamine (BBN), and several of them were maintained by serial transplantations into syngeneic rats and by tissue culture (*14*). We studied antigenic characteristics of these bladder cancers in order to know whether they have individually specific antigen or common antigen. This article summarizes the results and discusses the identity or difference between antigens detected by different immunological methods.

Tumors

Seven transplantation lines (BC12, BC31, BC35, BC41, BC43, BC47, and BC50) of BBN-induced cancers originating in different ACI rats were used at 10 to 20 passage generations. The primary tumors of the cancers showed similar histological patterns and all were diagnosed as transitional cell carcinoma. A single cell suspension was prepared from the tumor transplant by treating the well-minced tumor fragments with 0.25% trypsin solution containing 0.05% EDTA. Tissue culture lines (BC12TC, BC35TC, BC47TC, and BC50TC) were also employed for the target cells of *in vitro* tests following trypsinization with 0.125% trypsin solution. For immunofluorescence (IF) testing, trypsinized cells were preincubated in culture medium for 2 hr at 37°. In addition to bladder cancers, several ACI rat tumors including ascites hepatomas (AH3683, AH35TC2, AH3934A and HE 1), an MCA-induced ascites sarcoma (AMC60), and a nitrosourea-induced gastric sarcoma were used for the membrane IF test.

Cell Surface Antigen Detected by Antiserum Raised in Allogeneic Rat against ACI Rat Bladder Cancer

Donryu rats were immunized 4 times with BC47 bladder cancer. Serum from the immunized rats was highly cytotoxic to lymph node cells and thymocytes of an ACI rat in the presence of a guinea-pig complement, cytotoxic titers of which were 1/2,048 and 1/64, respectively, to the former and the latter cells. This cytotoxicity was abolished by repeated *in vitro* absorption of the serum with ACI rat lymphoid cells or with ACI rat hepatoma cells. These findings suggest that the immune serum contained an antibody against histocompatibility antigen of the ACI rat. *In vivo* absorption was also effective for removing the anti-histocompatibility antibody from the serum. Three milliliters of the serum was injected intraperitoneally into an ACI rat and serum was prepared from the blood which was collected 5 hr after the injection. The unabsorbed serum and absorbed serum were inactivated for 30 min at 56° and used for the IF tests.

Membrane IF testing was carried out by the method of Möller (*13*); target cells were treated with 1: 10 diluted unabsorbed serum or 1: 5 diluted absorbed serum and then with 1:20 diluted FITC-conjugated rabbit IgG anti-mouse IgG, each for 30 min at 37°.

The unabsorbed serum showed a positive IF to normal ACI rat cells including lymph node cells, trypsinized lung cells and bladder epithelial cells, and to cells of ACI rat tumors including bladder cancers, hepatomas, MCA-sarcoma and gastric sarcoma, while IF by the absorbed serum was negative against all cells examined except a few bladder cancer cell lines. Among 7 bladder cancer cell lines, BC47 cells showed strong IF by reacting with the absorbed serum, BC31 and BC50 cells showed weak IF, and BC12, BC35, BC41 and BC43 cells did not show IF. Cells of a transplantation line and of the corresponding tissue culture line gave a similar IF pattern. These findings suggest that bladder cancer cells of 3 lines share common TAA which is detected by an antibody present in the absorbed serum. This was substantiated by a further absorption of the absorbed serum with various normal tissues and tumor cells of ACI rats. The antibody present in the absorbed serum was absorbable by only the above 3 lines of bladder cancer cells, and not by other cells.

TSTA

The ligation-and-release method of Takeda *et al.* (*18*) was employed for the induction of transplantation immunity against syngeneic bladder cancers in ACI rats. This method is known to be a simple and effective method for inducing transplantation immunity against tumor cells in the syngeneic and autochthonous animals. When the tumor grew to about 2 cm in diameter, it was ligated tightly with a circular rubber string together with the overlaying skin. The rubber string was removed 24 hr later. At the time when the tumor regressed completely, the animals were challenged subcutaneously with 2 million cancer cells of the immunizing line at the contralateral flank, and the tumor growth was compared with that in untreated control rats. When the challenged cancer cells grew in the recipient animal, the newly developed tumor nodule was treated as above and the second challenge was undertaken. This procedure was repeated 3 times at most, then the growth of tumor was observed.

As shown in Fig. 1, rats acquired transplantation resistance after the first immunization with BC47 or BC35 cells and rejected the challenging cancer cells of the immunizing line. Whereas BC12, BC31, BC43, and BC50 cells grew in the rats which had been immunized 2 to 3 times with the respective cancers, the growth rate was similar to the rate in normal rats. These findings suggest that BC35 and BC47 cells have high antigenicity expressed as TSTA, but TSTAs of the other 4 bladder cancer cell lines are very low or undetectable.

In order to determine whether the present bladder cancers have common TSTA, the rats that had been immunized with BC47 or BC35 cells were challenged with cancer cells of each line. Those rats which had been immunized with BC47 cells rejected BC35 cells as well as rechallenged BC47 cells. However, they did not show transplantation resistance against BC12, BC31, BC43, or BC50 cells. Similar results were obtained with BC35-immune rats and they rejected BC47 as well as BC35 cells.

Taken together, the above results indicate that 2 out of 6 bladder cancer lines have high antigenicity in the TSTA, whereas the other 4 lines show little or no antige-

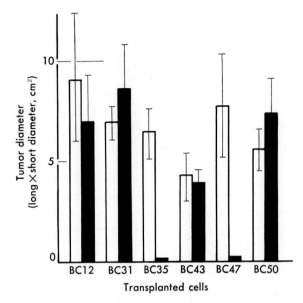

FIG. 1. Transplantation resistance against bladder cancers of the immunizing lines
     Immunized rats, which had been treated 2 to 3 times with the ligation-and-release
method, and unimmunized control rats, were injected with 2×10^6 cancer cells of the
immunizing line. The size of tumors was measured after 3 weeks, except BC43 and
BC50 tumors whose size was measured after 2 and 4 weeks, respectively. Size of tumor
in control rats (□) and in immunized rats (■).

nicity in the syngeneic animals, and 2 high antigenic cancers seem to have a common
TSTA. However, the presence of a common TSTA was not substantiated by the following *in vitro* cytotoxicity test using immune lymphoid cells.

Antigens Determined by In Vitro Cytotoxicity Tests

     ACI rats were repeatedly immunized with a high antigenic bladder cancer, BC47
or BC35 cells. Serum from the rat did not show complement-dependent cytotoxicity
to bladder cancer cells. IF testing by the serum against bladder cancer cells was also
negative. In contrast, as illustrated in Fig. 2, peritoneal exudate cells and spleen cells
of the immune rats demonstrated a marked cytotoxicity against cancer cells of the immunizing line, as assayed by the microtestplate method of Takasugi and Klein (*17*).
Since removal of adherent cells did not alter the cytotoxic activity of the aggressor cells,
the effector principle of the immune lymphoid cells were attributable to non-adherent
cells which were mainly lymphocytes. Testing of the cross reactivity of the immune
lymphoid cells to bladder cancers revealed that the immune lymphoid cells specifically
killed cancer cells of the immunizing line, *i.e.*, BC47- and BC35-immune lymphoid cells
killed BC47 and BC35 cells, respectively, but not the other cancer cells (Fig. 3), indicating that these 2 high antigenic cancers have individually specific antigen as dis-
tinguished by immune lymphoid cells.

     The above *in vitro* results were inconsistent with those of the transplantation ex-
periments by which cross resistance was observed between BC35 and BC47 cancer

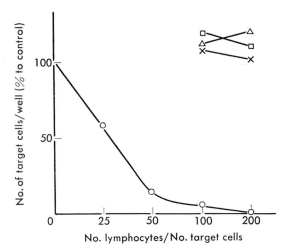

Fig. 2. *In vitro* cytotoxicity of BC47-immune lymphoid cells against ACI rat bladder cancer cells

Cytotoxicity of non-adherent peritoneal exudate cells from normal and BC47-immune rats was assayed with Falcon #3034 microtestplate. The number of cancer cells remaining in a well was counted after 24 hr. Target cells: BC47 (○), BC12 (△), BC35 (□), BC50 (×).

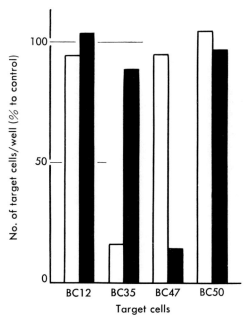

Fig. 3. *In vitro* cytotoxicity of spleen cells from normal, BC35-immune, and BC47-immune rats

Spleen cells were added to target cancer cells at the ratio of 100: 1, and the number of cancer cells remaining in a well was counted after 24 hr. Target cells with BC35-immune spleen cells (□), and with BC47-immune spleen cells (■) (percent of target cells to those with normal spleen cells).

cells. It seems possible, however, that immunization of an animal by a line of highly antigenic tumor cells induces not only the effector cells specific for those of the immunizing line but also stimulates an immune mechanism which is capable of eradicating the secondarily grafted, highly antigenic tumor cells of a different line without participation of a common antigen. This can be supported by the evidence obtained by Kobayashi *et al.* (*11*) and by Hosokawa *et al.* (*9*) that treatment of animals with allogeneic tumor cells or allogeneic normal tissues augments induction of transplantation immunity to subsequently inoculated tumor cells with antigen that is unrelated to the immunizing allogeneic cells.

CONCLUSIONS AND DISCUSSION

Antigenic characters of BBN-induced bladder cancers of ACI rats are summarized in Table I. A common antigen was detected in 3 cancer lines by an IF test using anti-BC47 serum which was induced in allogeneic rats and absorbed with normal ACI rat cells. However, this common antigen was not related to TSTA, suggesting that the antigen is TAA, but it may not act as an immunogen in the histocompatible host. By transplantation immunity in the syngeneic rats, 2 out of 6 cancer lines showed a high antigenicity, whereas the other 4 cancer lines had low or undetectable antigenicity. The 2 highly antigenic cancers gave rise to cross resistance in the immunized rats. However, this may not be due to the existence of a common antigen in the cancers as discussed above, since lymphoid cells from rats immunized with one cancer did not kill another cancer.

TABLE I. Antigens of BBN-induced ACI Rat Bladder Cancers
Detected by Different Methods

Cancer line	Cell surface antigen detected by absorbed Donryu anti-BC47 serum	Antigenicity (TSTA)	Cross reaction in transplantation immunity	Cytotoxicity of lymphocytes from rats of:	
				BC35-immune type	BC47-immune type
BC12	−	Low	−	−	−
BC31	+	Low	−	−	
BC35	−	High	+	+	−
BC43	−	Low	−		
BC47	+	High	+	−	+
BC50	+	Low	−	−	−

Acknowledgments

The author is most grateful to Drs. S. Odashima and M. Ishidate, Jr., of the National Institute for Hygienic Sciences, Tokyo, who donated the tumors used for this research.

The author is also grateful to Mrs. H. Kitagawa for her cooperation in this work. A part of the work has been done in the Tokyo Biochemical Research Institute, Tokyo, and I thank Dr. M. Okada, Director of the Institute. This work was supported by a Grant-in-Aid for Cancer Research from the Ministry of Education, Science and Culture of Japan.

REFERENCES

1. Baldwin, R. W. Immunological aspects of chemical carcinogenesis. *Adv. Cancer Res.*, **18**, 1–75 (1973).

2. Bauer, H. Virion and tumor antigens of C-type RNA tumor viruses. *Adv. Cancer Res.*, **20**, 275–341 (1974).

3. Bean, M. A., Pees, H., Fogh, J. E., Grabstald, H., and Oettgen, H. F. Cytotoxicity of lymphocytes from patients with cancer of the urinary bladder; detection by ^{3}H-proline microcytotoxicity test. *Int. J. Cancer*, **14**, 186–197 (1974).

4. Bubenik, J., Perlmann, P., Helmstein, K., and Moberger, G. Immune response to urinary bladder tumors in man. *Int. J. Cancer*, **5**, 39–46 (1970).

5. Bubenik, J., Baresová, M., Viklicky, V., Jakoubková, J., Sainerová, H., and Donner, J. Established cell line of urinary bladder carcinoma (T 24) containing tumor-specific antigen. *Int. J. Cancer*, **11**, 765–773 (1973).

6. Hellström, I., Hellström, K. E., and Pierce, G. E. *In vitro* studies of immune reactions against autochthonous and syngeneic mouse tumors induced by methylcholanthrene and plastic discs. *Int. J. Cancer*, **3**, 467–482 (1968).

7. Hellström, K. E. and Hellström, I. Cellular immunity against tumor antigens. *Adv. Cancer Res.*, **12**, 167–223 (1969).

8. Holmes, E. C., Morton, P. L., Schidlovsky, G., and Trahan, E. Cross-reacting tumor specific transplantation antigens in methylcholanthrene induced guinea pig sarcomas, *J. Natl. Cancer Inst.*, **46**, 693–700 (1971).

9. Hosokawa, M., Imamura, T., Oikawa, T., Nakayama, M., Gotohda, E., Sendo, F., Kodama, T., and Kobayashi, H. Inhibition of tumor growth in rats immunized with skin graft. *Int. J. Cancer*, **18**, 369–374 (1976).

10. Klein, E., Klein, G., Nadkarni, J. S., Nadkarni, J. J., Wigzell, H., and Clifford, P. Surface IgM-kappa specificity on a Burkitt lymphoma cell *in vivo* and in derived culture lines. *Cancer Res.*, **28**, 1300–1310 (1968).

11. Kobayashi, H., Gothoda, H., Kuzumaki, N., Takeichi, N., Hosokawa, M., and Kodama, T. Reduced transplantability of syngeneic tumors in rats immunized with allogeneic tumors. *Int. J. Cancer*, **13**, 522–529 (1974).

12. Mckhann, C. F. and Harder, F. H. Tumor-specific antigens of methylcholanthrene-induced sarcomas; *in vitro* studies. *Transplantation*, **6**, 655–656 (1968)

13. Möller, G. Demonstration of mouse isoantigens at the cellular level by the fluorescent antibody technique. *J. Exp. Med.*, **114**, 415–434 (1961).

14. Noda, M. and Hashimoto, Y. Transplantability of urinary bladder cancers induced in ACI/N rats by oral administration of butyl-(4-hydroxybutyl)nitrosamine and its acetate. *Japan. J. Urol.*, **64**, 397–401 (1973).

15. O'Toole, C., Perlmann, P., Unsgaad, B., Moberger, G., and Edsmyr, F. Cellular immunity to human urinary bladder carcinoma. I. Correlation to clinical stage and radiotherapy. *Int. J. Cancer*, **10**, 77–91 (1972).

16. O'Toole, C., Stejskal, V., Perlmann, P., and Karlsson, M. Lymphoid cells mediating tumor-specific cytotoxicity to carcinoma of the urinary bladder: Separation of the effector population using a surface marker. *J. Exp. Med.*, **139**, 457–466 (1974).

17. Takasugi, M. and Klein, E. The methodology of microassay for cell-mediated immunity. *Transplantation*, **9**, 219–223 (1970).

18. Takeda, K., Aizawa, M., Kikuchi, Y., Yamawaki, S., and Nakamura, K. Tumor autoimmunity against methylcholanthrene-induced sarcomas of the rat. *Gann*, **57**, 221–240 (1966).

19. Taranger, L. A., Chapman, W. H., Hellström, I., and Hellström, K. E. Immunological studies on urinary bladder tumors of rats and mice. *Science*, **176**, 1337–1340 (1972).
20. Thompson, D. M. and Alexander, P. A cross-acting embryonic antigen in the membrane of rat sarcoma cells which is immunogenic in the syngeneic host. *Br. J. Cancer*, **27**, 35–47 (1973).
21. Wahl, D. V., Chapman, W. H., Hellström, I., and Hellström, K. E. Transplantation immunity to individually unique antigens of chemically-induced bladder tumors in mice. *Int. J. Cancer*, **14**, 114–121 (1974).
22. Zbar, B., Wepsick, H. T., Rapp, H. G., Borsos, T., Kronman, B. S., and Churchill, W. H. Antigenic specificity of hepatomas induced in strain 2 guinea pigs by diethyl-nitrosamine. *J. Natl. Cancer Inst.*, **43**, 833–841 (1969).

GANN Monograph on Cancer Research 21, 1978

I REGION EXPRESSION ON CYTOTOXIC AND SUPPRESSOR T CELLS AGAINST SYNGENEIC TUMORS IN THE MOUSE

Shigeyoshi Fujimoto and Tomio Tada

*Laboratories for Immunology, School of Medicine, Chiba University**

The splenic thymus-derived lymphocytes (T cells) from animals bearing a growing syngeneic tumor specifically suppressed the activity of cytotoxic T cells (Tc) which were activated *in vivo* or *in vitro* by the homologous or cross-reactive tumor. The suppressor T cell (Ts) from the tumor-bearing host was killed by alloantisera against the product of the *I-J* subregion of the *H-2* histocompatibility complex. The Tc against some, but not all, tumor cell lines was also found to express Ia antigen coded for by a gene mapped in *I-A* subregion of the *H-2* complex. In general, those activated by newly established tumor cell lines possessed Ia antigen, while some other old cell lines, which were capable of growing across the *H-2* barrier, induced the Ia negative Tc. It was also found that Ts and Tc recognize different antigenic determinants present on the tumor cell, and that the Ts acts to suppress the Tc only in the presence of an antigen recognizable by Ts. These results give a clue for studying the multicellular interactions in the tumor immunity.

Our ideas on the multicellular response against tumor antigens evolves from the recent knowledge of the interactions of functionally different thymus-derived lymphocytes (T cells) which augment or suppress the immune response. One of the central issues in tumor immunology is concerned with the question of why normal animals usually do not exert strong immunological resistance against growing tumors, although these animals are potentially capable of doing so under certain circumstances. These are when the tumor has been surgically removed in the early phase of its growth, or when the host has been actively immunized with unreplicable live tumor cells. Recent reports from various laboratories including ours suggest that this apparent inability to develop immunity to the primary tumor is not due to the total lack of cellular response, but rather due to the induction of suppressor T cells (Ts) in the tumor-bearing host (TBH). The Ts appears to inhibit both the afferent and efferent limbs of tumor immunity, thus prevent the animals from active resistance against tumor growth (*4, 14*).

Fujimoto and his co-workers (*4, 5*) first demonstrated evidence that the spleen cells from TBH can inhibit the rejection of the secondary tumor implants upon transfer to the syngeneic immune host. The cell type responsible for this inhibition of tumor immunity has been determined to be a T cell which, by itself cannot kill the tumor cells but, nevertheless, is specifically generated by the growing homologous tumor. A similar

* Inohana 1-8-1, Chiba 280, Japan (藤本重義, 多田富雄).

observation has been reported by Takei *et al.* (*14, 15*) suggesting that the presence of such Ts inhibits the development of tumor immunity. Hence, it is apparent that a growing tumor activates a population of T cells by which the immunological resistance of the host to the tumor is paradoxically inhibited. These observations led us to study the nature of the above Ts involved in the prevention of tumor immunity, and the condition in which such cells are made active. One of our principal concerns is directed towards the mode of cellular interactions between Ts and other cell types which participate in the rejection of the tumor. Briefly reviewed in this paper are our recent studies on the characteristics of these subsets of T cells which interact to suppress tumor immunity, and some facets of these interactions which prevent the induction of tumor immunity are discussed.

Presence of Ts in the Spleen of Tumor-bearing Hosts

A 3-methylcholanthrene-induced sarcoma, S1509a, of the A/J mouse origin can grow in either syngeneic A/J or *H-2* histocompatible B10.A mice upon subcutaneous inoculation in the primary host, and generally kills the host within 40 days. However, if the animals were actively immunized with a subcutaneous injection of 1×10^6 cells of mitomycin C (MMC)-treated homologous tumor, they do not allow the growth of S1509a, leading to the rapid rejection of the secondary transplant.

This acquired immunity is also readily observed by neutralization of tumor growth

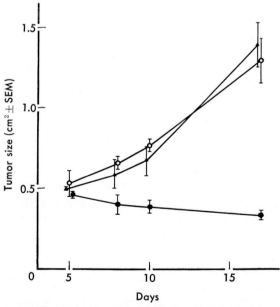

FIG. 1.   Growth of S1509a mixed with either immune lymphoid cells to S1509a (Tc) or Tc plus spleen cells of S1509a-bearing host (Ts)

In the control 5.0×10^5 S1509a were mixed with 2.5×10^7 Tc plus 2.5×10^7 normal spleen cells (●). Experimental groups received a subcutaneous injection of 5.0×10^5 S1509a cells mixed with 2.5×10^7 Tc plus 2.5×10^7 Ts (○), or with 2.5×10^7 normal spleen cells and 2.5×10^7 Ts (▲). Each group consisted of four animals.

with immune spleen and lymph node cells by the Winn test (16). S1509a (5×10^5 cells) was mixed with 2.5×10^7 immune or normal lymph node cells and inoculated subcutaneously into B10.A mice. Whereas the S1509a mixed with normal lymph node cells made a rapid growth in the primary host, the tumor growth was completely inhibited by concomitant inoculation of the lymph node cells obtained from S1509a-immune animals (Fig. 1). The neutralizing activity was found to be mediated by Thy 1 antigen-positive T cells (Tc) in the lymph node of immune animals. Such an activity was not found in the spleen cells of TBH in which S1509a was growing. If the tumor cells were admixed with 2.5×10^7 immune cells (Tc) and an equal number of spleen cells from TBH (Ts), the tumor growth was comparable to that without immune lymph node cells which contain cytotoxic T cells (Tc). The results indicate that the spleen cells from TBH suppressed the neutralizing activity of Tc directed to the homologous tumor. This suppressive effect of spleen cells of TBH on Tc was completely removed by treating the spleen cells with anti-Thy 1.2 and C, thus the suppressive effect was exerted by T cells (Ts) generated in TBH. The result is in accordance with the previous result that the suppression of tumor rejection in the immune hosts was mediated by Thy 1 antigen-positive spleen cells (Ts) from TBH (4).

Presence of I-J Subregion Gene Product on Ts in the Tumor-bearing Host

It has recently been demonstrated that the Ts observed in antigen-specific (13) and allotype-specific (10) suppressions carries a determinant coded for by gene(s) in the I-J subregion which was newly determined to be intercalated between the I-B and I-C subregions of the mouse H-2 complex. Therefore, we attempted to learn whether the Ts in TBH would have a similar determinant coded for by the I-J subregion.

The spleen cells from TBH, which had been shown to have a suppressive effect on tumor rejection, were treated with one of the two alloantisera directed to different subregions of the mouse H-2 complex. B10.A(3R) anti-B10.A(5R) is an antiserum specific for the I-J subregion of the H-2^k haplotype, and an antiserum (C3H.Q × B10.D2)F$_1$ anti-AQR is specific for the I-A, I-B, and I-J subregions. The latter antiserum was made specific for the I-A and I-B subregions of H-2^k by absorbing the antiserum with spleen cells of B10.A(5R) which has in common the I-J subregion of the H-2^k haplotype origin. Twenty million per milliliter spleen cells of S1509a-bearing A/J mice were treated with a 1:10 dilution of one of the above antiserum and C, and then were added to the 1:50 mixture of tumor cells and immune lymph node cells. The total mixture was injected subcutaneously into B10.A mice, and the growth of the implanted tumor was measured.

Figure 2 shows a representative result of the experiment. The control is the growth curve of S1509a mixed with immune lymph node cells and untreated TBH spleen cells (Tc+Ts), which shows no inhibition of tumor growth. This indicates that the dose of Ts in TBH spleen is sufficient to neutralize the cytotoxic activity of immune lymph node cells under this experimental condition. If the spleen cells of TBH (Ts) were pretreated with the antiserum 3R anti-5R, which was directed to the I-J subregion of H-2^k, the growth of S1509a was completely inhibited, indicating that the immunosuppressive activity of TBH spleen cells was abrogated by treatment with anti-I-J^k. On the contrary, treatment with antiserum directed to the I-A and I-B subregions did

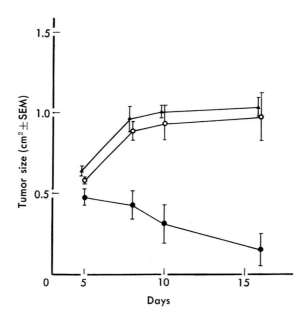

FIG. 2.   Presence of *I-J* subregion product on suppressor T cells from tumor-bearing host

S1509a (5.0×10^5 cells) were mixed with Tc and untreated spleen cells of TBH (Ts) at tumor/Tc/Ts ratio of 1 : 50 : 50 (control, ▲). In the experimental groups Ts was treated with B10. A(3R) anti-B10. A(5R) (anti-*I-J^k*) (●), or with (C3HQ×B10. D2)F$_1$ anti-AQR absorbed with B10. A(5R) (anti-*I-A^k*, *I-B^k*) and C (○).

not abolish the suppressive effect of TBH spleen cells, resulting in the normal growth of S1509a. These results indicate that spleen cells of TBH contain a population of lymphocytes which suppress the activity of Tc, thus inhibiting the neutralization of tumor growth by Tc against the homologous tumor. The results clearly demonstrate that the activity of Ts was completely removed by treating the cells with anti-*I-J* and C, but not with anti-*I-A* and *I-B*.

In Vitro Demonstration of Ia Antigens Determined by Different Loci in the H-2 Complex on Functionally Different Subsets of T Cells in Tumor Immunity

Since the above experiments indicate that the Ts generated in TBH can suppress the activity of Tc which acts to reject the syngeneic tumor, we are naturally interested in the phenotypic expressions on both cell types. It is obvious that the resistance to syngeneic tumors may well depend on the balance of these cell types generated in the host, and hence the examination of phenotypic differences between these cell types may be of importance in the study of the regulatory events in tumor immunity. To study this, we have utilized an *in vitro* culture system in which Tc was cultured with ^{51}Cr-labeled target cells, and the Ts from TBH was added at different doses.

The Tc specific for spontaneous lymphoma (L1117) of the A/J mouse origin was induced *in vitro* by the following procedure: A mixture of unprimed spleen and lymph node cells was cultured for 5 days with MMC-treated L1117 cells at a responder/

TABLE I. *I* Region Specificity Expressed on Ts for L1117

Tc specific for L1117	Ts treated with	*I* region specificity	Lysis (%)	Suppression
+	Control[a]	—	12.2	—
+	Untreated	—	0.5	+
+	A.TH anti-A.TL	*A, B, J, E, C*	11.4	—
+	(B10.HTT×A.BY)F₁ anti-A.TL	*A, B, J*	9.2	—
+	B10.A(3R) anti-B10.A(5R)	*J*	11.9	—
+	B10.S(7R) anti-B10.HTT	*E, C*	2.5	+
+	NMS	—	1.2	+

Effector/suppressor/target ratio=40 : 40 : 1.
[a] Normal spleen cells.

stimulator ratio of 100: 1. For the cytotoxic assay, the cultured lymphoid cells were mixed with 1.5×10^4 ^{51}Cr-labeled target L1117 cells, and were incubated for 6 hr in a microtestplate at an effector/target cell ratio of 40: 1. The cultured lymphoid cells with the tumor cells showed a significant specific cytotoxicity for L1117 cells, indicating that lymphoid cells from syngeneic animals can be activated to become Tc by *in vitro* incubation with MMC-treated L1117. To observe the *in vitro* suppression of this cyto-toxic killing by Tc, 6×10^5 spleen cells from an L1117-bearing host were added to the mixture of *in vitro* activated Tc and ^{51}Cr-labeled target cells, and the degree of specific ^{51}Cr release was likewise measured. It was found that the addition of spleen cells from L1117 TBH significantly suppressed the ^{51}Cr release of target cells induced by *in vitro* activated Tc (Table I).

The *I* region gene expression on the Ts from TBH was studied by treating the suppressive spleen cells with various alloantisera directed to restricted subregions of the *H-2* complex, and then added to the mixture of the target and Tc. The results are summarized in Table I. The antiserum A.TH anti-A.TL (anti-*I^k*) was always found capable of removing Ts activity. The other antiserum (B10.HTT×A.BY)F₁ anti-A.TL, which is specific for *I-A*, *I-B*, and *I-J* subregions had the ability to remove Ts. As was expected, the antiserum specific only for *I-J^k* (3R anti-5R) could also kill the Ts, and thus the antisera containing *I-J^k* specificity were constantly capable of remov-ing the Ts activity of spleen cells from an L1117-bearing host. On the other hand, an antiserum putatively reactive to the *I-E* and *I-C* subregions (7R anti-HTT) was not able to remove the Ts activity. These results collectively indicate that the Ts in L1117-bearing animals has an expression of the *I-J* subregion, and can suppress the cytotoxic killing of L1117 cells by *in vitro* activated Tc. Other experiments indicated that this suppression of Tc activity by Ts was strictly tumor-specific (see below), and thus in this *in vitro* system the tumor-specific Ts was found to carry determinants coded for by a gene in the *I-J* subregion.

A similar approach was made to determine cell surface markers on Tc for L1117. The activated lymphoid cells capable of killing L1117 cells were treated with various alloantisera and C, and then tested for their cytotoxic activity by mixing with ^{51}Cr-labeled L1117 cells. The Tc activity against L1117 was removed by treatment either with anti-Thy 1.2 or with anti-*I^k* and C, indicating that the Tc for L1117 is a T cell having the Ia determinant (data not shown). In order to map the gene which codes

TABLE II. *I* Region Specificity Expressed on Tc for L1117

Tc treated with	*I* region specificity	Lysis (%)	Cytotoxicity
Untreated	—	11.0	+
A.TH anti-A.TL	*A, B, J, E, C*	0.4	—
[A.TH×B10.S(9R)]F₁ anti-A.TL	*A, B, C*	0	—
(B10.HTT×A.BY)F₁ anti-A.TL	*A, B, J*	2.9	—
B10.A(4R) anti-B10.A(2R)	*B, J, E, C*	10.1	+
B10.A(3R) anti-B10.A(5R)	*J*	9.5	+
B10.S(7R) anti-B10.HTT	*E, C*	7.9	+
(B10.K×A.TL)F₁ anti-B10.A	*C*	9.5	+
NMS	—	10.7	+

Effector/target ratio=40:1.   Target: L1117 cell.

for the Ia antigen on Tc, the cells were treated with various alloantisera directed to restricted subregions of the *H-2* complex as listed in Table II. The results in Table II clearly indicate that only antisera having specificity against the *I-A* subregion can remove the Tc activity for L1117, whereas those lacking *I-A* subregion specificity are incapable of killing the Tc. The result is different from those of other investigators who showed that Tc against allogeneic target cells possesses no Ia determinant on it (*9*).

Based upon the above findings, we have attempted to learn whether or not the Tc against syngeneic and allogeneic tumors always have an *I* region determinant. Three tumor cell lines of the A/J origin were utilized to study this problem. In addition to L1117 and S1509a, another 3-methylcholanthrene-induced sarcoma, SaI was used as a stimulator of Tc. Lymphoid cells from syngeneic A/J and allogeneic C3H and SJL mice were stimulated *in vitro* with MMC-treated cell lines for 5 days; the Tc thus obtained were treated with appropriate anti-Ia antisera. These treated Tc were then

TABLE III. Presence of Ia Antigen on Tc to Some Tumor Cell
Lines of the A/J Mouse Origin

Strain	*H-2* haplotype	Tc treated with	Lysis (%)		
			L1117	S1509a	SaI
A/J	*H-2ᵃ*	None	12.0	6.3	9.1
		A.TH anti-A.TLᵃ	1.2	1.2	10.8
		A.TL anti-A.THᵇ	12.8	5.4	11.0
C3H	*H-2ᵏ*	None	11.4	14.3	13.2
		A.TH anti-A.TL	0	0	9.3
		A.TL anti-A.TH	14.8	NDᶜ	ND
SJL	*H-2ˢ*	None	12.7	ND	6.1
		A.TH anti-A.TL	15.7	ND	ND
		A.TL anti-A.TH	4.3	ND	6.8

[a] Anti-*Iᵏ*.
[b] Anti-*Iˢ*.
[c] ND: not done.

tested for their cytotoxic activity against the homologous tumor cells and their results are shown in Table III. It is clearly seen that Tc stimulated with L1117 and S1509a are killed by appropriate anti-*I* region antisera both in syngeneic and allogeneic systems, whereas the Tc activated by SaI was not affected by anti-Ia antisera. It was further shown that Tc of A/J activated by EL-4, an allogeneic tumor cell line of *H-2^b* mouse origin, was not killed by anti-Ia antisera (data not shown). These results indicate that the Ia antigen is not expressed on Tc against certain syngeneic and allogeneic tumors. Since the expression of Ia antigen on Tc is dependent on the cell lines used for stimulation regardless of their genetic origin, it is suggested that there exist two types of Tc, one having Ia antigen, and the other lacking this expression. It is not known at present what causes such a disparity in the expression of Ia antigen on Tc, but this may depend on the nature of the tumor cell lines. Both SaI and EL-4 have a long, established history, and can occasionally grow in allogeneic mice if the dose of tumor cells is high. On the other hand, L1117 and S1509a cannot grow across the major histocompatibility barrier. The contribution of a large amount of virus production in SaI and EL-4 should also be considered.

Tc and Ts Recognize Different Antigenic Determinants on Tumor Cells

A previous study by one of the authors (*3*) demonstrated that there exists a cross reactivity between two 3-methylcholanthrene-induced sarcomas, S1509a and SaI in the effector phase. This was shown by the fact that the animals immunized with S1509a could also reject SaI, and *vice versa*. However, this cross reactivity was not demonstrable at the level of Ts: the Ts obtained from S1509a-TBH was not able to suppress the cross-reactive rejection process against SaI, and *vice versa*, and thus it was suggested that Tc and Ts would recognize different antigenic determinants expressed on tumor cells. Similar but more definite findings were shown in the *in vitro* cytotoxic assay. The Tc stimulated with MMC-treated S1509a showed comparable cytotoxic activity for both homologous S1509a and cross-reactive SaI (see Table IV). The Ts specific for S1509a could suppress the cytotoxic activity against S1509a, but the same Ts was found inactive in suppressing the cross-reactive cytotoxic activity against SaI. On the other hand, Ts derived from an SaI-bearing host could suppress the cytotoxic activity against the homologous SaI regardless of the fact that this cytotoxicity was exerted by Tc induced by S1509a.

TABLE IV.   Recognition of Different Determinants on Closely-related
Tumor Cell Lines by Tc and Ts

Tumor cell	Tc specific for	Ts specific for	Lysis[b] (%)
S1509a	S1509a	—[a]	17.7
SaI	S1509a	—[a]	17.3
S1509a	S1509a	S1509a	0
SaI	S1509a	S1509a	26.3
SaI	S1509a	SaI	3.9

Effector/suppressor/target ratio=40 : 40 : 1.
[a] Normal spleen cells.
[b] ^{51}Cr-release assay was performed by 16-hr incubation.

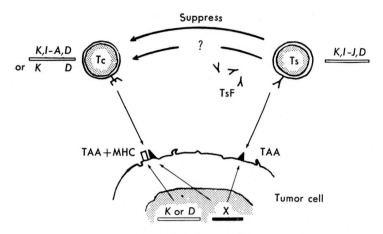

FIG. 3.   MHC gene expressions and possible recognition structures on Tc and Ts
     TAA, tumor-associated antigen; MHC, major histocompatibility complex; X,
gene(s) codes for tumor-associated antigen.

These results suggest that two closely related sarcomas, S1509a and SaI, possess two distinct types of antigenic determinants; one is shared by these two tumors and the other is unique to the individual tumor. Thus, the Tc would react with the cross-reactive determinants which have a common structure for both tumors, whereas the Ts can recognize only the individual tumor-associated antigens. Therefore, it seems that Ts can suppress the activity of Tc when the relevant antigen to Ts is present in the system.

From these results and those obtained by other investigators, we would suggest a possible mechanism in the regulation of the immune response against syngeneic tumors, as illustrated in Fig. 3. In this scheme, cross-reactive determinants which are recognized by the Tc are the complex of tumor-associated antigen and self-histocompatibility antigens determined by the *K* or *D* locus of the *H-2* complex, *i.e.*, "altered self" (*6*, *12*). The individual antigenic determinant recognizable by Ts is the tumor-associated antigen itself. The latter is highly probable, because the antigen-specific Ts cell can be generated in the absence of macrophages (*1*, *8*), and the Ts can be adsorbed to an antigen-coated column (*11*). In the observed suppression of cytotoxic killing of tumor cells, Ts and Tc would react with these different antigenic determinants, and the Ts would give a suppressive signal to the Tc, either by cell to cell contact or *via* specific factor released from Ts. The presence of such a soluble material has been reported previously (*2*, *7*). The expression of *I* region determinants on Ts and some of Tc may have some bearing on this cell-to-cell communication but the mechanism for it is still wide open for investigation.

CONCLUSION

The Tc against syngeneic tumors can be generated *in vitro* by culturing spleen and lymph node cells with unreplicable live tumor cells. They are capable of killing the target tumor cells *in vitro*, and can inhibit the tumor growth *in vivo* when they are admixed with homologous tumor cells at implantation. We have found that the Tc activated with some tumors (L1117 and S1509a) carry Ia antigen coded for by a gene in the *I-A* subregion of the *H-2* complex, while those activated with other tumors (SaI and EL-4) do not express this Ia antigen. At the moment it is not known what causes the difference in the *I* region expression on Tc against different tumors or what is the biological significance of Ia antigen on Tc. On the other hand, TBH was found to carry T cells (Ts) which are capable of suppressing the Tc activity, both in *in vivo* and *in vitro* experiments. The results indicate that Ts directly inactivates Tc. Thus, this suppression is one of the examples in which Ts acts in the efferent arm of the immune response.

Ts obtained from TBH carries an *I-J* subregion determinant on its cell surface, which is analogous to the situation in allotype and antigen-specific suppression. Although the role of Ia antigens expressed on Ts and Tc in tumor immunity is largely unknown, it is suggested that the induction of tumor immunity depends on the balance of activities between Tc and Ts, both of which are controlled by different subregions of the *H-2* complex. It seems to be of great importance to determine how the expression of genes in different *I* subregions is controlled, and how to activate or inactivate a specific subset of T cells by immunological means for the future development of cancer immunotherapy.

Acknowledgments

The authors wish to express their sincere thanks to Dr. A. H. Sehon for his kind supply of several tumor cell lines of A/J mouse origin, and to Drs. C. S. David and D. H. Sachs for their generous supply of alloantisera against restricted subregions of the *H-2* complex. The authors also extend their gratitude to the excellent experimental assistance of Drs. T. Matsuzawa and K. Nakagawa. They thank Miss Yoko Yamaguchi for the secretarial assistance. This work was supported by a Grant-in-Aid for Cancer Research from the Ministry of Education, Science and Culture of Japan.

REFERENCES

1. Feldmann, M. and Kontiainen, S. Suppressor cell induction *in vitro*. II. Cellular requirements of suppressor cell induction. *Eur. J. Immunol.*, **6**, 302–305 (1976).
2. Fujimoto, S., Greene, M. I., and Sehon, A. H. Immunosuppressor T cells in tumor-bearing hosts. *Immunol. Commun.*, **4**, 207–217 (1975).
3. Fujimoto, S., Greene, M. I., and Sehon, A. H. Immunosuppressor T cells and their factors in tumor-bearing hosts. *In* "Suppressor Cells in Immunity," ed. by S. K. Singhal and N.R.St.C. Sinclair, The University of Western Ontario Press, Ontario, pp. 136–148 (1975).
4. Fujimoto, S., Greene, M. I., and Sehon, A. H. Regulation of the immune response to tumor antigens. I. Immunosuppressor cells in tumor-bearing host. *J. Immunol.*, **116**, 791–799 (1976).
5. Fujimoto, S., Greene, M. I., and Sehon, A. H. Regulation of the immune response to tumor antigens. II. The nature of immunosuppressor T cells in tumor-bearing host. *J. Immunol.*, **116**, 800–806 (1976).
6. Germain, R. N., Dorf, M. E., and Benacerraf, B. Inhibition of T-lymphocyte mediated tumor-specific lysis by alloantisera directed against the *H-2* serological specificities of the tumor. *J. Exp. Med.*, **142**, 1023–1028 (1975).
7. Greene, M. I., Fujimoto, S., and Sehon, A. H. Regulation of the immune response to

tumor antigens. III. Characterization of immunosuppressive T cell factor(s). *J. Immunol.*, **119**, 757–764 (1977).

8. Ishizaka, K. and Adachi, T. Generation of specific helper cells and suppressor cells *in vitro* for the IgE and IgG antibody responses. *J. Immunol.*, **117**, 40–47 (1976).

9. Lonai, P. Genetic control of the stimulator and effector function in allogeneic lymphocyte interaction: The expression of *I* region gene products on T and B lymphocytes. *In* "Immune Recognition," ed. by A. S. Rosenthal, Academic Press, New York, pp. 683–704 (1975).

10. Murphy, D. B., Herzenberg, L. A., Okumura, K., Herzenberg, L. A., and McDevitt, H. O. A new *I* subregion (*I-J*) marked by a locus (Ia-4) controlling surface determinants on suppressor T lymphocytes. *J. Exp. Med.*, **144**, 699–711 (1976).

11. Okumura, K., Takemori, T., and Tada, T. Specific enrichment of suppressor T cells bearing the products of *I-J* subregion. *In* "Immune System: Genetics and Regulation," ed. by E. Sercarz, L. A. Herzenberg, and C. F. Fox, Academic Press, New York, pp. 533–538 (1977).

12. Schrader, J. W. and Edelman, G. M. Participation of the *H-2* antigens of tumor cells in their lysis by syngeneic T cells. *J. Exp. Med.*, **143**, 601–614 (1976).

13. Tada, T., Taniguchi, M., and David, C. S. Properties of the antigen-specific suppressive T-cell factor in the regulation of antibody response of the mouse. IV. Special subregion assignment of the gene(s) that codes for the suppressive T-cell factor in the *H-2* histocompatibility complex. *J. Exp. Med.*, **144**, 713–725 (1976).

14. Takei, F., Levy, J. G., and Kilburn, D. G. *In vitro* induction of cytotoxicity against syngeneic mastocytoma and its suppression by spleen and thymus cells from tumor-bearing mice. *J. Immunol.*, **116**, 288–293 (1976).

15. Takei, F., Levy, J. G., and Kilburn, D. G. Characterization of suppressor cells in mice bearing syngeneic mastocytoma. *J. Immunol.*, **118**, 412–417 (1977).

16. Winn, H. J. Immune mechanisms in homotransplantation. II. Quantitative assay stimulated by tumor homografts. *J. Immunol.*, **86**, 228–239 (1961).

XENOGENIZATION OF TUMOR CELLS

Hiroshi KOBAYASHI

Laboratory of Pathology, Cancer Institute,
Hokkaido University School of Medicine*

Since 1969 the authors have been using viable tumor cell vaccine for immunotherapy of cancer in rats. All lines of rat tumors infected with murine leukemia viruses, such as Friend, Gross, or Rauscher, became unable to grow; or even if they grew initially, they eventually regress in all normal adult rats (xenogenization of tumor cells). After the regression of tumors infected with a virus, strong immunizing effect is produced against identical types of tumor, so that the immunity produced by virus-infected tumor cells is specific. The strength of the immunity is superior to that obtained when using irradiated, glutaraldehyde-treated tumor cells, and ligation and released tumor cells. The strong immunizing effect produced by virus-infected tumor cells may be caused by viable cell immunization, in which tumors grow for a while and then regress immunologically in all cases. However, the immunity produced by virus-infected xenogenized tumor cells is limited in inhibiting the growth of tumor, if the tumor has already grown visibly. The tumor must be surgically removed and combined with viable cell immunization to produce a significant decrease in the recurrence and metastasis of the tumor. Combination of chemotherapy with immunotherapy resulted in a marked prolongation of survival days and decrease in lethal growth. In this paper the authors describe the grade of increase in antigenicity of tumor cells after infecting them with persistent virus compared with the results obtained with chemicals and irradiation.

Xenogenization is a word which I have coined to designate the spontaneous regression of tumors in rats after artificially infecting them with murine leukemia viruses (*7–10*). I am sure that this phenomenon is due to an immunological mechanism. First, I am going to relate how we were able to recognize xenogenization, and second, I will discuss the mechanism of xenogenization and its application to the problem of cancer immunotherapy.

Natural Xenogenization

Friend virus is lethally infectious to mice but not to rats. However, only newborn rats were susceptible to Friend virus infection and developed leukemia approximately 6 months later. Leukemia involved the spleen and liver in rats injected at birth with Friend virus.

---

* Kita 15, Nishi 7, Kita-ku, Sapporo 060, Japan (小林　博).

TABLE I. Growth of Friend Virus-induced Tumors (Inoculated i. p.)

Tumor	Lethal growth in	
	Friend-tolerant rat	Normal rat
WFT-1	128/129	3/38
WFT-2	113/113	0/53
WFT-3	84/84	0/26
WFT-4	25/25	0/9
WFT-5	9/12	—
WFT-6	9/9	0/4
WFT-7	7/13	0/3
WFT-8	11/11	0/5
WFT-9	13/13	0/4
WFT-10	2/2	—
WFT-11	2/2	—
WFT-12	2/2	—
WFT-13	50/50	0/26
	455/465 (97.8%)	3/168 (1.8%)

Friend virus-induced luekemia developed from the spleen reveals typical lymphosarcoma or reticulum cell sarcoma. However, tumors are very difficult to maintain in normal adult rats (6).

We now have more than 13 transplantable lines of tumors developed from the spleen of rats suffering from Friend virus leukemia which can be transplanted in 2–3 months old Friend virus-conditioned and the so-called tolerant rats injected at birth with Friend virus (Table I). In the normal rats, however, there was no successful growth of the tumors. This differed from the usual results in our transplantation experiments.

The question then arose as to why such histologically typical malignant tumors were not capable of growing and killing the normal adult host but only the Friend virus-tolerant host or immunologically suppressed host (14). The same is true in Gross virus-induced tumors and Rauscher virus-induced tumors (13, 27).

Artificial Xenogenization

As the second step in our experiments, we attempted to convert commonly transplanted rat tumors, induced by methods other than viruses, from lethal to non-lethal tumors after an artificial infection with Friend virus. The stimulus for the following experiments was derived from the previous finding in which rat Friend tumors originating in the rats injected at birth with Friend virus proliferated well and killed the syngeneic rat only when it was Friend virus-tolerant. However, they either failed to grow, or grew and then regressed later, if the host was not tolerant. Then more than 10 different transplantable lines of tumors were used which were divided into 5 groups according to the cause of the tumor. The 5 groups were spontaneously developed sarcomas, 3-methylcholanthrene (MCA)-induced sarcomas, N-nitrosobutylurea (NBU)-in-

TABLE II. Lethal Growth of Various Rat Tumors Artificially Infected with
Murine Leukemia Viruses in the Syngeneic or Autochthonous Rat

Tumors infected with virus		Lethal growth in	
Tumor	Virus	Normal rats (%)	Tolerant or immunosuppressed rats (%)
Spont. sarcoma (WST-5)	Friend	0/26 (0)	7/8 (88)
Spont. sarcoma (Takeda)	Friend	6/23 (23)	— —
MCA sarcoma (Primary)	Friend	0/4 (0)	4/4 (100)
MCA sarcoma (KMT-17)	Friend	0/43 (0)	30/30 (100)
MCA sarcoma (KMT-17)	Gross	0/9 (0)	12/12 (100)
MCA sarcoma (KMT-68)	Friend	0/24 (0)	28/28 (100)
NBU breast (KBT-1)	Friend	0/12 (0)	9/9 (100)
NBU breast (KBT-2)	Friend	0/8 (0)	10/10 (100)
4NQO lung (Sato-LT)	Friend	0/28 (0)	11/12 (92)
DAB hepatoma (AH109)	Friend	2/8 (25)	— —
Total		8/185 (4)	111/113 (98)

duced breast cancers, 4-nitroquinoline 1-oxide(4NQO)-induced lung cancer, and
4-dimethylaminoazobenzene (DAB)-induced liver cancers. As a result, these tumors
became incapable of growing and killing normal rats after they were infected with
Friend virus. Even if the tumors grew initially, most of them later regressed spontaneously (Table II).

That the tumors were actually neoplasms even after the virus infection is evidenced
by the fact that the virus-infected tumors were capable of growing and killing rats
tolerant to Friend virus and rats immunologically suppressed by chemicals or X irradiation. We tentatively referred to this phenomenon as "xenogenization."

Figure 1 is one of the examples of the growth curve of Friend virus-infected and

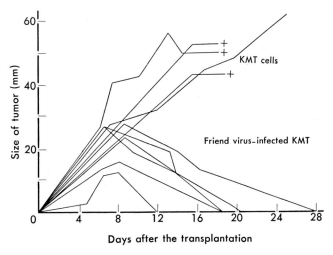

FIG. 1. Growth curve of Friend virus-infected KMT tumor in syngeneic rats

non-infected KMT tumor. Friend virus-infected tumors grow and regress in all cases, while non-infected tumors grow and kill the host. Most tumors infected with Friend virus do not grow as large as KMT tumor infected with Friend virus (*7, 33*).

Regression of Metastasis

Photo 1 is a picture of metastasis of a tumor xenogenized with Friend virus in the lumbar lymph nodes of rats 11 days after transplantation of KMT tumor in the foot-pad. KMT-17 tumor, most often used in our experiment, is a tumor growing rapidly and killing the host approximately 4 days after intraperitoneal (i.p.) transplantation and 2–3 weeks after subcutaneous (s.c.) transplantation. However, if the metastatic tumor, such as the one shown, was xenogenized, the metastasis regressed spontaneously (*23–25*).

Photo 2 shows an early stage of metastasis of KMT tumor infected with Friend virus growing in the regional lymph node and Photo 3 shows a late stage of metastasis of the same tumor beginning to regress accompanied with a number of reactive cells.

Figure 2 shows one of the methods for infection of rat tumors with Friend virus. There are several ways to infect the tumor with the virus, but this one is commonly used because of its simplicity and effectiveness. When the tumor is transplanted into the rats injected at birth with Friend virus for one or two generations, the tumor cells are infected with Friend virus while the tumor is growing in the host suffering from Friend virus leukemia. Cultured tumor cells are also easily infected with Friend virus (*18*).

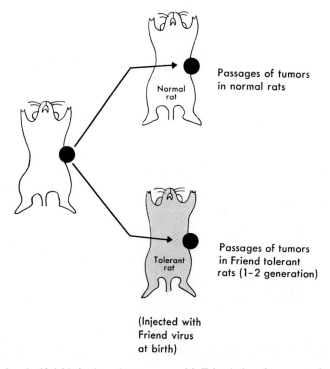

Fig. 2.   Artificial infection of rat tumors with Friend virus for xenogenization

Mechanism of Xenogenization

Photo 4 proves that the tumor cell was infected with Friend virus. The electron micrograph prepared by Dr. T. Kodama indicates budding of the Friend virus from the surface of the cell.

Fine ferritin granules of ferritin-labeled antibody can also be seen on the surface of the KMT-17 tumor cell revealing the virus-specific membrane antigen, which was newly formed by virus infection after xenogenization (Photo 4) (*20–22, 34*).

I will here explain the mechanism of xenogenization. I think that the major reason why the tumor cells infected with Friend virus are not capable of growing even in the normal syngeneic rat is because the virus-specific antigen (VSA), which appeared on the cell surface after xenogenization may be highly antigenic and easily recognized as foreign and thus be rejected by the rat. Note that the tumor cells in mice even after infection with Friend virus were not highly antigentic to the mouse. Thus, the Friend virus-infected mouse tumors did not regress spontaneously and were only slightly inhibited by a previous immunization with Friend virus (*12*). The experiments with the hamster were first conducted by Dr. Svet-Moldavsky and others using some other virus-infected mouse tumor system. In the rat system, however, the previous immunization with the virus is not necessary to make regress tumors infected with the virus: They regress spontaneously.

Another possible reason for regression of virus-infected tumors is that the tumor-specific antigen (TSA) existing on the cell surface, which is weakly antigenic before xenogenization, becomes moderately antigenic after xenogenization. This is because the immunosensitivity of tumor cells represented by the complement-dependent cyto-toxicity test increased after xenogenization. For example, anti-KMT-17 serum obtained from a rat immunized by the ligation-and-release method was highly cyto-toxic to virus-infected, xenogenized KMT-17 cells compared with non-infected, non-xenogenized KMT-17 (*3*).

Some results obtained by Dr. E. Gotohda in our laboratory will be described here on the cytotoxic immune sensitivity of KMT-17 tumor cells on successive days after i.p. transplantation of the tumor. The cytotoxic index of the tumor cells against anti-tumor serum decreased daily after transplantation of the tumor (Fig. 3) (*2*). In the early stages after transplantation, the cytotoxicity of the tumor cells was high. But in the later stages, which are the usual time for tumor transplantation, the cytotoxicity of the cell decreased. However, the cytotoxicity of the xenogenized tumor cell infected with Friend virus became stable and did not decrease even after transplantation, so that its immunosensitivity remained constantly at a high level even after the late stages of transplantation. Therefore, it can be said in this case the xenogenization prohibited the successive decrease of antigenicity after transplantation. In any event, the cytotoxicity remains high in the virus-infected, xenogenized tumor cell compared to the non-infected tumor cells, for an extended period after transplantation. Therefore, the rejection mechanism of xenogenized tumor cells may be explained by the high immunosensitivity of TSA in addition to the newly acquired VSA.

Photo 5 is a scanning electron micrograph showing an abundant number of irregular microvilli in the later stage of KMT-17 tumor cell. However, the cell infected with Friend virus (FV-KMT-17) was comparatively smooth and microvilli were not

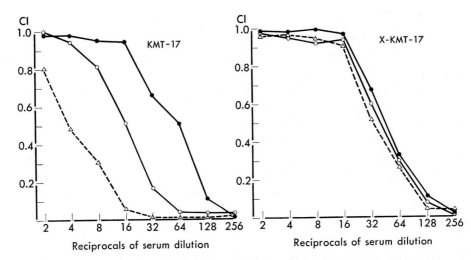

Fig. 3. Sensitivity of KMT-17 and X-KMT-17 cells to the cytotoxic effect of anti-KMT-17 serum by days after their i.p. transplantation
● 1-day-old; ○ 2-day-old; △ 3-day-old.

observed (Photo 6). The scanning electron micrograph of the cell surface of KMT-17 tumor correlated with the daily change in cytotoxicity of the cell infected or not infected with the virus. This suggests that the microvilli appearance reveals something about lateral mobility of the cell, which in turn may possibly be related to TSA distribution on the cell surface (*32*).

Immunotherapy Using Xenogenized Tumor Cells

Next, immunological treatment of cancer was attempted using the same type of xenogenized tumor cells infected with Friend virus which regressed later. VSA is neces-

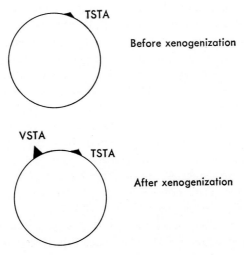

Fig. 4. Increase of antigenicity of tumor cell after xenogenization

TABLE III. Intensity of Immunity of DLT Cells Infected with Friend Virus on Growth of DLT Cells Compared with Other Conventional Immunization

Immunization with DLT cells treated by	Number of cells challenged (s.c.)	Lethal growth (temporary growth)
Inactivated immunity:		
^{60}Co irradiation (6,000 rads/10^7 cells, $\times 3$)	10^6	4/5 (5/5)
	10^5	0/5 (0/5)
Formalin (0.2%) treatment	10^6	3/5 (5/5)
(10^7–10^8 cells, $\times 3$)	10^5	3/5 (3/5)
Ligation-and-release	10^7	7/10 (9/10)
	10^6	1/4 (3/4)
Friend virus infection (10^7 cells)	10^8	0/13 (0/13)
	10^7	0/6 (3/6)
	10^6	0/6 (0/6)
	10^5	0/3 (0/3)
Not immunized	10^8	4/4 (—)
	10^7	5/5 (—)
	10^6	8/8 (—)
	10^5	2/2 (—)

sary to make the tumor regress, and TSA of the xenogenized cell may be capable of producing immunity against the same TSA of a non-infected cell. Immunization of the host with a viable and growing tumor cell is possible (Fig. 4).

It is probable that the previous immunization with living, growing cells will produce a much stronger immunizing effect than with inactivated cells or non-growing, viable cells (Table III). In fact, xenogenized tumor cells produce the strongest immunizing effect after regression of xenogenized tumor cells. As indicated in Table III, the immunizing effect was compared with that produced by other methods, such as ^{60}Co irradiation, Formalin treatment, and necrosis of tumor tissue by ligation and release (11). They were arranged so as to elicit the strongest immunizing effect obtainable. Immunization with ^{60}Co-irradiated or Formalin-inactivated DLT cells inhibited the 10^5 DLT cell inoculation, and none of 5 rats given the ^{60}Co treatment and only 3 of 5 given Formalin treatment died of tumor growth. Ligation-and-release inhibited the growth of 10^7 cells. However, lethal growth was observed in 7 of the 10 rats. On the other hand, immunization with DLT cells infected with Friend virus brought about strong resistance to the transplantation of non-infected DLT cells.

I think it is important to describe the qualitative increase of immunogenicity of killed tumor cells after xenogenization. In the experiment involving active immunization with virus-infected, xenogenized or non-infected tumor cells under the same conditions the growth of identical types of tumors was more evidently inhibited in the rats immunized with virus-infected xenogenized cells (11). For example, in the experiment using rats immunized with Formalin-treated tumor cells, the DLT tumor was more strongly inhibited in rats immunized with Formalin-treated, xenogenized tumor cells than in those immunized with Formalin-treated, non-xenogenized tumor cells. This suggests that the immunogenicity of tumor cells increases after xenogenization (Table IV). Therefore, it can be concluded that the strong immunizing effect of the

TABLE IV.   Immunogenicity of Friend Virus-infected Tumor Cells in Rats

Inactivation by	Lethal growth in rats immunized with	
	Friend virus-infected cells	Non-infected cells
Irradiation	3/20	10/20
Formalin	1/8	5/8
Ligation-and-release	0/6	7/10

virus-infected tumor cells may be attributed not only to the immunity caused by viable and growing tumor cells but also to the possibility that the inherently weak immunogenicity of the tumor cells has been strengthened by infection with Friend virus.

Immunotherapy with Surgery

To apply immunotherapy to cancer, surgical excision of the main tumor is first necessary, and subsequent immunization with an identical type of xenogenized tumor cells is also necessary to inhibit growth of the tumor which was already metastasizing. KMT-17 tumor is a rapidly-growing tumor and produces metastases in regional lymph nodes and kills the host in all cases (Fig. 5).

On the 3rd day after footpad transplantation, the tumor was removed by surgical excision. However, metastatic growth of the tumor in the lymph nodes resulted in the death of almost all of the rats and only 18 out of 56 rats (32%) survived, as shown in the No. 2 group. In the No. 3 group active immunization alone was not enough to prevent the growth of the previously transplanted tumor, and none of the rats survived. This suggests that immunotherapy alone, even when xenogenized viable tumor cells are used, is not effective in treating tumors already growing visibly. However, when

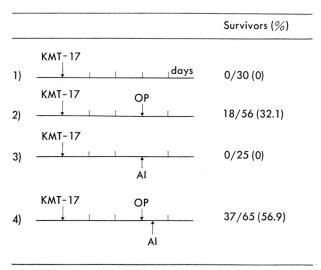

FIG. 5. Active immunization with xenogenized tumor cell against metastasis after surgical operation of KMT tumor in WKA rat

KMT-17: 1×10^6, footpad. AI: active immunization with xenogenized KMT-17 tumor, 1×10^6, s.c. OP: surgical excision of the footpad tumor.

surgical excision was combined with active immunization in the No. 4 group, a much higher survival rate (57%) was obtained (*15*).

Immunotherapy with Chemotherapy

In the second experiment for immunochemotherapy, mitomycin C (MMC) and xenogenized cells were used (Fig. 6). MMC was used on the 3rd day after the KMT tumor transplantation. It is necessary to begin immunotherapy at the earliest stage of tumor transplantation in order to achieve a high immunizing effect. Hence, both active immunization with xenogenized tumor cells and adoptive immunization with lymphocytes from rats immunized with xenogenized tumor cells within one day after tumor transplantation were employed. As shown in Fig. 6, 1) a control, 2) a single treatment of MMC, 3) active immunization with xenogenized cells, and 4) adoptive immunization with lymphocytes from the host immunized with xenogenized cells, were not satisfactory. However, when MMC treatment was combined with active immuni-

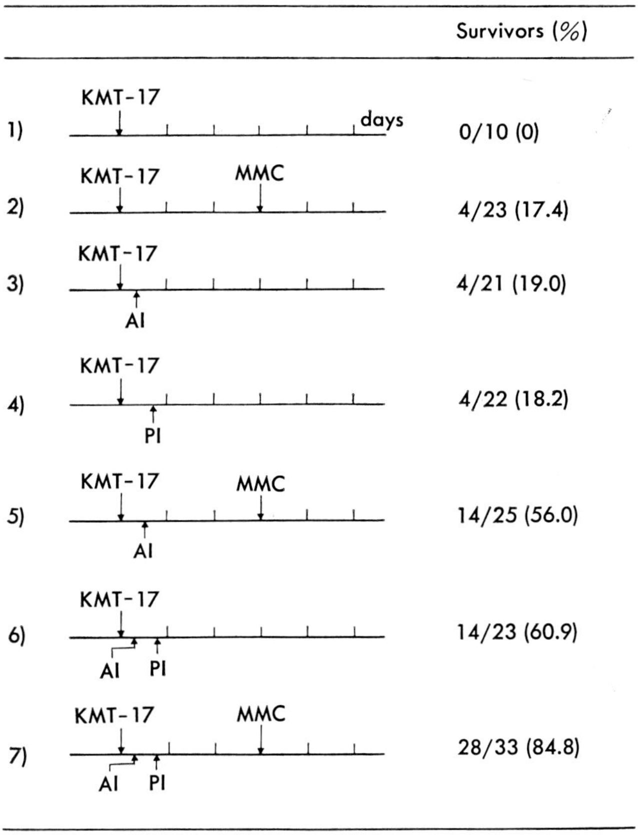

FIG. 6. Inhibitory effect to KMT-17 tumor in WKA rat by combination treatments of chemotherapy (MMC) and immunotherapy

MMC: 1 mg/kg, intravenously (i.v.). AI: active immunization of xenogenized KMT-17, s.c. PI: passive immunization with 5×10^7 lymphoid cells from WKA rats immunized with xenog-KMT-17, i.v. KMT-17: 1×10^4, s.c.

zation (No. 5 group), the inhibitory effect on the KMT tumor increased to 56%. The same was true in the No. 6 group using immunization combined with adoptive immunization, when 60% of the rats survived. Furthermore, when MMC treatment was combined with active immunization and adoptive immunization in the No. 7 group, the effect was the most satisfactory. More than 80% of the rats survived. Therefore, we have to recognize that there is a limit to the immunizing effect even when combined with other treatments. However, a definite increase in the antitumor effect can be expected (*1, 4, 5, 16*).

CONCLUSION

I have described the phenomenon of "xenogenization," in which tumors induced by Friend virus in rats cannot grow in syngeneic rats. Even if they do grow initially, they eventually regress. That the tumors are unable to grow in rats when the tumors are artificially infected with Friend virus was also noted. The former phenomenon is referred to as natural xenogenization, while the latter is referred to as artificial xenogenization; in both, the neoplasms regress immunologically without other treatments. As a sequel to the study of natural and artificial xenogenization of tumors, attention is being focused on the more detailed mechanisms of xenogenization and also the application of xenogenization to human cancer treatment.

REFERENCES

1. Gotohda, E., Sendo, F., Hosokawa, M., Kodama, T., and Kobayashi, H. Combination of active and passive immunization and chemotherapy to transplantation of methylcholanthrene-induced tumor in WKA rats. *Cancer Res.*, **34**, 1947–1951 (1974).
2. Gotohda, E., Sendo, F., Nakayama, M., Hosokawa, M., Kawamura, T., Kodama, T., and Kobayashi, H. Change of antigenic expression on rat tumor cells after their transplantation. *J. Natl. Cancer Inst.*, **55**, 1079–1083 (1975).
3. Gotohda, E., Moriuchi, T., Kawamura, T., Akiyama, J., Oikawa, T., Sendo, F., Hosokawa, M., Kodama, T., and Kobayashi, H. Stabilized expression of tumor-associated antigen on rat tumor cells by infection with Friend virus. Submitted to *J. Natl. Cancer Inst.* (1978).
4. Hosokawa, M., Sendo, F., Gotohda, E., and Kobayashi, H. Combination of immunotherapy and chemotherapy to experimental tumors in rats. *Gann*, **62**, 57–60 (1971).
5. Kaji, H., Sendo, F., Shirai, T., Saito, H., Kodama, T., and Kobayashi, H. Immunotherapy of rat tumors with tumor cells artificially infected with mouse Friend virus. *Mod. Med.*, **24**, 1329–1333 (1969) (in Japanese).
6. Kobayashi, H., Hosokawa, M., Takeichi, N., Sendo, F., and Kodama, T. Transplantable Friend virus-induced tumors in rats. *Cancer Res.*, **29**, 1385–1392 (1969).
7. Kobayashi, H., Sendo, F., Shirai, T., Kaji, H., Kodama, T., and Saito, H. Modification in growth of transplantable rat tumors exposed to Friend virus. *J. Natl. Cancer Inst.*, **42**, 413–419 (1969).
8. Kobayashi, H., Kodama, T., Shirai, T., Kaji, H., Hosokawa, M., Sendo, F., Saito, H., and Takeichi, N. Artificial regression of rat tumors infected with Friend virus (xenogenization): An effect produced by acquired antigen. *Hokkaido J. Med. Sci.*, **44**, 133–134 (1969).
9. Kobayashi, H. Growth of rat tumor cells infected with Friend virus: An approach to

the immunological treatment of cancer. Immunity and tolerance in oncogenesis. *IV Perugia Quadrenn. Int. Conf. on Cancer* 1969, 637–659 (1970).

10. Kobayashi, H., Shirai, T., Takeichi, N., Hosokawa, M., Saito, H., Sendo, F., and Kodama, T. Antigenic variant (WFT-2N) of a transplantable rat tumor induced by Friend virus. *Eur. J. Clin. Biol. Res.*, **15**, 426–428 (1970).

11. Kobayashi, H., Sendo, F., Kaji, H., Shirai, T., Saito, H., Takeichi, N., Hosokawa, M., and Kodama, T. Inhibition of transplanted rat tumors by immunization with identical tumor cells infected with Friend virus. *J. Natl. Cancer Inst.*, **44**, 11–19 (1970).

12. Kobayashi, H., Takeichi, N., Hosokawa, M., and Kodama, T. Characteristics of Friend virus-induced tumors in the rat compared with those in the mouse. *GANN Monogr. Cancer Res.*, **12**, 73–92 (1972).

13. Kobayashi, H., Kuzumaki, N., Gotohda, E., Takeichi, N., Sendo, F., Hosokawa, M., and Kodama, T. Specific antigenicity of tumors and immunological tolerance in the rat induced by Friend, Gross and Rauscher viruses. *Cancer Res.*, **33**, 1598–1603 (1973).

14. Kobayashi, H. Relationship between carcinogenesis and immunity. *In* "Analytic and Experimental Epidemiology of Cancer," ed. by W. Nakahara *et al.*, Japan Scientific Societies Press, Tokyo, pp. 381–388 (1973).

15. Kobayashi, H., Gotohda, E., Hosokawa, M., and Kodama, T. Inhibition of metastasis in rats immunized with xenogenized autologous tumor cells after excision of the primary tumor. *J. Natl. Cancer Inst.*, **54**, 997–999 (1975).

16. Kobayashi, H., Kodama, T., Hosokawa, M., Sendo, F., Takeichi, N., Kuzumaki, N., Gotohda, E., Oikawa, T., Nakayama, M., and Imamura, M. Xenogenized cell and allogeneic cell: Possible relation of immunotherapy for cancer. *In* "Host Defense against Cancer and Its Potentiation," ed. by D. Mizuno *et al.*, Japan Scientific Societies Press, Tokyo, pp. 199–211 (1975).

17. Kobayashi, H. Lymphomas and immunological tolerance in the rat induced by murine leukemia viruses. *In* "Comparative Leukemia Research 1973," ed. by Y. Ito and R. M. Dutcher, Japan Scientific Societies Press, Tokyo, pp. 291–300 (1975).

18. Kodama, T., Kobayashi, H., Saito, H., Shirai, T., and Matsumiya, H. Electron microscopic studies on the cultured human cells infected with Friend virus. *Gann*, **61**, 219–221 (1970).

19. Kodama, T., Takeichi, N., Gotohda, E., and Kobayashi, H. Electron microscopic studies on the sialoglycoprotein layer of rat Friend tumor cells. *Gann*, **64**, 613–616 (1973).

20. Kodama, T., Kuzumaki, N., and Takeichi, N. Immuno-electron microscopic studies on cell surface antigens of Friend virus-induced tumor in the rat. *Gann*, **64**, 273–276 (1973).

21. Kodama, T., Gotohda, E., and Kobayashi, H. Immuno-electron microscopic studies on surface antigens of rat tumor cells infected with Friend virus. *Gann*, **64**, 475–479 (1973).

22. Kodama, T., Gotohda, E., and Kobayashi, H. Morphological aspects of xenogenization of tumors by artificial infection with virus. *GANN Monogr. Cancer Res.*, **16**, 167–181 (1974).

23. Kodama, T., Gotohda, E., Takeichi, N., Kuzumaki, N., and Kobayashi, H. Histopathology of immunologic regression of tumor metastasis in the lymph nodes. *J. Natl. Cancer Inst.*, **52**, 931–939 (1974).

24. Kodama, T., Gotohda, E., Takeichi, N., Kuzumaki, N., and Kobayashi, H. Histopathology of regression of tumor metastasis in the lymph nodes. *Cancer Res.*, **35**, 1628–1636 (1975).

25. Kodama, T. Pathology of immunologic regression of tumor metastasis in the lymph nodes. *GANN Monogr. Cancer Res.*, **20**, 83–91 (1977).

26. Kojima, K., Takeichi, N., Kobayashi, H., and Maekawa, A. Electrokinetic charge of

transplantable Friend virus-induced tumors in rats. *Nagoya Med. J.*, **16**, 7–13 (1970) (in Japanese).

27. Kuzumaki, N., Takeichi, N., Sendo, F., Kodama, T., and Kobayashi, H. Correlation between various cell-surface antigens induced by murine leukemia virus in the rat: Serological analysis. *Int. J. Cancer*, **11**, 575–585 (1973).

28. Kuzumaki, N., Kodama, T., Takeichi, N., and Kobayashi, H. Friend lymphatic leukemia virus-induced autoimmune hemolytic anemia with glomerulonephritis in the rat. *Int. J. Cancer*, **14**, 483–492 (1974).

29. Kuzumaki, N. and Kobayashi, H. Cell-surface antigens induced by Friend and Rauscher virus complexes and their associated lymphatic leukemia viruses in the rat. *Cancer Res.*, **35**, 1718–1722 (1975).

30. Kuzumaki, N., Moriuchi, T., Kodama, T., and Kobayashi, H. Xenogenization of rat erythroid cells by lymphatic leukemia virus: Its role in induction of autoimmune hemolytic anemia. *J. Immunol.*, **117**, 1250–1255 (1976).

31. Kuzumaki, N. and Kobayashi, H. Reduced transplantability of syngeneic mouse tumors superinfected with membrane viruses in nu/nu mice. *Transplantation*, **22**, 545–550 (1976).

32. Moriuchi, T., Gotohda, E., Hosokawa, M., Kodama, T., and Kobayashi, H. Correlation between concanavalin A agglutinability and cytotoxic sensitivity to antiserum against tumor-associated antigen infibrosarcoma cells. Submitted to *J. Natl. Cancer Inst.* (1978).

33. Sendo, F., Kaji, H., Saito, H., and Kobayashi, H. Antigenic modification of rat tumor cells artificially infected with Friend virus in the primary autochthonous host. *Gann*, **61**, 223–226 (1970).

34. Shirai, T., Kaji, H., Takeichi, N., Sendo, F., Saito, H., Hosokawa, M., and Kobayashi, H. Cell surface antigens detectable by cytotoxic test on Friend virus-induced and Friend virus-infected tumors in the rat. *J. Natl. Cancer Inst.*, **46**, 449–460 (1971).

35. Takeichi, N., Kuzumaki, N., Kodama, T., Sendo, F., Hosokawa, M., and Kobayashi, H. Runting syndrome in rats inoculated with Friend virus. *Cancer Res.*, **32**, 445–449 (1972).

36. Takeichi, N. Comparative studies of immunological disorders in rats infected with Friend or Gross virus. *Acta Pathol. Japon.*, **23**, 953–962 (1973).

37. Takeichi, N., Kuzumaki, N., and Kobayashi, H. Immunological studies of runting syndrome in rats inoculated with Friend virus. *Cancer Res.*, **33**, 3096–3102 (1973).

38. Takeichi, N., Kuzumaki, N., and Kobayashi, H. Suppression of specific and nonspecific immune responses in rats infected with Friend or Gross virus. *GANN Monogr. Cancer Res.*, **16**, 27–35 (1974).

EXPLANATIONS OF PHOTOS

PHOTO 1. Metastasis of KMT-17 tumor xenogenized with Friend virus in the lumbar lymph nodes that regressed later spontaneously.

PHOTO 2. Early stage of KMT-17 tumor metastasis growing in the regional lymph node.

PHOTO 3. Late stage of KMT-17 tumor metastasis accompanied with a number of reactive cells.

PHOTO 4. Electron micrograph indicates the budding of the Friend virus and VSA witn fine ferritin granules.

PHOTO 5. Scanning electron micrograph shows an abundant number of microvilli in KMT-17 cells.

PHOTO 6. Scanning electron micrograph shows a comparatively smooth surface of xenogenized KMT-17 cells infected with Friend virus.

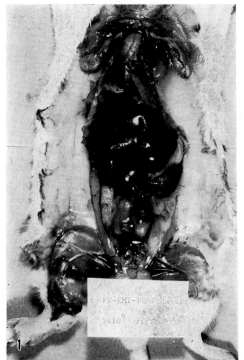

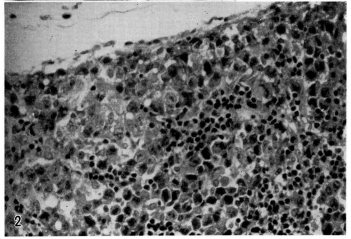

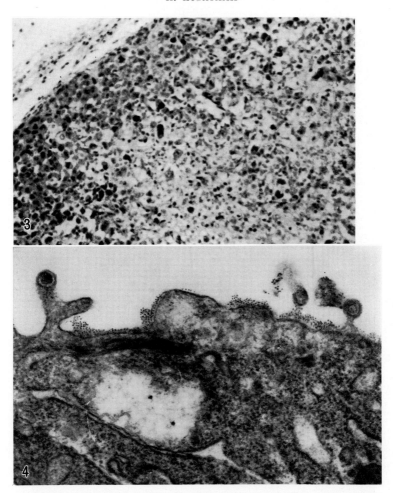

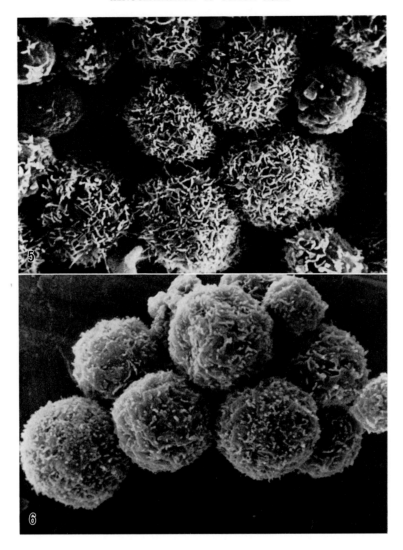

GANN Monograph on Cancer Research 21, 1978

T CELL FUNCTION IN THE INDUCTION OF IMMUNE RESISTANCE AGAINST SYNGENEIC MURINE TUMOR

Masayasu Kitagawa,*[1] Hiromi Fujiwara, Toshiyuki Hamaoka, Hiroshi Yamamoto, and Kumiko Teshima

Institute for Cancer Research, Osaka University Medical School[2]

The mechanism of immune response of C3H/He mice against syngeneic X5563 plasmacytoma was analyzed and specific immunopotentiation against this tumor was attempted by utilizing supplementary immune mechanisms deficient in this tumor system.

When C3H/He mice were inoculated with viable X5563 cells followed by tumor resection, tumor-specific T cell-mediated immunity was successfully elicited. While killer T cells against tumor-associated transplantation antigens (TATA) were detected in those immunized animals, these TATA did not induce any significant helper T cell activity against TATA. On the other hand, lymphoid cells from allogeneic C57BL/6 mice immunized with viable X5563 cells revealed both killer and helper T cell activities against alloantigens, thus indicating that the immune response to TATA of X5563 tumor was different from that to alloantigens both qualitatively and quantitatively.

It may be reasonable to assume that helper T cells are involved in the augmentation of the killer T cell generation. Therefore, the augmentation of tumor-specific immunity by supplementation of the helper T cell system was carried out. This was accomplished by immunizing with hapten-modified tumor cells along with introducing a helper T cell system against the hapten. The hapten-reactive helper T cells were generated by immunization with hapten-mouse γ globulin; this activity was further amplified through the selective elimination of hapten-reactive suppressor T cells by treatment with hapten conjugates of D-glutamic acid and D-lysine. When the mice were immunized with hapten-substituted tumor cells in the presence of the augmented helper T cell activity, the tumor-specific immunity against TATA was significantly enhanced.

Thus, the supplementation of a helper T cell system may provide an intriguing model for immunopotentiation in the helper T cell deficient syngeneic tumor system.

The presence of tumor-associated transplantation antigens (TATA) on tumor cell surfaces (*10*) and positive immune responses to these TATA (*8*) have been demonstrated in many experimental systems, raising the question as to why immunogenic tumors

---

*[1] Deceased.

*[2] Fukushima 1-1-50, Fukushima-ku, Osaka 553, Japan (北川正保, 藤原大美, 浜岡利之, 山元 弘, 豊島久美子).

escape the host's immune surveillance (7). This was, indeed, contrasted to the phenomenon that animals can easily reject transplanted allogeneic tumors by eliciting strong immune responses to alloantigens. Regarding these established, rather contradictory phenomena, the question needs to be solved of how the response mechanisms of immunocompetent cells in syngeneic tumor systems are different from those in allogeneic tumor systems, qualitatively and quantitatively. One of the difficulties of solving this question may be that the magnitude or strength of syngeneic tumor rejection is not so striking as that of allogeneic tumor graft rejection. However, if one could establish a model system for effective rejection of a syngeneic tumor system, and further analyze the immune mechanisms to the syngeneic tumor with reference to the allogeneic tumor, the differences, if any, may explain in part the difficulty in rejection of the syngeneic tumor. It might also provide us with a potential approach to immunopotentiation in the syngeneic tumor system.

The present paper will review typical differences in immune mechanisms between syngeneic and allogeneic tumor systems. Based on these differences the augmentation of syngeneic tumor immunity was attempted by the supplementation of immune mechanisms deficient in the syngeneic tumor system.

T Cell Responses of C3H/He Mice to Syngeneic X5563 Plasmacytoma (PC)

When viable X5563 PC cells were inoculated into syngeneic C3H/He mice followed by surgical resection of the tumor, tumor-specific cell-mediated immunity was induced (3). This was demonstrated in the spleens of these mice by means of the *in vitro* cytotoxicity test (Table I) and *in vivo* tumor neutralization assay (3). In addition to the evidence that this immunity could not be developed in T cell-deprived mice induced by treatment with rabbit anti-thymocyte serum subsequent to adult thymectomy, a striking increase in *in vitro* tumor killing and *in vivo* tumor neutralizing activity in a T cell-enriched population (passed through nylon wool column of the immune spleen cells and T cell content of more than 90%) indicated the involvement of T cells in this tumor immunity (3).

TABLE I. *In Vitro* Cytotoxicity Test[a] with Spleen Cells or Sera from Immune Mice (3)

Type of cytotoxicity (culture period)	Effector cell type (Effector-to-target ratio)		Sera (final dil.)	Complement	Specific killing (%)
Cell-mediated (24 hr)	Normal	(50:1)	—	—	—
	Immune[b]		—	—	70.0
	Normal	(25:1)	—	—	—
	Immune		—	—	45.7
Antibody-mediated complement-dependent (1.5 hr)	—		Normal (×4)	+	—
	—		Immune[b] (×4)	+	0.0
	—		Hyperimmune[c] (×4)	+	0.0

[a] *In vitro* cytotoxicity test was performed according to that described previously (4).

[b] Spleen cells or sera from the mice resistant to intraperitoneal (i.p.) challenge with 10^6 X5563 cells after the surgical resection of intradermally (i.d.) implanted tumor.

[c] Sera from the mice resistant to consecutive i.p. challenges with 10^6, 3×10^6, and 5×10^6 X5563 cells after the surgical resection of i.d. implanted tumor.

Despite positive killer T cell-mediated immunity, no antibody activity against tumor was detected (Table I). These observations are consistent with the reports of Röllinghoff *et al.* (*11*) that, in the combination of BALB/c mice and syngeneic myeloma, T cell-mediated immunity was detected, but tumor-specific antibody was not. This failure to detect tumor-specific antibody suggested the unsuccessful triggering of helper T cells against the TATA of X5563 tumor. To examine helper T cell activity against TATA of X5563 cells, dinitrophenyl-keyhole limpet hemocyanin (DNP-KLH)-primed spleen cells were transferred intravenously (i.v.) into 600R X-irradiated syngeneic recipients as a source of DNP-primed B cells, along with the above spleen cells immunized with syngeneic X5563 cells or unprimed spleen cells, and stimulated by i.v. inoculation of 5×10^6 mitomycin C (MMC)-pretreated and trinitrophenylated X5563 cells (TNP-PC). Seven days after the cell transfer and antigenic stimulation, indirect anti-DNP plaque-forming cells (PFC) were assayed in the spleens of those recipients. As shown in Table II, no significant helper T cell activity was detected in the spleens of syngeneic C3H/He mice in both the tumor-bearing and hyperimmune state, despite positive killer T cell activity, as confirmed in the same donor pool.

In contrast to the negative response of anti-tumor antibody in X5563 plasmacytoma system, a potent anti-tumor antibody has been demonstrated in the MM102 tumor system (*12*) of the same C3H/He origin. Therefore, it was determined whether in such a tumor system, helper T cell activity against TATA can be successfully detected by the assay system used in the present study. The helper T cell activity was determined in the spleen cells immunized with MM102 tumor (MM) cells by the same

TABLE II. Failure to Detect Helper T Cell Activity against Syngeneic X5563 Cells in the Spleen from C3H/He Mice Immunized with X5563 Cells (*4*)

Exp. No.	B cells	Spleen cell types tested for helper T cell activity	2nd antigen	Helper T cell activity against X5563 cells[a]	
				Anti-DNP PFC/spleen	Helper index
1	DNP-KLH-primed cells	Normal	5×10^6 TNP-PC	2,755 (1.34)	1.00
		PC-tumor bearer[b]		1,744 (1.38)	0.63
		PC-hyperimmune[c]		872 (1.38)	0.32
2	DNP-KLH-primed cells	Normal	5×10^6 TNP-PC	<120	1.00
		PC-tumor bearer[b]		<120	1.00
		PC-hyperimmune[c]		<120	1.00

[a] Helper T cell ativity was measured by anti-DNP antibody response of transferred DNP-KLH-primed cells (30×10^6) at the stimulation of TNP-X5563 cells (5×10^6) in the presence of the spleen cells (50×10^6) from mice immunized with syngeneic X5563 cells or from normal mice. Helper index represents a ratio of mean value of PFC in experimental group to that in normal group of each 3 to 4 animals.

[b] Mice inoculated i.d. with 10^6 X5563 cells (PC) 10 days before: mean cytotoxic activity as confirmed 3 days before the helper T cell assay in the same donor pool was 39.7 and 32.4% in Exp. 1 and Exp. 2, respectively, at an effector-to-target cell ratio of 100:1.

[c] Mice resistant to consecutive i.p. challenges with 10^6, 3×10^6, and 5×10^6 viable X5563 cells after the surgical resection of i.d. implanted tumor: mean cytotoxic activity as confirmed 3 days before the helper T cell assay in the same donor pool was 46.9 and 31.3% in Exp. 1 and Exp. 2, respectively, at effector-to-target cell ratio of 100:1.

TABLE III. Helper T Cell Activity against MM102-associated Antigens in the Spleens of C3H/He Mice Immunized with Syngeneic MM102 Tumor Cells (4)

Exp. No.	B cells	Spleen cell types tested for helper T cell activity	2nd antigen	Helper T cell activity against MM or PC cells	
				Anti-DNP PFC/spleen	Helper index
1	DNP-KLH-primed cells	Normal		649 (1.51)	1.00
		MM-tumor bearer[a]	5×10^6 TNP-MM	7,692 (1.05)	11.85
		MM-immune[b]		8,544 (1.07)	13.16
		MM-hyperimmune[c]		14,312 (1.19)	22.05
2	DNP-KLH-primed cells	Normal	5×10^6 TNP-MM	120 (1.00)	1.00
		MM-tumor bearer[a]	5×10^6 TNP-MM	3,515 (1.33)	29.29
		Normal	5×10^6 TNP-PC	294 (1.45)	1.00
		PC-immune[d]	5×10^6 TNP-PC	120 (1.00)	0.41

[a] Mice inoculated i.d. with 10^6 MM102 cells (MM) 13 and 14 days before, in Exp. 1 and 2, respectively.

[b] Mice which resisted i.p. challenge with 10^6 MM102 cells after the surgical resection of i.d. implanted tumor.

[c] Mice which resisted consecutive i.p. challenges with 10^6, 3×10^6, and 5×10^6 MM102 cells after the surgical resection of i.d. implanted MM102 tumor.

[d] Mice which resisted i.p. challenge with 10^6 X5563 cells (PC) after the surgical resection of i.d. implanted X5563 tumor.

experimental procedure as in the X5563 tumor system, except for the challenge with TNP-MM. The results in Table III indicate that in the MM102 tumor system, an ample helper T cell activity was detected and furthermore in Exp. 2, which was conducted in parallel with the X5563 PC system, a significant helper T cell activity was again detected in the spleens of MM102 tumor-bearing mice, whereas the helper T cell activity against X5563 TATA was not detected. Thus, it can be concluded that X5563 tumor cannot develop helper T cell activity against its TATA.

While these results established that C3H/He mice preferentially generated killer T cell activity to TATA without inducing any helper T cell activity, the T cell responses were next compared with allogeneic mice against X5563 tumor cells with respect to killer and helper T cell activities. The T cell responses of allogeneic C57BL/6 mice against X5563 tumor are summarized in Table IV. These allogeneic mice were found to generate doth killer and helper T cell activities against alloantigens in parallel. This was in contrast to the results in the syngeneic combination as listed in Tables II and III. This qualitative difference between T cell responses in syngeneic and allogeneic systems seems to be of vital importance in the following aspects: firstly, the X5563 syngeneic tumor system fails to provide the double defense mechanisms of both cell-mediated and humoral immunity relating to killer and helper T cell generation. Furthermore, failure to induce helper T cell activity against X5563 TATA may have some relation to the lower level of the generation of killer T cell activity to syngeneic tumor cells in general.

In fact, the selective generation of killer T cells indicates that the generation of helper T cell activity against TATA may not be an absolute prerequisite for the effective development of killer T cell responses. However, these results do not exclude the

TABLE IV. T Cell Responses of C57BL/6 Spleen Cells Immunized
with Allogeneic X5563 Plasmacytoma Cells (PC) (4)

Spleen cell types tested[a]	Cytotoxic activity against PC[b] Specific killing (%)	Helper T cell activity against PC[c] Anti-DNP PFC/spleen
Normal	0.0	1,697
PC-primed ($\times$1)	73.1	9,158
Normal	0.0	5,250
PC-primed ($\times$4)	67.3	59,342

[a] C57BL/6 mice were i.p. immunized 1 to 4 times with 10^7 X5563 cells (PC) and spleen cells were submitted to cytotoxicity and helper T cell assays 10 days after the last immunization.

[b] Cytotoxicity assay was performed at an effector-to-target cell ratio of 100:1.

[c] Helper T cell activity was measured by anti-DNP antibody response of transferred DNP-KLH-primed cells (30×10^6) to stimulation with TNP-X5563 cells (5×10^6) in the presence of spleen cells from mice immunized with X5563 cells.

possibility of the augmenting effect of helper T cells on the generation of killer T cell activity. Cantor and Boyse (1, 2) reported that killer T cell development against allogeneic tumor cells was augmented by collaboration with another subset of amplifier T cells which carries the Ly specificity, distinct from the killer T cells, and recognizes alloantigens different from those recognized by prekiller cells. At present, although it is not known whether these T cells are equivalent to the helper T cells responsible for humoral immune responses in the present study, it is conceivable that if the collaborative response of helper T cells with the prekiller cells can be successfully induced in the syngeneic tumor system, the T cell response against killer determinants may be potentiated.

In this context, if animals were immunized with tumor cells modified by additional antigenic determinants with which the helper (amplifier) T cells might be capable of reacting, augmentation of the specific T cell response against killer determinants could be predicted. In our experiments, hapten was introduced as additional determinants because hapten-reactive helper T lymphocyte activity can be easily generated in mice by immunization with hapten-mouse γ-globulin (MGG) (14), and the amplifying effect of helper T cells on killer T cell generation can be analyzed by utilizing hapten-conjugated tumor cells. In the following section, the method for effective induction of helper T lymphocyte activity against hapten is summarized.

Generation of Helper T Cell Activity against Haptenic Determinants

It has been established that hapten-reactive helper T cells are developed along with hapten-specific B cells by immunization with hapten-isologous carrier conjugate, and that the former cells can exhibit their helper activity on anti-hapten antibody production against another haptenic group on the same carrier (14). As shown in Fig. 1, *p*-azobenzoate (PAB)-reactive helper cell activity was detected by cotransferring DNP-specific B lymphocytes with PAB-MGG-primed spleen cells and stimulating with a double hapten-conjugated isologous protein, DNP-MGG-PAB. Futher, it is also shown in Fig. 1 that the hapten (PAB)-reactive cell activity was susceptible to treatment with

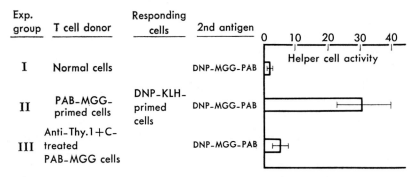

Fig. 1.   The induction of PAB-reactive helper cell activities by immunization with PAB-MGG and the susceptibility of those cells to the treatment with anti-Thy. 1 antiserum plus complement (*13*)

Spleen cells (50×10^6) from donor mice primed 10 weeks earlier with 100 μg of DNP-KLH in Freund's complete adjuvant (CFA), were used as responding cells, and transferred intravenously (i.v.) into 600R X-irradiated recipients together with spleen cells from either unprimed mice or PAB-MGG-primed mice. The PAB-MGG-primed mice had been immunized intraperitoneally (i.p.) with 100 μg of PAB-MGG in CFA 3 weeks before the cell transfer. Secondary antigenic challenges were performed by i.p. injection of 100 μg of DNP-MGG-PAB immediately after the cell transfer. Geometric means and standard errors of anti-DNP PFC responses in the spleens of the recipients 7 days after the cell transfer are illustrated.

anti-Thy-1.2 antiserum plus C, thus indicating that these helper cells are T lymphocytes (Fig. 1).

More recent studies about this system revealed that the above immunization regimen generated not only helper T cell activity but also suppressor T cell activity against the same haptenic determinants (*13*). This was demonstrated by measuring the inhibiting activity of PAB-MGG-primed cells on the anti-DNP antibody response of

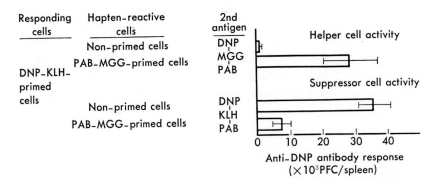

Fig. 2.   Detection of both PAB-reactive helper and suppressor cell activity in a single experimental system (*13*)

The experimental protocol is essentially the same as for Fig. 1. Secondary antigenic challenges were made by i.p. injection of 100 μg of hapten-carrier conjugates, as indicated, immediately after the cell transfer. Geometric means and standard errors of anti-DNP PFC responses in the spleens of the recipients 7 days after the cell transfer are illustrated.

transferred DNP-KLH-primed cells to stimulation with DNP-KLH-PAB (Fig. 2). The evidence that helper and suppressor T cell activity against the same haptenic determinants coexist in the spleen cells from a single donor pool indicates that the true helper T cell activity may be lessened by the presence of suppressor T cell activity. These results lead to the possibility that, if the suppressor T cell activity could be selectively eliminated, the true helper T cell activity would be restored to the original level, or apparently augmented. Therefore, further study was carried out to augment the helper T cell activity by eliminating the suppressor T cell activity coexsisting in the spleen cell suspensions.

The specific inactivation of hapten-specific B cell activity was easily accomplished by pretreatment with the haptenic determinant coupled to nonimmunogenic synthetic polypeptides, copolymer of D-glutamic acid and D-lysine (D-GL) (9). In the same way, specific unresponsiveness or inactivation could be induced exclusively at the level of the hapten T cells (5). Thus, the induction of B cell and T cell tolerance by the hapten-conjugated D-GL complex has been firmly established. Furthermore, the experimental conditions have been developed to selectively inactivate hapten-reactive suppressor T cell activity by the appropriate administration of hapten-D-GL conjugate (6). One of the typical examples of the selective inactivation of hapten-reactive suppressor T cell activity is shown in Fig. 3. As is evident from Fig. 3, when PAB-D-GL conjugate was administered to mice 4 days before the PAB-MGG priming, significantly augmented helper T cell activity was generated in those mice compared with an untreated group.

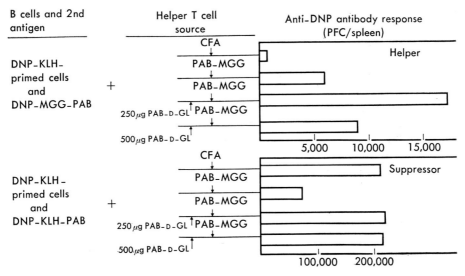

FIG. 3. Differential effect of PAB-D-GL pretreatment on the generation of PAB-reactive helper and suppressor T cells (6)

Normal animals were either pretreated with PAB-D-GL 3 days before PAB-MGG immunization or not pretreated. The PAB-reactive helper and suppressor T cell activities generated in these PAB-MGG-primed animals were measured 3 weeks after the PAB-MGG immunization by transferring them into 600R X-irradiated recipient mice together with DNP-KLH-primed cells and stimulating with 100 μg of DNP-MGG-PAB or DNP-KLH-PAB. The DNP-KLH-primed cells came from other donor mice which had been immunized 9 weeks previously.

The specific inactivation of suppressor T cell activity by PAB-D-GL pretreatment was
further confirmed by the results of suppressor T cell activity, as detected by the protocol shown in the lower panel of Fig. 3.

Thus, the experimental system to develop augmented helper T cell activity was
established against the haptenic determinant, and such a system was applied to the
augmentation of the generation of an effector T cell population responsible for syngeneic tumor immunity. This system is the first trial of the application of a hapten-
reactive T lymphocyte system to the immunotherapy model through T-T cell interaction *in vivo*.

Augmented Generation of Effector T Cell Activity by T-T Cell Interaction

Firstly, it seems to be important to select a suitable type of hapten for the modification of tumor cells. Trinitrophenol (TNP) was chosen because trinitrophenylation
brought about little damage on the viability of X5563 tumor cells. TNP-reactive T lymphocytes were induced by immunization with TNP-MGG, and the helper T cell activity was tested according to the helper T cell assay used in the PAB-helper system.
As shown in Fig. 4, TNP-reactive helper T cells were generated by TNP-MGG priming, and the augmenting effect of these TNP-reactive helper T cell activity on the
generation of killer T cells to TATA on X5563 was next detected.

This was accomplished by immunization with TNP-substituted tumor cells in the
presence of TNP-reactive helper T lymphocytes which had been generated through
immunization with TNP-MGG. The animals preimmunized with TNP-MGG exhibited significantly enhanced killer T cell activity against TATA of X5563 cells after
immunization with TNP-substituted X5563 cells (Fig. 5).

However, the amplifying activity of such a TNP-reactive helper T cell population
was not so striking. It is conceivable that hapten (TNP)-reactive suppressor cells gen-

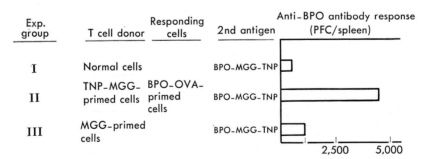

FIG. 4.   Generation of TNP-reactive helper T cell activity by immunization with
TNP-MGG

Spleen cells (50×10^6) from donor mice primed 10 weeks earlier with 100 μg of
BPO-OVA in CFA, were used as responding cells, and transferred i.v. into 600R X-
irradiated recipients together with spleen cells from either unprimed mice, TNP-
MGG-primed, or MGG-primed mice. The TNP-MGG-primed mice had been im-
munized i.p. with 100 μg of TNP-MGG in CFA 4 weeks before the cell transfer.
Secondary antigenic challenges were performed by i.p. injection of 100 μg of BPO-
MGG-TNP immediately after the cell transfer. Anti-BPO PFC responses in the
spleens of the recipients 7 days after the cell transfer are illustrated.

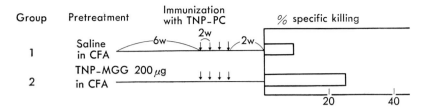

FIG. 5. Augmentation of killer T cell generation against X5563 TATA by hapten-TATA cooperation

Unprimed C3H mice or mice preimmunized with TNP-MGG were inoculated with 3×10^7 of TNP-PC (PC cells were pretreated with MMC), 4 times i.p. at 2-week intervals. Cytotoxic activity of X5563 cells against TATA was tested by using uncoupled X5563 cells as target cells 2 weeks after the last immunization. Effector-to-target cell ratio in the cytotoxicity test was 100: 1.

erated together with TNP-reactive helper cells by immunization with TNP-MGG may reduce the apparent helper T cells activity, as observed in the PAB-T cell system. Accordingly, if TNP-reactive suppressor T cell activity could be selectively eliminated from the system beforehand, the generation of TNP-reactive helper T cell activity may

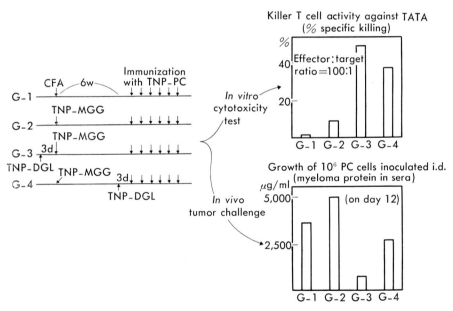

FIG. 6. Amplifying effect of TNP-D-GL treatment on generation of killer T cells and development of *in vivo* resistance against tumor in the helper T to killer T cell interaction

C3H/He mice were immunized with 100 μg of TNP-MGG (Groups 2, 3, and 4). Five hundred micrograms of TNP-D-GL were inoculated i.p. 3 days before (Group 3) or 6 weeks after TNP-MGG immunization (Group 4). These groups of mice and unprimed mice were inoculated i.p. with 10^7 of TNP-PC (MMC-treated), 6 times at 1-week intervals. One week after the final immunization, each group of mice were submitted to the *in vitro* cytotoxicity test and the rest of mice were challenged intradermally with 10^6 viable PC cells. Cytotoxic activity against X5563-TATA was tested by using uncoupled X5563 cells as target cells.

be augmented and a potent induction of tumor-specific immunity could be expected by providing augmented TNP-reactive helper T cell activities. C3H/He mice were inoculated intraperitoneally (i.p.) with 500 μg of TNP-DGL 3 days before TNP-MGG priming or 3 days before immunization with TNP-PC, *i.e.*, 6 weeks after TNP-MGG priming. Either unprimed mice or mice which received TNP-MGG priming with or without TNP-D-GL treatment, were then immunized with 10^7 TNP-PC (MMC-treated) cells, 6 times at 1-week intervals. One week after the final tumor immunization, the development of *in vitro* cytotoxic T cell activity against X5563 cells and T cell-mediated immune resistance against the challenge with 10^6 viable tumor cells were determined. As illustrated in Fig. 6, the mice pretreated with TNP-D-GL, especially when pretreated before TNP-MGG priming, were found to generate the stronger *in vitro* and *in vivo* antitumor immunity when compared with the TNP-D-GL untreated group.

Thus it is concluded that the augmentation of syngeneic tumor immunity can be accomplished by the supplemention of helper T cell activity against the additional determinant which was introduced onto the viable tumor cell surface. Further applicability of this hapten-reactive helper T cell activity to various tumor systems, including autochthonous tumor, is now under investigation.

Acknowledgment

This work was supported in part by Grants-in-Aid for Scientific Research from the Ministry of Education, Science and Culture and from the Ministry of Health and Welfare, Japan.

REFERENCES

1. Cantor, H. and Boyse, E. A. Functional subclasses of T lymphocytes bearing different Ly antigens. I. The generation of functionally distinct T-cell subclasses in a differentiative process independent of antigen. *J. Exp. Med.*, **141**, 1376–1389 (1975).
2. Cantor, H. and Boyse, E. A. Functional subclasses of T lymphocytes bearing different Ly antigens. II. Cooperation between subclasses of Ly$^+$ cells in the generation of killer activity. *J. Exp. Med.*, **141**, 1390–1399 (1975).
3. Fujiwara, H., Hamaoka, T., Nishino, Y., and Kitagawa, M. Inhibitory effect of tumor-bearing state on the generation of *in vivo* protective immune T cells in a syngeneic murine tumor system. *Gann*, **68**, 589–601 (1977).
4. Fujiwara, H., Hamaoka, T., Teshima, K., Aoki, H., and Kitagawa, M. Preferential generation of killer or helper T lymphocyte activity directed to the tumor-associated transplantation antigens. *Immunology*, **31**, 239–248 (1976).
5. Hamaoka, T., Yamashita, U., Takami, T., and Kitagawa, M. The mechanism of tolerance induction in thymus-derived lymphocytes. I. Intracellular inactivation of hapten-reactive helper T lymphocytes by hapten-nonimmunogenic copolymer of D-amino acids. *J. Exp. Med.*, **141**, 1308–1328 (1975).
6. Hamaoka, T., Yoshizawa, M., Yamamoto, H., Kuroki, M., and Kitagawa, M. Regulatory functions of hapten-reactive helper and suppressor T lymphocytes. II. Selective inactivation of hapten-reactive suppressor T cells by hapten-nonimmunogenic copolymers of D-amino acids and its application to the study of suppressor T cell effect on helper T cell development. *J. Exp. Med.*, **146**, 91–106 (1977).

7. Hellström, K. E. and Hellström, I. Lymphocyte-mediated cytotoxicity and blocking serum activity to tumor antigens. *Adv. Immunol.*, **18**, 209–277 (1974).
8. Herberman, R. B. Cell-mediated immunity to tumor cells. *Adv. Cancer Res.*, **19**, 207–263 (1974).
9. Katz, D. H., Hamaoka, T., and Benacerraf, B. Immunological tolerance in bone marrow-derived lymphocytes. I. Evidence for an intracellular mechanism of inactivation of hapten-specific precursors of antibody-forming cells. *J. Exp. Med.*, **136**, 1404–1429 (1972).
10. Klein, G. Tumor antigens. *Annu. Rev. Microbiol.*, **20**, 223–252 (1966).
11. Röllinghoff, M., Rouse, B. T., and Warner, N. L. Tumor immunity to murine plasma cell tumors. I. Tumor-associated transplantation antigens of NZB and BALB/c plasma cell tumors. *J. Natl. Cancer Inst.*, **50**, 159–172 (1973).
12. Takizawa, K., Yamamoto, T., and Mitsui, H. Transplantation resistance and potent antibody production induced in C3H/He mice against C3H/He mammary tumor by continuous infusion of solubilized antigen. *Gann*, **65**, 541–544 (1974).
13. Yamamoto, H., Hamaoka, T., Yoshizawa, M., Kuroki, M., and Kitagawa, M. Regulatory functions of hapten-reactive helper and suppressor T lymphocytes. I. Detection and characterization of hapten-reactive suppressor T cell activity in mice immunized with hapten-isologous protein conjugate. *J. Exp. Med.*, **146**, 74–90 (1977).
14. Yamashita, U. and Kitagawa, M. Induction of anti-hapten antibody response by hapten-isologous carrier conjugate. I. Development of hapten-reactive helper cells by hapten-isologous carrier. *Cell. Immunol.*, **14**, 182–192 (1974).

GANN Monograph on Cancer Research 21, 1978

SYSTEMIC AND LOCAL RESPONSE OF IMMUNOCYTES TO HUMAN CANCER

Kokichi Kikuchi, Hiroshi Yamaoka, Kiminobu Uchizawa,
and Susumu Iguchi

*Department of Pathology, Sapporo Medical College**

Cancer-specific immune responsiveness in cancer patients was evaluated with lymphoblastogenesis in mixed lymphocyte-tumor cell culture (MLTC). About one-third of cancer patients studied showed more than three-fold higher reactivity of lymphocytes to autochthonous cancer cells than to normal cells. Three M KCl extract of autologous cancer cells was also stimulative to lymphocytes of cancer patients.

Blastogenic responsiveness in MLTC was inversely proportional to the clinical stages of cancer patients. A follow-up study of these patients revealed that those who had died within 20 months after operation were all non-responders to autologous cancer antigen. Studies with anti-human T cell serum (ALS-T) and anti-human B cell serum (ABS) indicated that cancer-specific blastogenesis was involved with T cells.

The mononuclear cell reaction in the site of cancer proliferation was well correlated to *in vitro* lymphoblastogenesis in MLTC. Immunofluorescence studies using ALS-T and ABS revealed that there was a tendency for B cells to cluster in the stroma, and for T cells to infiltrate diffusely into cancer nests attaching to cancer cells.

These results suggest that T cells are responsible for resistance against the autochthonous cancer, and that lymphoblastogenesis in MLTC is useful as a parameter of specific immunity in human cancer.

We have previously reported that lymphoblastogenesis to phytohemagglutinin (PHA) in cancer patients was markedly depressed and there was a significant relationship between stimulation index (SI) in lymphoblastogenesis and the clinical stage and prognosis of cancer (*2, 6*). In spite of their depressed immune reactivity some cancer patients have specific responsiveness to their autochthonous tumors.

In this paper, the systemic cancer-specific immune reaction in cancer patients is demonstrated and compared with local response to cancer tissue. To evaluate immune reactivity to the autochthonous cancer cells, mixed lymphocyte-tumor cell culture (MLTC) was applied. Details of the method have been described elsewhere (*3, 8*). In this test, lymphocytes of cancer patients were cultured with mitomycin C-treated autologous cancer cells or normal cells and the uptake of ^{3}H-thymidine into lymphocytes was measured. The ratio of radioactivity with tumor cells to that with normal cells was expressed as the cancer-specific stimulation index. Lymphoblastogenesis was determined before surgical operation, when the patients had not been given any chemo-

* Minami 1, Nishi 17, Chuo-ku, Sapporo 060, Japan (菊地浩吉, 山岡 博, 内沢公伸, 井口 進).

therapy or radiation therapy. Patients with cancer of the stomach, breast, colon, and thyroid gland were selected.

Lymphocyte Blastogenesis in MLTC in Cancer Patients

Subjects included 24 gastric, 13 breast, 10 colon, and 10 thyroid cancer patients. As shown in Fig. 1, normal cells did not stimulate the autologous lymphocytes with few exceptions. About 30% of cancer patients studied showed a more than three-fold higher reactivity of lymphocytes to the autochthonous cancer cells than to normal cells. Cancer-specific stimulation index (SI) of various kinds of cancer is shown in Fig. 2. Colon cancer patients tended to be low responders to their own cancer cells. The blastogenic reactivity of lymphocytes to the autochthonous tumor cells is considered to indicate recognition of tumor antigen by cancer patients. Cancer-specific lympho-blastogenesis was also obtained with 3M KCl extract from cancer cells of several of the 30 patients, although the value of the index was somewhat lower than that with whole cells. This made it possible to measure the response to autologous cancer antigen in patients during their clinical course.

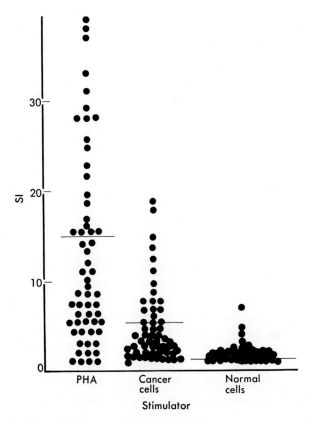

FIG. 1. Lymphoblastogenesis with autochthonous cancer or normal cells

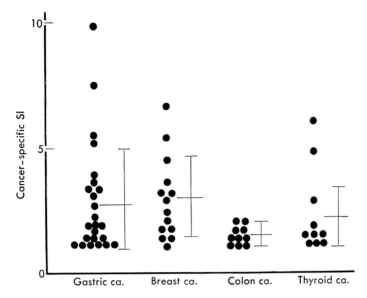

FIG. 2. Cancer-specific SI (SI with autochthonous cancer cells/SI with autochthonous normal cells) in various cancers

Relationship between Cancer-specific and General Cell-mediated Immunity as Expressed by Lymphoblastogenesis and Skin Reaction

MLTC lymphoblastogenesis was compared with PHA lymphoblastogenesis, which is considered to express non-specific cell-mediated immunity (Fig. 3). There was a significant correlation between cancer-specific SI and SI with PHA. Cancer-specific SI also correlated significantly with skin reactions to PHA or *Candida* antigen. These facts

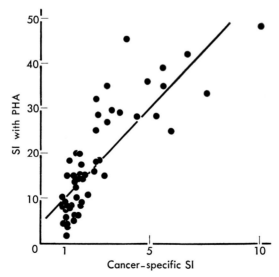

FIG. 3. Relationship between MLTC and PHA lymphoblastogenesis
$y = 5.3x + 4.2, r = 0.84, p < 0.05.$

suggest that the elevation of non-specific cell-mediated immunity may contribute to the specific immune reactions to cancer.

Cancer-specific Lymphoblastogenesis and Clinical Status of Cancer

The most important point is whether the cancer-specific lymphoblastogenesis is correlated to the resistance of patients to their own cancer. Figure 4 indicates the relationship between cancer-specific blastogenic response and the clinical stage of the cancer. In gastric cancer patients, high responders to autologous cancer tended to be in stage II, and low responders were in stage III. Non-responders were all in stage IV.

A follow-up study of these patients revealed that those who had died within 20 months after operation were all non-responders, and high responders were all alive more than 20 months (Fig. 5). These facts strongly indicate that the reactivity of cancer patients' lymphocytes to cancer-specific antigen, determined by MLTC, is related to the patients' resistance against autochthonous cancers.

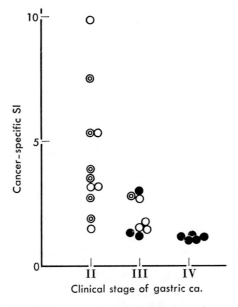

FIG. 4.   MLTC blastogenesis and clinical stage of gastric cancer
● dead<20 months; ○ alive>20 months; ◎ alive>36 months.

Local Mononuclear Cell Reaction in Cancer Tissue and Systemic Lymphocyte Reaction with Cancer Cells In Vitro

Previously, it was reported that PHA blastogenesis did not always parallel mononuclear cell reaction to cancer tissue (6). The next problem is whether the local mononuclear cell reaction at the site of cancer cell proliferation is correlated to in vitro lymphoblastogenesis in MLTC.

We graded and classified the histological appearance of mononuclear cell infiltration in the marginal part of the tumor mass, as no, slight, moderate, and marked

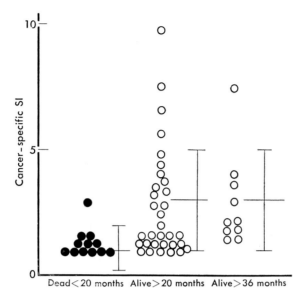

FIG. 5. Lymphocyte blastogenesis with autochthonous cancer cells (20-month fol-low-up data)

Vertical bars show mean±SD.

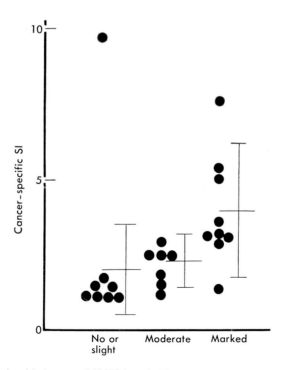

FIG. 6. Relationship between MLTC lymphoblastogenesis and local mononuclear cell response in gastric cancer

according to the predominant picture. Cellular reactions, mostly of polymorphs, to necrosis or infection were neglected and attention was concentrated on the marginal part of the tumor protrusion. Two trained pathologists were independently engaged in evaluating and classifying the histology without knowing the value of MLTC blastogenesis in the patients. Figure 6 shows the relationship between lymphoblastogenesis in MLTC and local mononuclear cell reaction in gastric carcinoma. There are some exceptions but it appears that there is some histological correlation between MLTC blastogenesis and mononuclear cell reaction. The same tendency was observed in breast cancer. There was no significant relationship between MLTC blastogenesis and histological types of cancer. Care is needed to interpret the histology of human cancer as significant because in the human there are so many factors that produce the histological appearance. The reason why we attach importance to the cellular reaction in human cancer tissue is based on animal experiments using an autochthonous tumor system (4, 5). Time course studies of tumor autograft rejection in a highly antigenic tumor strain by optical and electron microscopy revealed the massive infiltration of lymphocytes into the tumor tissue and close adherence of lymphocytes to tumor cells which subsequently degenerated and died (5). On the other hand, autografts of low antigenic tumor or syngeneic tumor grafts showed less lymphocyte reaction and grew progressively until the hosts died. Significance of mononuclear cell reaction was obvious in the experimental systems. Results in human cancer tissues, together with the animal experiments, suggest that *in vivo* and *in vitro* lymphocyte responsiveness are correlated and that both reflect resistance against the autochthonous cancer.

Identification of Cells Responsible for Reaction to Cancer

In order to analyze the lymphoid cells involved in recognition or in effector mechanisms, heterologous rabbit anti-human T cell serum (ALS-T) and anti-human B cell serum (ABS) were developed. The methods for preparation and evidence for specificity of these sera have been described previously (1, 7). Pretreatment of lymphocytes with ALS-T and complement strongly reduced the lymphoblastogenesis in MLTC, however, pretreatment with ABS did not (Table I). This finding indicates that cancer-specific blastogenesis involves T cells. In other words, T cells are relevant to the recognition of autologous cancer cells.

In order to identify cells reacting to cancer tissue, indirect immunofluorescence using ALS-T and ABS was applied. It was found that there was a tendency for B cells to cluster in the stroma, while T cells infiltrated diffusely into cancer nests attaching to cancer cells. The histological manifestations of host resistance in human cancer are not

TABLE I. Effects of ALS-T and ABS Plus Complement on
MLTC or PHA Lymphoblastogenesis

Treatment	Exp. 1 (Δ cpm)		Exp. 2 (Δ cpm)	
	MLTC	PHA	MLTC	PHA
Medium+C	661	14,551	2,714	36,850
ABS+C	983	12,549	3,032	29,840
ALS-T+C	83	7,477	21	10,765

simple, since there are numerous factors including infection or necrosis. In the model system, in which rejection mechanisms of autochthonous 3-methylcholanthrene-induced rat tumors were investigated, it was found, using the immunofluorescence technique and neutralization test, that T cells played a major role in tumor destruction (4). The animal experiments support the idea that T cells demonstrated immunohistochemically in human cancer are an important part of the immunological resistance to cancer.

CONCLUSIONS

It is evident that some, but not all, cancer patients are reacting immunologically to their own cancer antigen. The reactivity is parallel to the resistance against cancer estimated by clinical stages and survivals of these patients. The intensity of mononuclear cell reaction in cancer tissues seems to be proportional to responsiveness of peripheral blood lymphocytes to cancer antigen. There was a significant relationship between cancer-specific and general cell-mediated immunity as expressed by lymphoblastogenesis and skin reaction. The results suggest that the elevation of non-specific cell-mediated immunity may contribute to the specific immune reaction to cancer. Evidence was presented that T cells are involved in the above-mentioned cancer-specific immune reactions in human cancer patients.

REFERENCES

1. Ishii, Y., Koshiba, H., Ueno, H., Maeyama, I., Takami, T., Ishibashi, F., and Kikuchi, K. Characterization of human B lymphocyte specific antigens. *J. Immunol.*, **114**, 466–469 (1975).
2. Kanaya, T. Studies on cell-mediated immunity in cancer patients. Part 1. Blastogenic transformation of peripheral lymphocytes of cancer patients with PHA. *Sapporo Med. J.* **43**, 48–59 (1974).
3. Kanaya, T. Studies on cell-mediated immunity in cancer patients. Part 2. Specific blastogenic transformation of lymphocyte with autochthonous cancer antigen. *Sapporo Med. J.* **43**, 60–67 (1974).
4. Kikuchi, K., Ishii, Y., Ueno, H., and Koshiba, H. Cell-mediated immunity involved in autochthonous tumor rejection in rats. *Ann. N. Y. Acad. Sci.*, **276**, 188–206 (1976).
5. Kikuchi, K., Ishii, Y., Ueno, H., Kanaya, T., and Kikuchi, Y. Analysis of tumor-specific cell-mediated immune reactions in the primary autochthonous host. *GANN Monogr. Cancer Res.*, **16**, 99–116 (1974).
6. Kikuchi, K., Kanaya, T., Yamaoka, H., Suzuki, T., and Ishii, Y. Lymphoblastogenesis with Phytohemagglutinin, local response of mononuclear cells and prognosis of cancer patients. *Tumor Res.*, **10**, 12–19 (1975).
7. Koshiba, H., Ishii, Y., Yamanaka, N., and Kikuchi, K. Identification of human peripheral T cell antigens. *J. Immunol.*, **118**, 625–629 (1977).
8. Yamaoka, H. Studies on cancer-specific cell-mediated immunity in cancer patients. *Sapporo Med. J.* **46**, 341–353 (1977).

EXPERIMENTAL STUDY. II. IMMUNOPOTENTIATORS AND THEIR MODES OF ACTION

GANN Monograph on Cancer Research 21, 1978

MODE OF ANTITUMOR ACTION OF BCG

Tohru Tokunaga, Tetsuro Kataoka, Reiko M. Nakamura,
Saburo Yamamoto, and Kiyoko S. Akagawa

Department of Tuberculosis, National Institute of Health*

Both the effector mechanisms against cancer and the inhibitor mechanisms against the effectors are multiple; the host responses to BCG are also multiple. The mode of antitumor action of BCG is, therefore, very intricated and dynamic depending on many variable factors. This review focuses on the mode of action in "local immunotherapy" with BCG.

The effector mechanisms in local BCG therapy are composed of 3 different ones which arise sequentially after BCG administration. Mechanism A is an immediate-type inflammation caused by BCG. The effector cells in this mechanism are macrophages (Mp) activated directly by BCG without T cell participation. The *in vivo* significance of this event was indicated by the results of therapeutic trials of athymic nude mouse tumors with BCG. Mechanism B is a tuberculin-type inflammation, in which the effector cells are Mp activated by lymphokines (Lk). The first step of this mechanism is proliferation of BCG-specific T cells, accompanying polyclonal proliferation of T cells. Lk production of BCG-sensitized T cells seems to require stimulation by histocompatible Mp ingesting BCG. On the other hand, activation of Mp with Lk was found to require a prestimulation of Mp with BCG. Contact of viable, activated Mp with tumor cells was necessary for target cell destruction. Mechanism C is the induction of tumor-specific immunity. The interaction of the BCG-stimulated, polyclonally proliferating T cells with the Mp that have ingested both BCG and tumor cell debris may be important for the effective induction of tumorspecific killer T cells.

Genetic control of prophylactic and therapeutic effects of BCG in mice has been clarified to some extent. A major gene controlling the host response to BCG is transmitted according to Mendel's laws, and expressed as a dominant trait. Other miscellaneous problems, such as immune depression by intravenous injection with BCG, comparison of living and dead BCG, oral administration of BCG, and systemic, nonspecific effects of BCG, are discussed.

The effector cell mechanism against tumor cells is known to be multiple; killer T cells (*4*), activated macrophages (*1, 7*), polymorphonuclear cells (*6, 11*), K cells with antibody (*28*), and N cells (*15*) are all possible effector cells. Antibody itself with com-

---

* Kamiosaki 2-10-35, Shinagawa-ku, Tokyo 141, Japan (徳永　徹，片岡哲朗，中村玲子，山本三郎，赤川清子).

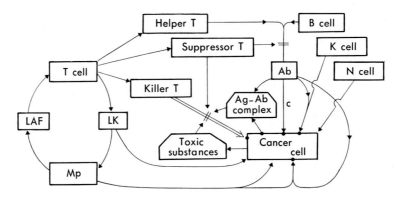

Fig. 1. Multiple effector mechanism against tumor cells

Lk, lymphokines; LAF, lymphocyte-activating factor; Ag, antigen; Ab, antibody; Mp, macrophages; c, complement; ●, tumor-specific antigen.

plement and lymphotoxin (*13*), produced by T cells is also reported to be cytotoxic *in vitro*. On the other hand, some factors, such as suppressor T cells (*10, 39*), antigen-antibody complexes (*31*), and toxic substances produced by tumor cells (*17*) inhibit or block these effector mechanisms. These multiple effector and inhibitor mechanisms are shown schematically in Fig. 1.

Mycobacterium bovis BCG (BCG) is, at present, the most widely employed immunotherapeutic agent against cancer (*2, 23*); its mode of action has been studied by many investigators (*9, 14, 21, 43, 44*). It is known that the host response to BCG is multiple and varies according to the route, dose, timing, *etc.* of BCG administration.

This review will focus on the mode of action of BCG in "local immunotherapy" (*44*), where BCG is introduced into the tumor site, because the most convincing therapeutic effect of BCG in human cancer has been reported in "local immunotherapy" and because the mechanisms of action of BCG have been clarified relatively well in "local" administration.

In addition to BCG, we used *Mycobacterium smegmatis* strain ATCC607 (Smeg) as an immunopotentiator, because it is a rapidly growing, non-pathogenic myco-bacterium, convenient to handle, and it suppresses the growth of various syngeneic tumors *in vivo* as BCG, at least under certain conditions (*36, 37, 41*).

Multiple Mechanisms of BCG in Local Immunotherapy

In order to clarify the theme of this presentation, we will show first a comprehensive scheme (Fig. 2) of cellular mechanisms related to the antitumor action of BCG. This illustration was based on the extensive studies of the cellular response to BCG infection in mice by Mackaness and his co-workers (*3, 20*), on the local immunotherapy with BCG of metastatic tumors in guinea pigs by Zbar and his co-workers (*42, 44*), and on our own data in mice and guinea pigs.

This illustration shows that the 3 different effector mechanisms resulted from the response to BCG to attack tumor cells. These 3 mechanisms, A, B, and C in Fig. 2, occur sequentially after "local" infection with BCG. Mechanism A means an im-

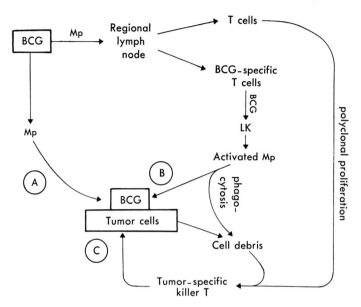

FIG. 2. Mechanisms of anti-tumor action of BCG in "local immunotherapy"

mediate-type inflammation by cutaneous infection with BCG, the effector cells in which are macrophages (Mp) as described later. Mechanism B is the reaction called tuberculin-type or Koch's phenomenon, the effector cells in which Mp are activated by T cell products. Mechanism C indicates the induction process of tumor immunity, in which the effector cells may be killer T cells. Mechanism A is completely non-specific, B is specific to BCG but not to the tumor, and C is specific to the tumor.

The In Vivo Role of Non-specific Augmentation of Step A Mechanism

Within 3–5 hr after injection of living BCG into a murine cutaneous tumor nodule, we observed a large number of polymorphonuclear cells (PMN) and mononuclear cells (MN) appearing at the injection site. In order to study the *in vivo* role of this type of inflammation, that arises independent of T cell functions contrary to the other 2 mechanisms, B and C, we thought that athymic nude mice which lack the immunological functions usually associated with T cells would be suitable animals. The following experiments on "local immunotherapy" of nude mouse tumors with BCG were carried out.

Exp. 1. Previously we found that 2 intraperitoneal (i.p.) injections with 10^7 Smeg cells 5 days before and 3 days after i.p. inoculation with 10^4 Ehrlich ascites tumor cells completely inhibited tumor growth in ddY mice (*36*). This experiment was repeated using BALB/c (nu/nu and nu/+) mice (*37*). All of the untreated controls received Ehrlich cells alone were died within 20 days in both nu/nu and nu/+. All mice treated with Smeg, however, completely suppressed their tumor growths.

Exp. 2. Pimm and Baldwin (*27*) showed that intradermal (i.d.) growth of xenogeneic rat tumor cells mixed with BCG was suppressed in nude mice. This type of experiment was carried out using both syngeneic KKN-1 fibrosarcoma cells that were originally induced in a male nu/nu with 3-methylcholanthrene (MCA) by A. Goda and T. Suzuki (Kitasato Institute, Tokyo) and K. Nomoto (Kyushu University, Medical School, Fukuoka), and allogeneic Ehrlich tumor cells. Growth of both tumors was inhibited in nu/nu as well as in nu/+ when the tumor cells were injected together with either BCG or Smeg, while tumor only controls grew progressively and killed the hosts.

Exp. 3. Nu/nu and nu/+ were injected i.d. with 10^5 KKN-1 or Ehrlich tumor cells. One week later, 10^7 BCG or Smeg cells were injected directly into the tumor nodules. The tumors regressed gradually in nu/+ mice, however they continued to grow in nu/nu mice.

These experiments suggest that (a) the host defence mechanism independent from T cell function (step A mechanism) works strongly against tumors if they are activated by BCG (or Smeg) injected adjacent to the place where a relatively small number of tumor cells exist, and (b) augmentation of this mechanism has a strict limitation; established, growing solid tumors did not regress if a single dose of BCG (or Smeg) was given directly into the regions. In this case T cell functions are required (*37*).

The activity of Smeg to elicit the step A mechanism seems to be stronger than BCG (data not shown).

Effector Cells of Step A Mechanism

Peritoneal exudate cells (PEC) harvested from nu/nu mice given 10^7 Smeg cells i.p. 4 days before, inhibited ^{3}H-TdR incorporation into KKN-1 tumor cells *in vitro* at an effector-to-target cell ratio of 5 (*40*). Resident peritoneal cells (PC) of nu/nu were not cytotoxic at this ratio. Similar phenomena were observed in various syngeneic tumor systems of mice and guinea pigs as shown in Table I.

The effector cells in the PEC were determined using the following 2 syngeneic systems: KKN-1 tumor cells and PEC from nu/nu, and EL4 leukemia cells and PEC from C57BL/6J. Time course analysis on cell population of the PEC from mice that had received 10^7 Smeg cells i.p. revealed that early after i.p. injection with Smeg (such

TABLE I. Inhibition of ^{3}H-TdR Uptake of Various Tumor Cells by Syngeneic Peritoneal Exudate Cells Stimulated by Smeg

Tumor cells	Animals	^{3}H-TdR incorporation (%)	
		PC	Smeg PEC
EL4 leukemia	C57BL/6J	81.7	7.3
P815 mastocytoma	DBA/2	94.0	2.0
B16 melanoma	C57BL/6J	96.0	3.0
K5 fibrosarcoma	SWM/Ms	60.0	13.0
KKN-1 fibrosarcoma	BALB/c (nu/nu)	76.2	6.8
Line-10 hepatoma	Strain 2 guinea pig	84.6	40.0

PC were harvested from normal donors. Smeg PEC were collected from the animals given 10^7 Smeg i.p. 4 days before. Target tumor cells (10^5) were inoculated with PC or Smeg PEC (5×10^7) for 40 hr at $37°$ in a CO_2 incubator. ^{3}H-TdR (0.1 μCi) was added 16 hr before the end of the incubation.

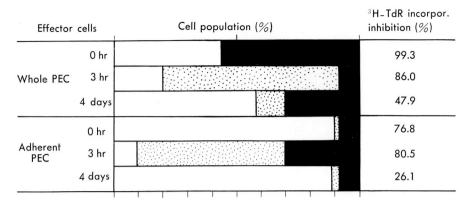

FIG. 3. *In vitro* cytotoxicity of Mp-rich and PMN-rich PEC against EL4 cells
☐ large and small MN; ▦ PMN; ■ lymphocytes.

as 3 hr) more than 60% of the PEC were PMN, but at a later period (such as 4 days) PMN decreased, and MN increased to about 60%.

In order to check the possibility that PMN are the effector cells (*6, 11*), the *in vitro* cytotoxicity of the PMN-rich PEC, harvested 3 hr after Smeg injection, were compared with those of the PMN-poor PEC, harvested 4 days after Smeg. Cytotoxicity of their adherent and non-adherent fractions was also compared. Figure 3 shows the cell populations (%) of the whole and adherent PEC from C57BL/6J mice. The inhibition (%) of ^{3}H-TdR incorporation into EL4 cells with these PEC is also shown in Fig. 3. The PMN-rich fractions showed weaker cytotoxicities than the PMN-poor but MN-rich fractions. The results from nu/nu PEC against KKN-1 were similar. It was suggested strongly that PMN are not the effector cells in these systems.

Further searches for the effector cells in the PEC indicated that these cells possess the following characteristics (*41*): a) Adherent to plastic or glass surfaces, b) not affected by anti-*θ* or anti-lymphocyte serum, c) inactivated by *in vivo* or *in vitro* treatment with carageenan, trypan blue, or cytochalasin B, d) inducible in the peritoneal cavity of nu/nu mice, e) more cytotoxic in the Mp-rich fraction than in the PMN-rich one, as stated above, and f) show Mp-like morphology in electron micrographs.

These facts suggest that the effector cells in these systems are Mp activated directly by Smeg, and probably by BCG also, without the help of T cells.

Activation of T Cells (1st Step of Mechanism B)

1) Proliferation of BCG-sensitized T cells

Mackaness (*3, 20*) and Zbar (*44*) showed that BCG is rapidly disseminated to regional lymph nodes after i.d. or intratumoral (i.t.) injection of living BCG, and leads to a local proliferation of BCG-sensitized T cells that are released into the systemic circulation about 4–5 days after BCG inoculation. The cell proliferation in regional nodes increased for about 14 days and remained elevated for 28 days or more.

TABLE II. Effects of BCG on Anti-SRBC and Anti-TNP PFC Production

Guinea pig strain	BCG treatment	Anti-SRBC PFC		Anti-TNP PFC	
		/10⁷ cells	/spleen	/10⁷ cells	/spleen
2	−	19	912	22	1,083
	+	316	30,924	504	49,164
JY-1	−	47	846	9	162
	+	181	7,167	613	24,275

Guinea pigs received 10^7 BCG i.v., and 2×10^8 TNP-SRBC were injected i.v. 14 days later. The spleen cells were harvested 7 days after TNP-SRBC and counted for PFC.

2) Polyclonal increase of T cells

Not only the proliferation of BCG-sensitized T cells but also polyclonal increase of T and B cells in the regional nodes was reported. Table II shows a part of our own data (K. S. Akagawa and T. Tokunaga, unpublished). Two inbred strains of guinea pig were given intravenous (i.v.) injection with 10^7 living BCG 14 days before i.v. injection with 2×10^8 trinitrophenylated-sheep erythrocytes (TNP-SRBC). Seven days after that, the number of plaque-forming cells (PFC) in the spleen was counted by the direct method. Both anti-SRBC and anti-TNP PFC increased by pretreatment with BCG in both strains. Similar results were reported in mice using T-dependent and -independent antigens (8, 9, 24).

The reason for polyclonal increase of lymphocytes after BCG is not clear yet. However, it is probable that the lymphocyte-activating factor (LAF) (25) released from Mp activated directly by BCG, and/or the mitogenic activity of BCG to T and B cells, may play an important role in this event.

The clones increased polyclonally with BCG may contain a clone of the tumor antigen-specific killer T cells. This clone may be selected and proliferate further by a stimulation of processed tumor antigen associated with BCG-activated Mp.

Activation of Mp with Lymphokines (Lk) (2nd Step of Mechanism B)

1) Genetic regulation of functional Mp-lymphocyte interaction

BCG-sensitized T cells released into the systemic circulation produced Lk at the sites of tumor infiltrated with BCG or lymph nodes containing BCG. It was reported by Rosenthal and Shevach (29) using strain 2 and 13 guinea pigs that activation of T cell DNA synthesis by Mp bearing complex protein antigens requires identity of histocompatibility-linked gene products on both Mp and lymphocyte.

A similar experiment was performed using inbred guinea pig strains, JY-1, JY-2, and strain 2 immunized with living BCG. Mixed lymphocyte reaction (MLR) between these strains showed that they are histoincompatible (T. Kataoka and T. Tokunaga, unpublished). Table III shows the results. BCG-sensitized lymphocytes were activated only by histocompatible Mp pulsed with PPD (T. Kataoka and T. Tokunaga, unpublished).

2) Lk susceptibility of Mp

Pathological sectioning of a murine solid tumor prepared 14 days after i.t. injection of BCG and stained by Ziehl-Neelsen staining showed that a great number of Mp

TABLE III. Requirement for Histocompatible Macrophages in Antigen-mediated DNA
Synthesis in BCG-immune Guinea Pig Lymph Node Lymphocytes

| Macrophage | | ³H-TdR incorporation (cpm) | |
Strain	PPD pulse	Strain JY-1	Strain JY-2
JY-1	−	1,844	2,283
	+	23,525	2,233
JY-2	−	6,295	1,335
	+	7,310	9,574
2	−	2,601	2,494
	+	3,004	2,580

Peritoneal macrophages (10^6) induced by oil were pulsed with 100 μg/ml PPD for 60 min at 37°,
washed and mixed with an equal number of syngeneic or allogeneic lymph node lymphocytes from
animals immunized with living BCG. Lymphocyte blast formation was assessed after 72 hr of culture;
1 μ Ci ³H-TdR was added for the last 18 hr.

that had ingested BCG accumulated and surrounded necrotic tumor tissue (R. Taka-
hashi, T. Kataoka and T. Tokunaga, unpublished). It is conceivable that BCG-sensitized
T cells stimulated by the Mp-associated BCG release Lk and activate Mp, resulting in
tumor cell destruction. In this context, we recently found that Mp activation with Lk
seems to require a preliminary stimulation of Mp. A crude Lk fraction was obtained
from serum of C57BL/6J mice immunized with BCG and challenged with old tuberculin
(OT) (30), or from culture supernatant of the spleen cells of a BCG-immunized guinea
pig incubated with purified protein derivatives (PPD). Resident PC and the PEC induced
by i.p. injection with protese peptone 4 days before, were obtained from C57BL/6J
mice and incubated for 24 hr with either the mouse or guinea pig Lk fraction. As
controls, medium alone, serum of normal C57BL/6J injected i.v. with OT, or culture
supernatant of normal guinea pig spleen cells plus PPD, were added to the PC and
the PEC. The mixtures were then washed and tested for cytotoxicity against EL4
leukemia cells. The results are shown in Table IV (S. Yamamoto and T. Tokunaga,
unpublished). Both Lk fractions from syngeneic and xenogenic animals gave cytotoxicity to the peptone-induced PEC but not to the resident PC. Similar results were
observed when BCG was employed instead of protese peptone (S. Yamamoto and
T. Tokunaga, unpublished).

TABLE IV. *In Vitro* Activation of Cytotoxic PC with Lk

| Effector cells | Preincubation for 60 min with | ³H-TdR incorporation into EL4 (%) | |
		Exp. A	Exp. B
Resident PC	Medium	118.7	100.3
	Control of Lk	117.6	103.5
	Lk	99.0	92.7
Peptone-induced PC	Medium	106.8	116.9
	Control of Lk	123.0	115.5
	Lk	18.8	10.6

Exp. A: Lk from syngeneic mice immunized with BCG was employed.
Exp. B: Lk from guinea pigs was employed.

These facts suggest the sequence of events that BCG administered locally stimulates Mp first at the injection site, and renders them susceptible to Lk released from BCG-sensitized lymphocytes. Studies on possible Mp subsets, including Mp wit or without the surface receptor for Mp-activating factor contained in Lk, are under way.

3) Target cell destruction with activated Mp

The process of target tumor cell destruction with activated Mp has been elucidated morphologically by other investigators (5, 16, 32, 38). Direct contact between activated and target cells is required for tumor cell killing. During the period of contact, a process of cell membrane fusion occurs and Mp lysosomes are passed through this cell junction into the tumor cells which are destroyed as a consequence. According to our own data on the interaction of PEC activated by Smeg with EL4 cells, viable Mp were required for the cytotoxicity; γ-ray irradiated or freeze-thawed Mp were ineffective (41). Electron micrographs of ultrathin sections of mixtures of EL4 and the PEC showed that activated Mp do not engulf intact tumor cells but rapidly phagocytize tumor cell debris (41). This is also reported in the other tumor systems (5, 7).

Induction of Tumor-specific Immunity (Step C Mechanism)

We showed that i.t. injection of BCG into KKN-1 and Ehrlich solid tumors resulted in regression of the tumors in nu/+ mice but not in nu/nu mice. This indicates clearly that T cell function is necessary for tumor regression. This T function seems to include both the mechanisms of B and C; the relative role of these 2 mechanisms in vivo is not clearly understood.

The fact that timing of administrations of tumor antigen and BCG is an important factor for an effective induction of tumor-specific immunity was indicated (14). It was shown that potentiation seemed to occur only when tumor antigen reached the regional node where lymphocytes in the T area are proliferating in response to BCG injection.

We confirmed this idea with our own system (R. M. Nakamura and T. Tokunaga, unpublished). A syngeneic fibrosarcoma of SWM/Ms, K5 (33), is weakly immunogenic, and an inoculum of ^{60}Co-irradiated K5 cells mixed with BCG into the mouse footpad cannot induce immunity against a challenge with live K5. However, if SWM/Ms mice were injected first with BCG into the footpad and 8 days later with ^{60}Co-irradiated K5 cells at the same site, they acquired systemic immunity against challenge with the tumor cells. In this context, living BCG was much stronger than dead organisms.

T lymphocytes increasing polyclonally in the regional lymph node responding to BCG may contain a clone of tumor-specific killer T cells. If so, this time interval between administration of BCG and tumor antigen, about 8 days, seems to be reasonable; the polyclonally increasing tumor-specific clone can proliferate further by selected stimulation of Mp-associated tumor antigen.

A stable form of delayed-type hypersensitivity (DTH) to SRBC in BCG-sensitized mice was reported (19, 22). Our preliminary experiment suggested that the DTH to SRBC in BCG-sensitized mice was resistant to passive transfer of suppressor T cells, resulting in stable DTH (K. S. Akagawa and T. Tokunaga, unpublished). Whether the tumor immunity produced by BCG-modulated primary response is subject to suppressor cells or not may be of importance.

Genetic Background of BCG Immunotherapy

Prophylactic and therapeutic effects of BCG on tumors are influenced greatly not only by the individual tumor's character, such as antigenicity, growth rate, and malignancy (*33, 34*), but also by the genetic background of the host. Clear experimental evidence of the latter problem has been presented (*34, 38*). Tumor incidence, 35 weeks after subcutaneous (s.c.) injection with MCA, was less than 90% in SWM/Ms mice, while it reached 100% within 12–15 weeks in C3H/He. BCG injection 2 weeks before 3-MCA significantly protected SWM/Ms from the tumors but not C3H/He. Thereapeutic effects of i.t. injections with BCG were also observed in the former strain but not in the latter.

DTH to BCG in SWM/Ms and C3H/He mice immunized with BCG 2 weeks previously was assessed by the footpad reaction, the Mp disappearance test, and the spleen cell blast formation test (*26*). SWM/Ms mice were high responders and C3H/He mice were low responders in all the tests. The footpad reactions to PPD of F_1 hybrids, (C3H×SWM) F_1, were all high, as shown in Fig. 4. The PPD reactions of both the F_2 from the brother-sister matings of the F_1 mice and the backcross mice (BC) between female F_1 and male C3H/He, were distributed over a wide range, as shown

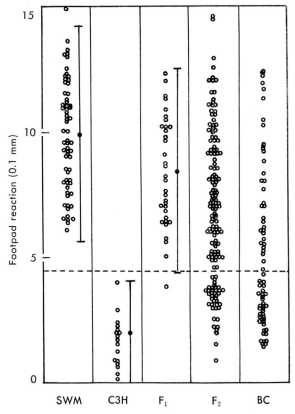

FIG. 4.   Footpad reactions of SWM/Ms, C3H/He and their F_1, F_2 and BC mice
Mice were given 10^7 BCG cells s.c. and footpad reactions with 10 μg PPD were tested 14 days later. Vertical bars indicate mean value $\pm$ 2SD.

in Fig. 4. χ^2 test of the results in F_2 and BC mice indicates that the difference of the responsiveness to PPD between SWM/Ms and C3H/He is controlled by a major gene transmitted by Mendel's law, although a possibility of polygene control is not completely excluded. The high responsiveness is expressed as a dominant trait. Partially purified non-adherent cells of the spleen from C3H/He mice immunized with BCG 2 weeks previously did not respond specifically to PPD *in vitro*, while those from SWM/Ms did (*26*). Preliminary studies at a cellular level on the host response to BCG indicated that suppressor T cells specific for BCG were induced in C3H/He mice of after i.v. injection with BCG.

Miscellaneous Problems

1) Immune depression with BCG

As stated before, the host response to BCG varies depending on the route, dose, and timing of BCG administration. It was reported that i.v. apministration of BCG, especially at high doses, inhibited the spleen cells in concanavalin A response (*9*), in PFC formation to T-dependent and -independent antigens (*8, 9*), and in a graft *vs.* host reaction or a mixed lymphocyte reaction (*12*).

We injected various doses of BCG i.v. into C57BL/6J mice and gave 10^8 SRBC 14days later. Four days after SRBC, direct PFC to SRBC in the spleens were counted. The PFC in control mice without BCG were $351,478\pm23.956$/spleen and $1,621\pm11/10^6$ spleen cells. The PFC in mice injected with 10^5 BCG cells were almost the same as in the controls, while those with 10^6 BCG cells decreased to one-half, and those with 10^8 BCG cells were only $17,275\pm7,494$ and 18 ± 9, respectively (K. Akagawa and T. Tokunaga, unpublished).

2) Active cell components

Physical and chemical requirements for cell components active in immunotherapy are important, and will be discussed by Azuma in this book.

3) Living and dead BCG

As an immunotherapeutic agent of human malignant diseases, living BCG, especially the relatively virulent BCG strains, has some disadvantages, such as BCG infection in immuno-depressed cancer patients. Experimentally, however, it is apparent that living BCG is stronger than dead BCG in the activation of both Mp and lymphocytes and in antitumor effects. From the standpoint of not only academic interest but also reconstitution of purified bacterial components for practical use, it would be worthwhile knowing the reason(s) why living BCG is stronger.

With regard to BCG, the following points in living BCG differ from dead BCG: (i) An increase of total dose of antigen(s) and adjuvant-active substance(s), (ii) a configuration of cell components in intact cells, such as covering with 3 lipid layers, that may be adequate for intracellular persistence and indigestibility of antigen, (iii) appearance of new cell components, such as "pili" which we detected by electron microscopy in naturally growing mycobacteria only (*35*), (iv) production and release of cell metabolites, and (v) integration of host substances, such as cholesterol esters, on the BCG surface during bacterial growth (*18*), that may moidfy BCG to resemble "self." From the host point of view: (vi) possible surface complex of Mp-MHC (major histocompatibility complex) with antigen may be produced more easily in intracellularly replicating antigen, and (vii) formation of many "point sources" of infection distributed through various lymphoid tissues may provide an adequate antigen gradient *in vivo*. Further basic studies are required.

4) Oral administration of BCG

The oral route of BCG has been clinically interesting, but there is little experimental evidence to support this approach. We attempted to treat several allogeneic and syngeneic tumors of mice and guinea pigs by oral BCG (T. Tokunaga, S. Taguchi, and T. Murohashi, unpublished). Weekly administration of 5 mg of lyophilized BCG (Japanese strain) per mouse, or 80 mg per guinea pig, showed some effects on some allogeneic tumors but not on several others. After daily administration of BCG for 4 days, living BCG was isolated only from Peyer's patches and mesenteric nodes in both mice and guinea pigs, while BCG was isolated from the spleens and the livers but not from Peyer's patches and mesenteric nodes in the animals that received single s.c. injections of BCG. Positive tuberculin skin reaction was observed within 10 days after single s.c. BCG, while it took about 2 months after the start of weekly oral BCG. Pathological observation of Peyer's patches after oral BCG showed a remarkable proliferation of lymphocytes in both T- and B-areas and a strong infiltration with Mp in the patches. The significance of these phenomena is under study.

5) Systemic, non-specific effects of BCG

Contrary to the local effects of BCG, systemic effects of BCG are not remarkable, at least in animal models. It seems apparent that Mp can be activated by BCG. However, it is not clear whether systemically activated Mp can attack a localized tumor or whether they can attack it only by a call-sign of Lk that are produced at the tumor site. It was reported, on the other hand, that BCG is a good producer of Lk and LAF, not only *in vitro* but also *in vivo*. However, systemic injections with these fractions showed little effect on tumors. It is also unknown whether differentiation of T cells after BCG administration is selective to, for instance, helper T or killer T, or non-selective.

Natural killer cells induced by BCG that were reported recently (40) should be one of the important problem to investigate in the future. It may be important to note, as a systemic role of BCG, that reticuloendothelial system activated by BCG may clear immune depressants, such as tumor antigen-antibody complexes and toxic substances released from tumor cells, shown in Fig. 1, and thus strengthen the antitumor effector mechanisms as a consequence.

It may also be important from the clinical standpoint that step A, B, and C mechanisms, shown in Fig. 2, should work against not only tumor cells but also infectious agents. Non-specific augmentation of resistance to such microbial infection with BCG should prolong survival time of the tumor bearers.

REFERENCES

1. Alexander, P. Activated macrophages and the antitumor action of BCG. *In* "Conference on the Use of BCG in Therapy of Cancer," ed. by T. Borsos and H. J. Rapp, N.l.H., Bethesda, pp. 127–133 (1973).

2. Bast, R. C., Jr., Zbar, B., Borsos, T., and Rapp, H. J. BCG and cancer. *N. Engl. J. Med.*, **290**, 1413–1420, 1458–1469 (1974).

3. Blanden, R. V., Lefford, M. J., and Mackaness, G. B. The host response to Calmette-Guérin Bacillus infection in mice. *J. Exp. Med.*, **129**, 1079–1101 (1969).

4. Brunner, K. T. and Cerottini, J. C. Cytotoxic lymphocytes as effector cells of cell-mediated immunity. *In* "Progress of Immunology," ed. by B. Amos, Academic Press, New York, pp. 385–398 (1971).

5. Bucana, C., Hoyer, L. C., Hibbs, B., Breeman, S., McDaniel, M., and Hanna, M. G. Morphological evidence for the translocation of lysosomal organelles from cytotoxic macrophages into the cytoplasm of tumor target cells, *Cancer Res.*, **36**, 4444–4458 (1976).

6. Burton, R. C., Holmes, M. C., Warner, N. L., and Woodruff, M.F.A. Mechanisms of resistance to syngeneic tumors in athymic (nude) mice. *In* "Proc. 2nd Workshop on Nude Mice," Gustuv Fischer Verlag, Stuttgart, West Germany, pp. 511–524 (1977).

7. Cleveland, R. P., Meltzer, M. S., and Zbar, B. Tumor cytotoxicity *in vitro* by macrophages from mice infected with *Mycobacterium bovis* strain BCG. *J. Natl. Cancer Inst.*, **52**, 1887–1895 (1974).

8. Doft, B. H., Merchant, B., Johannessen, L., and Chaparas, S. D. Contrasting effects of BCG on spleen and lymph node antibody response in nude and normal mice. *J. Immunol.*, **117**, 1638–1643 (1976).

9. Florentin, I., Huchet, R., Bruley-Rosset, M., Halle-Pannenko, O., and Mathé, G. Studies on the mechanisms of action of BCG. *Cancer Immunol. Immunother.*, **1**, 31–39 (1976).

10. Fujimoto, S., Greene, M. I., and Sehon, A. H. Regulation of the immune response to tumor antigen. I. Immunosuppressor cells in tumor-bearing hosts. *J. Immunol.*, **116**, 791–799 (1976).

11. Gale, R. P. and Zighelboim, J. Polymorphonuclear leukocytes in antibody-dependent cellular cytotoxicity. *J. Immunol.*, **114**, 1047–1051 (1975).

12. Geffard, M. and Orbach-Arbouys, S. Enhancement of T suppressor activity in mice by high doses of BCG. *Cancer Immunol. Immunother.*, **1**, 41–43 (1976).

13. Granger, G. A. and Kolb, W. P. Lymphocyte *in vitro* cytotoxicity: Mechanism of immune and non-immune small lymphocyte-mediated target L-cell destruction. *J. Immunol.*, **101**, 111–120 (1968).

14. Hawrylko, E. and Mackaness, G. B. Immunopotentiation with BCG. III. Modulation of the response to a tumor-specific antigen. *J. Natl. Cancer Inst.*, **51**, 1677–1682 (1973).

15. Herberman, R. B., Nunn, M. E., and Lavrin, D. H. Natural cytotoxic reactivity of mouse lymphoid cells against syngeneic and allogeneic tumors. II. Characterization of effector cells. *Int. J. Cancer*, **16**, 230–239 (1975).

16. Hibbs, J. B., Jr. Heterocytolysis by bacillus Calmette-Guérin activated macrophages by lysosome exocytosis into tumor cells. *Science*, **184**, 468–471 (1974).

17. Kennedy, J. C. *In vitro* and *in vivo* effects of immunosuppressive and toxic material produced and released by cancer cells. *In* "Host Defense against Cancer and Its Potentiation," ed. by D. Mizuno *et al.*, Japan Scientific Societies Press, Tokyo, pp. 67–79 (1975).

18. Kondo, E., Kanai, K., Nishimura, K., and Tsumita, T. Analysis of host-originated

lipids associating with "*in vivo* grown tubercle bacilli." *Japan. J. Med. Sci. Biol.*, **24**, 345–356 (1971).

19. Lagrange, P. H. and Mackaness, G. B. A stable form of delayed-type hypersensitivity. *J. Exp. Med.*, **141**, 82–96 (1975).
20. Mackaness, G. B. The influence of immunologically committed lymphoid cells on macrophage activity *in vivo*. *J. Exp. Med.*, **129**, 973–992 (1969).
21. Mackaness, G. B., Auclair, D. J., and Lagrange, P. H. Immunopotentiation with BCG. I. Immune response to different strains and preparations. *J. Natl. Cancer Inst.*, **51**, 1655–1667 (1973).
22. Mackaness, G. B., Lagrange, P. H., and Ishibashi, T. The modifying effect of BCG on the immunological induction of T cells. *J. Exp. Med.*, **139**, 1540–1552 (1974).
23. Mathé, G. Surviving in company of BCG. *Cancer Immunol. Immunother.*, **1**, 3–5 (1976).
24. Miller, T. E., Mackaness, G. B., and Lagrange, P. H. Immunopotentiation with BCG. II. Modulation of the response to sheep red blood cells. *J. Natl. Cancer Inst.*, **51**, 1669–1676 (1973).
25. Mitchell, M. S., Kirkpartrick, D., Makyr, M. B., and Gery, I. On the mode of action of BCG. *Nature New Biol.*, **243**, 216–218 (1973).
26. Nakamura, R. M. and Tokunaga, T. Strain difference of delayed-type hypersencitivity to BCG and its genetic control in mice. *Infec. Immun.*, in press (1978).
27. Pimm, M. V. and Baldwin, R. W. BCG immunotherapy of rat tumors in athymic nude mice. *Nature*, **254**, 77–78 (1975).
28. Pollack, S., Happner, G., Brawn, R. J., and Nelson, K. Specific killing of tumor cells *in vitro* in the presence of normal lymphoid cells and sera from hosts immune to the tumor antigens. *Int. J. Cancer*, **9**, 316–323 (1972).
29. Rosenthal, A. S. and Shevach, E. M. Function of macrophages in antigen recognition by guinea pig T lymphocytes. *J. Exp. Med.*, **138**, 1194–1212 (1973).
30. Salvin, S. B., Younger, J. S., Nishio, J., and Neta, R. Tumor suppression by a lymphokine released into the circulation of mice with delayed hypersensitivity. *J. Natl. Cancer Inst.*, **55**, 1233–1235 (1975).
31. Sjögren, H. O., Hellström, I., Bansal, S. C., and Hellström, K. E. Suggestive evidence that the "blocking antibodies" of tumor-bearing individuals may be antigen-antibody complexes. *Proc. Natl. Acad. Sci. U.S.*, **68**, 1372–1375 (1971).
32. Sondgrass, M. J. and Hanna, M. G., Jr. Ultrastructural studies of histiocyte-tumor cell interactions during tumor regression after intralesional injection of *Mycobacterium bovis*. *Cancer Res.*, **33**, 701–716 (1973).
33. Tokunaga, T., Kataoka, T., Nakamura, R. M., Yamamoto, S., and Tanaka, T. Tumor immunity induced by BCG-tumor cell mixtures in syngeneic mice. *Japan. J. Med. Sci. Biol.*, **26**, 71–85 (1973).
34. Tokunaga, T., Yamamoto, S., Nakamura, R. M., and Kataoka, T. Immunotherapeutic and immunoprophylactic effects of BCG on 3-methylcholanthrene-induced autochthonous tumors in Swiss mice. *J. Natl. Cancer Inst.*, **53**, 459–463 (1974).
35. Tokunaga, T. and Mizuguchi, Y. Mycobacterial pili. *Rinsho to Saikin*, **1**, 8–10 (1974) (in Japanese).
36. Tokunaga, T., Yamamoto, S., Nakamura, R. M., Mizuguchi, Y., Suga, K., Nitta, M., Taguchi, S., Kataoka, T., and Murohashi, T. Anti-tumor activity of *Mycobacterium smegmatis* and BCG. *In* "Proc. 10th Joint Conference Tuberculosis," U.S.-Japan Cooper. Med. Sci. Progr., N.I.H., pp. 444–459 (1975).
37. Tokunaga, T. and Yamamoto, S. Augmentation of host defence of nude mice against cancer. *In* "Proc. 2nd Workshop on Nude Mice," Gustuv Fischer Verlag, Stuttgart, West Germany, pp. 525–531 (1977).

38. Tokunaga, T., Yamamoto, S., Nakamura, R. M., Kurosawa, A., and Murohashi, T. Mouse-strain difference in immunoprophylactic and immunotherapeutic effects of BCG on carcinogen-induced autochthonous tumors. *Japan. J. Med. Sci. Biol.*, **31**, 143–154 (1978).

39. Treves, A. J., Cohen, I. R., and Feldman, M. Suppressor factor secreted by T-lymphocytes from tumor-bearing mice. *Eur. J. Immunol.*, **4**, 722–727 (1974).

40. Wolfe, S. A., Tracey, D. E., and Henney, C. S. BCG-induced murine effector cells. II. Characterization of natural killer cells in peritoneal exudates. *J. Immunol.*, **119**, 1152–1158 (1977).

41. Yamamoto, S. and Tokunaga, T. *In vitro* cytotoxicity of peritoneal macrophages activated with *Mycobacterium smegmatis*. *Microbiol. Immunol.*, **22**, 27–40 (1977).

42. Zbar, B., Bernstein, I. D., Bartlett, G. L., Hanna, M. G., Jr., and Rapp, H. J. Immunotherapy of cancer: Regression of intradermal tumors and prevention of growth of lymph node metastases after intralesional injection of living *Mycobacterium bovis*. *J. Natl. Cancer Inst.*, **49**, 119–130 (1972).

43. Zbar, B., Wepsic, H. T., Borsos, T., and Rapp, H. J. Tumor graft rejection in syngeneic guinea pigs: Evidence for a two-step mechanism. *J. Natl. Cancer Inst.*, **44**, 473–481 (1970).

44. Zbar, B., Ribi, E., Kelly, M., Granger, D., Evans, C., and Rapp, H. J. Immunologic approaches to the treatment of human cancer based on a guinea pig model. *Cancer Immunol. Immunother.*, **1**, 127–137 (1976).

GANN Monograph on Cancer Research 21, 1978

ANTITUMOR ACTIVITY OF BCG CELL-WALL SKELETON AND RELATED MATERIALS

Ichiro Azuma,[*1] Mikio Yamawaki,[*1] Takeshi Ogura,[*1] Takahiko Yoshimoto,[*1] Reiko Tokuzen,[*2] Fumio Hirao,[*1] and Yuichi Yamamura[*1]

*Third Department of Internal Medicine, Osaka University Medical School,[*1] and National Cancer Center Research Institute[*2]*

The antitumor activity of BCG cell-wall skeleton was examined in experimental tumor systems. BCG cell-wall skeleton treated with a light mineral oil (Drakeol 6VR) showed potent activities on (a) the rise of cell-mediated cytotoxicity depressed in tumor-bearing mice to a normal level (b) suppression and regression of tumor growth in syngeneic and autochthonous mice and rats, and prevention of metastasis in the hosts, and (c) the prevention of carcinogenesis with chemical carcinogens in mice, rats, and rabbits.

It was also shown that the cell-wall skeleton of *Nocardia rubra* attached to oil droplets was effective as an immunotherapeutic agent. Efficacy of the synthetic adjuvants, N-acetylmuramyldipeptide and its derivatives, as immunoadjuvants is also discussed.

It has been shown that the principal chemical structure of the cell-wall skeleton of *Mycobacterium bovis* BCG and related microorganisms such as other mycobacteria, nocardia, and corynebacteria is a "mycolic acid-arabinogalactan-mucopeptide" complex and the detailed chemical properties of each component have been examined (*2, 4*). We have reported that the cell-wall skeletons of mycobacteria, nocardia, and corynebacteria have a potent adjuvant activity on immune responses (*2, 3, 5, 10, 21, 24, 25, 29–31*), mitogenic activity on mouse lymphocytes (*7, 9, 27*), and antitumor activity in experimental tumor systems (*8, 10, 11, 19, 21, 28, 32, 33, 45, 46, 48*). Since 1974, the BCG cell-wall skeleton has been applied in the immunotherapy of human cancer, such as lung cancer (*13, 22, 36, 37, 40, 41, 43, 44*), leukemia (*16, 20, 35*), malignant melanoma (*23, 42*), gastric and colo-rectal cancer (*26*), uterine cervical cancer (Jimi *et al.*, unpublished data), and other neoplastic diseases in Japan.

In this review, we summarize the antitumor activity of BCG cell-wall skeleton and related materials in experimental tumor systems, and the mode of action of these materials is discussed.

[*1] Fukushima 1-1-50, Fukushima-ku, Osaka 553, Japan (東 市郎, 山脇幹夫, 小倉 剛, 吉本崇彦, 平尾文男, 山村雄一).

[*2] Tsukiji 5-1-1, Chuo-ku, Tokyo 104, Japan (徳善玲子).

Purification and Biochemical Properties of Cell-wall Skeletons of Mycobacteria, Nocardia, and Corynebacteria

The cell-wall skeletons of mycobacteria and related bacteria were prepared by the following procedures (*4, 11*). The cells were suspended in distilled water and disrupted with Sorvall cell fractionator (Model RF-1) at 35,000 lb/in² at 5–10°, or with Dynomill (Model KDL) at 3,000 rpm with glass beads (0.1–0.2 mm in diameter) for 15 min at 5–10°. The latter disruption procedure was repeated 2 or 3 times if necessary. The disrupted product was centrifuged at $800 \times g$ for 15 min to remove unbroken cells and cell debris, after which the whole cell-wall fraction was obtained by centrifugation at $20,000 \times g$ for 60 min. This fraction was treated repeatedly with DNase, RNase, trypsin, chymotrypsin, and then pronase, followed by sequential extractions with acetone, ether-ethanol (1: 1), chloroform, and chloroform-methanol (2: 1). The residual fraction, obtained in yields of 5–10% of whole cells was designated "cell-wall skeleton."

The cell-wall skeletons of mycobacteria, nocardia, and corynebacteria have been shown to be a "mycolic acid-arabinogalactan-mucopeptide" complex (Fig. 1), and the biochemical properties of each of the components were examined in detail. Mycolic acids were defined as "α-branched β-hydroxylated fatty acids." Their biochemical analyses have shown that mycobacterial cell-wall skeletons contain mycolic acids of about C_{70}–C_{86}, nocardia cell-wall skeletons contain nocardomycolic acids of C_{34}–C_{60} and corynebacteria cell-wall skeletons contain corynomycolic acids of C_{28}–C_{38}. The length of α-branches are C_{22} and C_{24} in mycolic acids and C_8–C_{16} in nocardomycolic acids and corynomycolic acids. These mycolic acids, nocardomycolic acids, and corynomycolic acids are bound by ester linkage to the 5-hydroxy group of the non-reducing termi-

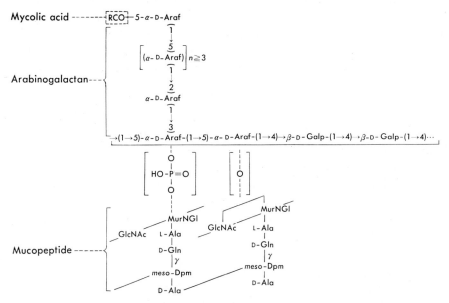

FIG. 1.   Principal chemical structure of BCG cell-wall skeleton (BCG-CWS)

    Araf, D-arabinofuranose; Galp, D-galactopyranose; GlcNAc, N-acetylglucosamine; MurNGl, N-glycolylmuramic acid; Dpm, α, ε-diaminopimelic acid; RCO, mycolic acid residue.

nal of D-arabinofuranose residue of arabinogalactan (polysaccharide) of cell-wall skeletons. A tetrapeptide, L-alanyl-D-isoglutaminyl-*meso*-diaminopimelyl-D-alanine was identified as the common subunit of the peptide moiety of mucopeptide fractions of mycobacteria, nocardia, and corynebacteria. N-acetylglucosaminyl-β-1,4-N-glycolyl-muramic acid was found as a subunit of the glycan moiety of the mucopeptide fraction of the cell-wall skeletons of mycobacteria and nocardia, whereas N-acetylglucosaminyl-β-1,4-N-acetylmuramic acid was found to be a subunit of the glycan of the cell-wall skeleton of corynebacteria. The presence of cross linkages between L-alanine and *meso*-diaminopimelic acid has been reported. The mode of linkage between arabinogalactan and mucopeptide fractions was proposed to be a phosphodiester linkage. The presence of a glycosidic linkage was also suggested.

Adjuvant Activity of Cell-wall Skeletons of Mycobacteria, Nocardia, and Corynebacteria

In previous papers (*2, 3, 31*), we have reported that cell-wall skeletons of mycobacteria, nocardia, and corynebacteria have a potent adjuvant activity for enhancing the humoral immune response against bovine serum albumin, sheep erythrocytes, and hapten-protein conjugate in both *in vivo* and *in vitro* immune systems. It was also shown that oil-attached cell-wall skeletons of mycobacteria, nocardia, and corynebacteria enhanced the generation of cell-mediated cytotoxic effector cells in allogeneic mice (*30*) and in syngeneic mice (*15*) by Brunner's assay system (*12*). In this review, the adjuvant activity of the cell-wall skeletons of mycobacteria, nocardia, and corynebacteria on the cell-mediated cytotoxicity in allogeneic mice are described.

1) Preparation of oil-attached cell-wall skeletons

Oil-attached cell-wall skeleton was prepared briefly as follows (*8, 19*): 10 mg of mineral oil (Drakeol 6VR, Pennsylvania Refining Co., Ltd., Butler, Pa.) was added to 4 mg of BCG cell-wall skeleton and ground to a smooth paste in a tissue homogenizer. One milliliter of saline containing 0.2% Tween 80 was added and grinding was repeated to make a homogenous suspension, which was sterilized by incubation at 60° for 30 min before use.

2) Adjuvant activity of oil-attached cell-wall skeletons on cell-mediated cytotoxicity in allogeneic mice

C57BL/6J mice were immunized intraperitoneally with mastocytoma P815-X2 cells (10^4), with or without 100 μg of oil-attached BCG cell-wall skeleton. The cytotoxic activity of the spleen cells in mice treated with oil-attached BCG cell-wall skeleton was measurable on day 6 and reached a maximum from day 11 to 14 after immunization with alloantigen. The enhancing effect persisted for 55 days or longer. As in the case of oil-attached BCG cell-wall skeleton, the oil-attached skeletons of *Nocardia rubra* and *Corynebacterium diphtheriae* PW8 were shown to be potent stimulators of allogeneic cell-mediated cytotoxicity in mice (Table I).

To examine the correlation between humoral response and cell-mediated cytotoxicity against mastocytoma cells, mice were immunized with mastocytoma P815-X2 cells (10^4) with or without 100 μg of oil-attached BCG cell-wall skeleton. Eleven days later, cytotoxic activity of the spleen cells was determined by chromium release assay and,

TABLE I. Effect of Oil-attached Cell-wall Skeletons (CWS) of *Mycobacterium*, *Nocardia*, and *Corynebacterium* on Cell-mediated Cytotoxicity (*30*)

Group	C57BL/6J mice were immunized with[a]	Specific cell lysis (%)
	Mastocytoma P815-X2 (1×10^4)	
1	+oil-attached BCG-CWS (100 μg)	65.9
2	+oil-attached *N. rubra*-CWS (100 μg)	94.0
3	+oil-attached *C. diphtheriae* PW8-CWS (100 μg)	66.2
4	+oil droplets	48.0
5	+medium (MEM[b])	15.3

[a] Mice of C57BL/6J were immunized intraperitoneally with a mixture of mastocytoma P815-X2 cells (10^4) and oil-attached CWS, oil droplets, or medium. Eleven days later, cell-mediated cytotoxicity of spleen cells of immunized mice was determined by incubation of spleen cells (effector cells) and ^{51}Cr-labeled mastocytoma P815-X2 cells (target cells) at ratio of 100:1 for 20 hr.

[b] Minimal essential medium.

at the same time, antimastocytoma antibody in the sera was measured by Wigzell's method (*34*). Cytotoxic activity of the spleen cells from the mice treated with mastocytoma cells and oil-attached BCG cell-wall skeleton reached almost 100%, whereas those of spleen cells from the mice immunized with mastocytoma cells and oil droplets or medium alone were 84 and 13%, respectively. However, the titers of antimastocytoma antibody produced in mice treated with mastocytoma cells and 100 μg of oil-attached BCG cell-wall skeleton were almost similar to those treated with either oil droplets or medium alone (*30*). These results were confirmed by the immunization of C57BL/6J mice with trinitrophenylated (TNP)-mastocytoma P815-X2 cells and determination of plaque-forming cells against TNP group and generation of cell-mediated cytotoxicity using immunized mouse spleen cells (*30*) suggesting that oil-attached BCG cell-wall skeleton is an excellent adjuvant for potentiating cell-mediated immunity rather than the humoral response to mastocytoma cells in mice. The above conclusion was supported by the results of Ohno *et al.* (*24*) and of Okuyama *et al.* (*25*).

3)   Effect of oil-attached BCG cell-wall skeleton on cell-mediated cytotoxicity in tumor-bearing mice

Recently, it has been established that the function of immune responses, especially T cell functions were suppressed in tumor-bearing hosts compared to normal mice (*29*). We have found that depressed function of an immune response, cell-mediated cytotoxicity, in tumor-bearing mice could be raised to a normal level by treatment with oil-attached BCG cell-wall skeleton. Age-matched C57BL/6J mice were divided into 7 groups.

Mice in groups II to VII were inoculated intradermally with viable melanoma B16 cells (2×10^5) on day 0. Group I was injected with medium alone and used as the control. On day 19, all mice were immunized intraperitoneally with mastocytoma P815-X2 cells (5×10^6) with or without oil-attached BCG cell-wall skeleton. Mice in group II were injected with oil-attached BCG cell-wall skeleton (100 μg) and with alloantigen intraperitoneally on day 19 and those in group V intradermally on days 19, 22, and 26. The cell-mediated cytotoxicity of the spleen cells of immunized mice was determined

TABLE II. Improvement of Depressed Cell-mediated Cytotoxicity of Spleen Cells from Tumor-bearing Mice with Oil-attached BCG Cell-wall Skeleton (BCG-CWS) (29)

Exp.	Group No.	C57BL/6J mice inoculated with	Alloantigen[a]	Adjuvant	Route of adjuvant[b]	Tumor size (mm)[c]	Specific target cell lysis[d]	
							Mean±SE (%)	p value[e]
		Day 0	Day 19	Day 19			Day 30	
A	I	Medium	P815 (5×10^6)	Medium	i.p.	0	86.9±3.8	
	II	Melanoma B16[f]	P815 (5×10^6)	Medium	i.p.	22.3±1.8	30.4±3.7	<0.01
	III	Melanoma B16	P815 (5×10^6)	Oil droplets	i.p.	20.3±2.0	54.2±3.3	<0.01
	IV	Melanoma B16	P815 (5×10^6)	BCG-CWS (100 μg)	i.p.	20.8±2.4	85.2±6.3	<0.01
		Day 0	Day 19	Days 19, 22, 26			Day 30	
B	V	Melanoma B16	P815 (5×10^6)	Medium	i.d.	16.3±1.9	20.4±1.9	
	VI	Melanoma B16	P815 (5×10^6)	Oil droplets (3×)	i.d.	16.2±0.9	50.4±5.1	<0.01
	VII	Melanoma B16	P815 (5×10^6)	BCG-CWS (3×, 100μg)	i.d.	15.5±1.0	73.6±1.7	<0.01

[a] Nineteen days after melanoma inoculation, all mice were immunized intraperitoneally with alloantigen (mastocytoma cells).

[b] i.p., intraperitoneally with mastocytoma cells; i.d., intradermally.

[c] Tumor size was determined as a diameter with calipers, and results indicate the average size±SE.

[d] Cell-mediated cytotoxicity of spleen cells was determined as shown in Table I.

[e] Student's t-test.

[f] Mice were inoculated intradermally with 2×10^5 viable melaoma cells on day 0.

on day 30 by using chromium release assay. As shown in Table II, the cell-mediated cytotoxicity of spleen cells obtained from solid tumor-bearing mice immunized with alloantigen and oil-attached BCG cell-wall skeleton (group II) was similar to those obtained from normal, control mice (group I). The differences in the tumor size in groups II, III, and IV were not statistically significant. Furthermore, the cytotoxicity of the spleen cells obtained from tumor-bearing mice treated with oil-attached BCG cell-wall skeleton separately (intradermally) by alloantigenic immunization was similar to that of spleen cells from normal mice. These results indicate that the impaired cell-mediated cytotoxicity of spleen cells from solid tumor-bearing mice could be elevated to a normal level when treated with oil-attached BCG cell-wall skeleton together with, or separately from, alloantigen. It was also found that treatment of tumor-bearing mice with oil-attached BCG cell-wall skeleton did not influence the tumor size in groups of IV and VII, compared to those of II and III, or V and VI, respectively.

Kitagawa et al. (17) have reported that a depressed immunological state, as determined by the function of carrier-specific helper T cells in mice that bore tumor or were treated with cell-free Ehrlich ascites, was raised to normal levels by intravenous injection with oil-attached BCG cell-wall skeleton.

4) Mitogenic activity

More recently, we have shown that the cell-wall skeletons of M. bovis BCG, N. rubra, and C. diphtheriae PW8 were active as mitogens on normal spleen cells, anti-θ serum-treated spleen cells and cortisone-resistant thymocytes of C57BL/6J mice and spleen cells of congenitally athymic (nude) mice (BALB/c-nu/nu) (45). From these results, it was concluded that the cell-wall skeletons of mycobacteria, nocardia, and corynebacteria acted as mitogens on both thymus-derived lymphocytes (T cells) and bone marrow-derived lymphocytes (B cells). It was proved that the cell-wall skeleton of N. rubra could not act as a mitogen on purified T cells at any concentration, however, mitogenic activity of the cell-wall skeleton of N. rubra was restored if the pure splenic T cells were reconstituted with X-irradiated peritoneal exudate cells of syngeneic mice (27). These results suggest the requirement of macrophages for T cell activation by the cell-wall skeleton as well as phytohemagglutinin or concanavalin A.

The chemical components of the cell-wall skeleton of mycobacteria responsible for the mitogenic activity on the mouse spleen cells are mycolic acid and its derivatives, such as arabinose-mycolates, mycoloyl-arabinogalactan and its methyl ester, and the mucopeptide fraction; arabinogalactan was inactive in this respect (7).

Antitumor Activity of Cell-wall Skeletons of Mycobacteria, Nocardia, and Corynebacteria

It has been shown that oil-attached BCG cell-wall skeleton shows suppression of tumor growth (8) and regression of established line 10 hepatoma in the syngeneic strain-2 guinea pigs (48). Systemic and specific tumor immunity was induced in the guinea pigs in which such tumor suppression or regression occurred. In this review, the experimental results of the antitumor activity of the cell-wall skeletons of mycobacteria, nocardia, and corynebacteria in mice, rats and rabbits are described.

1) Suppression of tumor growth in syngeneic mice

The suspension of tumor cells, mastocytoma P815-X2, melanoma B16, or EL4 leukemia, was mixed with oil-attached cell-wall skeleton, and 0.05 ml of this mixture was inoculated intradermally into the flank of each mouse. As shown in Table III, oil-

TABLE III. Suppression of Tumor Growth with Oil-attached Cell-wall Skeletons Prepared from *Mycobacterium* sp. (8)

Cell-wall skeletons of	Dose (μg)	No. of mice tested	Mastocytoma P815[a] (Exp. 730713)	Mastocytoma P815[a] (Exp. 730929)	EL-4 leukemia[b] (Exp. 730930)	Melanoma B16[c] (Exp. 730726)
M. bovis BCG (lot 181)	100	10	9/9	10/10	2/6	9/10[d]
(lot 182)	100	10	4/4	6/6	2/6	
M. kansasii	100	10	4/4	8/8	0/1	9/10
M. tuberculosis H37Rv	100	10	4/4	5/6	2/8	3/8
M. smegmatis	100	10	5/5	6/7	1/8	9/10
Control (oil droplets)	—	10	0/0	0/0	0/0	0/0

[a] A mixture of mastocytoma P815 (2×10^4) and oil-attached mycobacterial cell-wall skeleton was inoculated intradermally in F_1 hybrid mice (C57BL/6J $\times$ DBA/2). Values are the results 43 days after inoculation.

[b] A mixture of EL-4 leukemia (5×10^4) and oil-ottached mycobacterial cell-wall skeleton was inoculated intradermally in C57BL/6J mice. Values are the results 35 days after inoculation.

[c] A mixture of melanoma B16 (10^5) and oil-attached mycobacterial cell-wall skeleton was inoculated intradermally in C57BL/6J mice. Values are the results 35 days after inoculation.

[d] No. of tumor-free mice/No. of mice that survived.

attached cell-wall skeletons prepared from *Mycobacterium kansasii*, *Mycobacterium tuberculosis* H37Rv and H37Ra, and *Mycobacterium smegmatis* were as effective at a dose of 100 µg as that of *M. bovis* BCG, for suppression of transplantable tumor growth in syngeneic or semisyngeneic mice. Oil-attached cell-wall skeletons of *Nocardia asteroides* 131, *N. rubra*, *C. diphtheriae* PW8, and *Corynebacterium fermentans* also suppressed the growth of mastocytoma P815-X2 and EL4 leukemia in semisyngeneic and syngeneic mice (8). When tumor growth was suppressed in mice by intradermal injection of oil-attached cell-wall skeleton mixed with the tumor cells, mice showed systemic and specific resistance to subsequent challenge by tumor cells. Systemic tumor immunity was induced in mice by inoculation of a mixture of mitomycin C-treated or irradiated mastocytoma P815-X2 and oil-attached BCG cell-wall skeleton in semisyngeneic mice. However, it was shown that the inoculation of oil-attached BCG cell-wall skeleton separately from irradiated tumor cells could not induce systemic resistance to subsequent challenge by tumor cells. More recently, Tanaka *et al.* (28) reported that oil-attached BCG cell-wall skeleton suppressed the growth of 3-methylcholanthrene-induced fibrosarcoma in inbred SWM/Ms mice. It was also shown that oil-attached cell-wall skeletons of BCG and *N. rubra* suppressed the growth of 3-methylcholanthrene-induced fibrosarcoma in the footpads of syngeneic BALB/c-nu/nu mice (45).

2) *Effect of BCG cell-wall skeleton on experimental malignant pleurisy in mice*

Yoshimoto *et al.* (46) reported local immunotherapy with oil-attached BCG cell-wall skeleton of experimental pleural effusion using a transplantable pleural fibrosarcoma (MC-106) in ddO mice. All mice in the control group, which intrapleurally received saline solution 24 hr after the intrapleural injection of tumor cells (3×10^5), died within

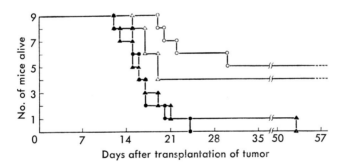

FIG. 2. Effect of oil-attached BCG cell-wall skeleton on experimental neoplastic pleural effusion in mice (46)

Viable cells (3×10^5) of MC-106 suspended in 0.1 ml of minimum essential medium were injected into the right pleural cavity of the mice on day 0. Group 1 (○), CWS i.pl., CWS s.c. −14, −7, +7, +14 days; group 2 (▲), od i.pl., CWS s.c. −14, −7, +7, +14 days; group 3 (△), CWS i.pl., CWS s.c. +7, +14 days; group 4 (●), NaCl sol. i.pl., NaCl sol. s.c. +7, +14 days.

CWS: 100 µg of oil-attached BCG cell-wall skeleton. od: oil droplets in diluent without BCG cell-wall skeleton. NaCl sol.: 0.1 ml of saline solution. i.pl., intrapleural; s.c., subcutaneous. i.pl. injections were made 24 hr after i.pl. injection of tumor cells. s.c. injections were made 7 and 14 days before and/or after i.pl. injection of tumor cells.

24 days (mean survival time 16.9±3.4 days). On the other hand, 50% of the mice which received 100 μg of oil-attached BCG cell-wall skeleton intrapleurally 24 hr after the injection of tumor cells, remained alive on day 95 and no malignant lesions of the pleura were observed upon histological examination except for residual changes in inflammatory reactions (Fig. 2). Similarly, the oil-attached cell-wall skeleton of *N. rubra* was active for the regression of experimental pleural effusion in mice (Yoshimoto *et al.*, unpublished data).

3) Effect of oil-attached cell-wall skeletons of mycobacteria and nocardia on autochthonous tumor and tumor grafts

Tokuzen *et al.* have shown that an autograft of autochthonous tumors, 3-methyl-cholanthrene-induced fibrosarcoma in ICR, and spontaneous mammary adenocarcinoma in SHN female mice, could be suppressed when implanted mixed with oil-attached cell-wall skeleton of BCG or *N. rubra* (*32*). Presensitization of mice with oil-attached cell-wall skeleton of *N. rubra* enhanced the suppression of autografts of fibrosarcoma and mammary adenocarcinoma with oil-attached cell-wall skeleton of *N. rubra* in respective mice (*33*). It was shown that intralesional injection of oil-attached cell-wall skeleton of *N. rubra* (100 μg, 5 times every week) was effective for the prolongation of survival period of ICR mice bearing 3-methylcholanthrene-induced fibrosarcoma (Table IV).

TABLE IV. Effect of Intralesional Injection of Oil-attachted Cell-wall Skeleton of *N. rubra* on Spontaneous Mammary Adenocarcinoma in SHN Mice and 3-Methylcholanthrene-induced Fibrosarcoma in ICR Mice (*33*)

Mice were treated	No. of mice	Survival period days±SE (survival ranges)	p value[c]
Spontaneous mammary adenocarcinoma			
Untreated	40	46.9± 2.5 (20–96)[b]	0.05< p <0.1
Cell-wall skeleton of *N. rubra*[a]	10	59.3± 5.7 (29–86)	
Fibrosarcoma induced by 3-methylcholanthrene			
Untreated	6	56.5± 6.5 (29–85)	
Saline	8	52.0± 7.5 (30–88)	0.02< p <0.05
Cell-wall skeleton of *N. rubra*	13	98.8±11.1 (30–244)	

[a] Oil-attached cell-wall skeleton of *N. rubra* (150 μg) was injected intralesionally into spontaneous mammary adenocarcinoma and 3-methylcholanthrene-induced fibrosarcoma (tumor sizes 3–5 mm) in mice, weekly, 5 times.

[b] Survival periods were calculated from the start of intralesional injection of *N. rubra* cell-wall. skeleton.

[c] Student's *t*-test.

4) Effect on lymphocyte trapping and prevention of metastatic spread of tumors

Oil-attached BCG cell-wall skeletons of BCG and *N. rubra* were demonstrated to have an activity of inducing lymphocyte trapping in the draining lymph node in rats when injected into the growing syngeneic transplantable tumor (*21*, and Ogura *et al.*, unpublished data). Repeated intratumor injections of oil-attached cell-wall skeleton of BCG or *N. rubra* resulted in the regression of tumor growth in primary tumor sites as well as in metastatic sites. Even in the case where the primary tumor had not regressed, prolongation of the survival period and inhibitory effect on metastatic spread were attained by treatment with oil-attached cell-wall skeletons of BCG or *N. rubra*.

Prevention of Carcinogenesis in Rabbits and Mice with Oil-attached BCG Cell-wall Skeleton

1) Prevention of experimental lung cancer

Hirao *et al.* (*14*) reported that experimental lung cancer was induced in rabbits by the instillation of chemical carcinogens (3-methylcholanthrene and 4-nitroquinoline l-oxide) into the lower bronchus with the aid of a specially designed bronchoscope. The effect of oil-attached BCG cell-wall skeleton on the prevention of lung cancer in rabbits was examined. As shown in Table V, in rabbits that received an intravenous injection of oil-attached BCG cell-wall skeleton (5 mg) at the start of the experiment (group C), the incidence of lung cancer was 50%, a figure almost identical to that of the control (group A). On the other hand, no lung cancer occurred in rabbits that received 5 mg of oil-attached BCG cell-wall skeleton at the start of the experiment and 2 mg of oil-attached BCG cell-wall skeleton every 30–40 days; these animals survived more than 300 days (group D) or 200–300 days (group F) after the instillation of carcinogens. The control groups (groups A and E) experienced a 47.2 and 28% incidence, respectively, of lung cancer. The thymectomized rabbits (group B) developed lung cancer by the instillation of carcinogens, at an incidence of 80.0%, compared to 47.2% in the control (group A) (Table V).

TABLE V. Effect of Oil-attached BCG Cell-wall Skeleton (BCG-CWS) on the Incidence of Lung Cancer in Rabbits by the Instillation of Chemical Carcinogens (*14*)

Group		Intravenous injection of oil-attached BCG-CWS[a]	Survival period (days)	Lung cancer incidence (%)
A	Normal	No treatment (control 1)	>300	17/36 (47.2)
B	Thymectomized	No treatment	>300	32/40 (80.0)
C	Normal	5 mg (once)	>300	5/10 (50.0)
D	Normal	5 mg (once) and 2 mg (every 30–40 days)	>300	0/20 (0)
E	Normal	No treatment (control 2)	200–300	7/25 (28.0)
F	Normal	5 mg (once) and 2 mg (every 30–40 days)	200–300	0/24 (0)

[a] Rabbits were instillated intrabronchially with a mixture of 3-methylcholanthrene (40 mg) and 4-nitroquinoline 1-oxide (0.4 mg) in rabbit plasma every 30–40 days by use of a specially designed bronchoscope.

2) Prevention of the induction of pleural fibrosarcoma in mice

Yoshimoto *et al.* (*47*) described a method for the induction of pleural fibrosarcoma by substernal injection of 3-methylcholanthrene into the thoracic cavity of mice. Beginning one week after the injection of carcinogen, 100 μg of oil-attached BCG cell-wall skeleton was injected subcutaneously, once a week for 10 weeks. The incidence of pleural fibrosarcoma at the end of 130 days was 67% in the control group, whereas it was 39% in the group that received oil-attached BCG cell-wall skeleton. The latent period of tumor induction was prolonged in the mice treated with BCG cell-wall skeleton.

Recently, Kitagawa *et al.* (unpublished data) have shown that the intravenous administration of oil-attached BCG cell-wall skeleton partially prevented carcinogenesis induced with 2,4-dimethylbenzanthracene in mice of strains C57BL/6, BALB/c, and C3H, but not in strain BTK. Kuwamura (personal communication) has also shown that the incidence of hepatoma induced by feeding 3'-methyl-4-dimethylaminoazobenzene to Donryu rats was suppressed to 26% by the subcutaneous administration of oil-attached BCG cell-wall skeleton, compared to 50% in the control group.

Other Immunotherapeutic Agents Purified from Bacterial Fractions and Synthetic Compounds

1) Cell-wall skeleton of N. rubra and other bacterial fractions

Recently, the authors have reported that the cell-wall skeletons of *Nocardia* have potent adjuvant activity in the immune response (*2, 30, 31*), and antitumor activity, especially by the cell-wall skeleton of *N. rubra* has been shown to be most effective in the immunotherapy of experimental syngeneic transplantable tumors (*8, 10, 11*) and autochthonous systems (*32, 33*). As shown in Fig. 3, the principal chemical structure of *N. rubra* cell-wall skeleton (Fig. 3) consists of nocardomycolic acid, arabinogalactan, and mucopeptide, which are almost similar to that of BCG cell-wall skeleton except for the molecular weight and content of nocardomycolic acid. The cell-wall skeleton of *N. rubra* has various advantages as an immunotherapeutic agent compared with BCG cell-wall skeleton. The strain of *N. rubra* is non-pathogenic and easily cultivated in synthetic and semisynthetic media within a few days, and the cell-wall skeleton of *N. rubra* is obtained by the same method as that of BCG cell-wall skeleton. The adjuvant and antitumor activities of the cell-wall skeleton of *N. rubra* are more potent than those of BCG cell-wall skeleton; the cell-wall skeleton of *N. rubra* is also less toxic. The cell-wall skeleton of *N. rubra* is now being applied to the immunotherapy of human cancer, such as lung cancer and acute leukemia, in Japan.

The cell-wall skeletons of *Propionibacterium* species such as *Propionibacterium acnes* C7, *Propionibacterium granulosum*, *Propionibacterium avidum*, as well as *Corynebacterium parvum* were purified, and their biochemical and immunological properties were investigated in detail (*5*). These cell-wall skeletons of anaerobic coryneforms

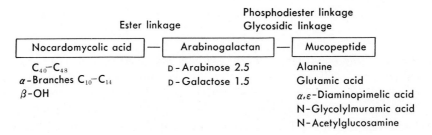

FIG. 3. Principal chemical structure of the cell-wall skeleton of *N. rubra* (*10*)

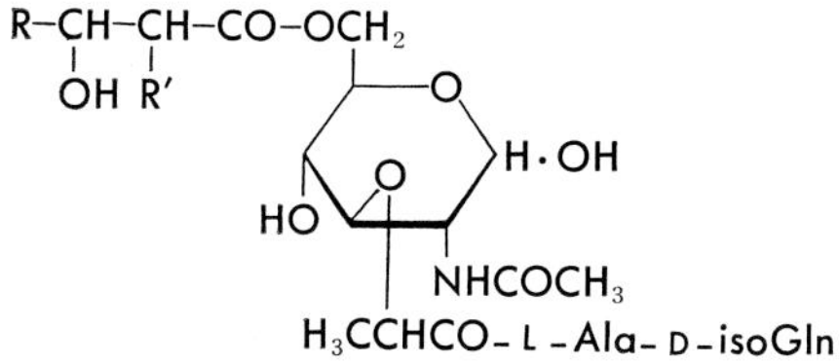

R–CH–CH–CO–OCH$_2$
  | |
 OH R'

H·OH

HO

NHCOCH$_3$

H$_3$CCHCO– L –Ala– D –isoGln

Mycolic acid residue : R–CH–CH–CO
                         | |
                        OH   R'

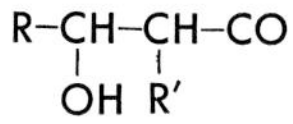

Mycolic acid (*M.tuberculosis* Aoyama B) R=C$_{43-57}$ R'=C$_{24}$

Nocardomycolic acid (*N.asteroides* 131) R=C$_{31-43}$ R'=C$_{10-14}$

Corynomycolic acid (*C.diphtheriae* PW8) R=C$_{11-15}$ R'=C$_{10-14}$

FIG. 4. Chemical structure of 6-O-mycoloyl-N-acetylmuramyl-L-alanyl-D-isoglutamine (*39*)

especially *P. acnes* C7 have been shown to have potent antitumor activity in transplantable tumor systems in syngeneic mice and guinea pigs (I. Azuma *et al.*, unpublished data).

2) Synthetic N-acetylmuramyldipeptide derivatives

It has been shown that the minimal adjuvant-active subunit of bacterial cell wall is N-acetylmuramyl-L-alanyl-D-isoglutamine (*1, 6*). This conclusion was confirmed by the study using synthetic N-acetylmuramyldipeptide and related compounds. These synthetic N-acetylmuramyldipeptides have potent adjuvant activity in immune systems, however, they were shown to have no antitumor activity in any experimental tumor systems in which we tested them.

More recently, the authors (*18, 39*) have synthesized the hydrophobic derivatives of N-acetylmuramyldipeptide by the introduction of mycolic acid into the 6-O-position of muramic acid of N-acetylmuramyl-L-alanyl-D-isoglutamine (Fig. 4). The results of its immunological study indicated that 6-O-mycoloyl-N-acetylmuramyldipeptide showed potent adjuvant activity for the cell-mediated immune response rather than in enhancing a circulating antibody formation (*38*). Synthetic 6-O-mycoloyl-N-acetylmuramyldipeptide showed suppression of tumor (MH134) growth in syngeneic mice (C3H/He) (*39*), and the prolongation of survival time of those with malignant pleurisy by using pleural fibrosarcoma (Yoshimoto *et al.*, unpublished). Synthesis of muramylpeptide derivatives is now being carried out.

Acknowledgements

This work was supported by Grants-in-Aid for Cancer Research from the Ministry of Education, Science and Culture and from the Ministry of Health and Welfare of Japan, and from the Princess Takamatsu Cancer Research Fund.

REFERENCES

1. Adam, A., Ciorbaru, R., Ellouz, F., Petit, J.-F., and Lederer, E. Adjuvant activity of monomeric bacterial cell wall peptidoglycans. *Biochem. Biophys. Res. Commun.*, **56**, 561–567 (1974).

2. Azuma, I., Kanetsuna, F., Taniyama, T., Yamamura, Y., Hori, M., and Tanaka, Y. Adjuvant activity of mycobacterial fractions. I. Purification and *in vivo* adjuvant activity of cell wall skeletons of *Mycobacterium bovis* BCG, *Nocardia asteroides* 131 and *Corynebacterium diphtheriae* PW8. *Biken J.*, **18**, 1–13 (1975).

3. Azuma, I., Kishimoto, S., Yamamura, Y., and Petit, J.-F. Adjuvanticity of mycobacterial cell walls. *Japan. J. Microbiol.*, **15**, 193–197 (1971).

4. Azuma, I., Ribi, E., Meyer, T. J., and Zbar, B. Biologically active components from mycobacterial cell walls. I. Isolation and composition of cell wall skeleton and component P_3. *J. Natl. Cancer Inst.*, **52**, 95–101 (1974).

5. Azuma, I., Sugimura, K., Taniyama, T., Aladin, A. A., and Yamamura, Y. Chemical and immunological studies on the cell walls of *Corynebacterium parvum* ATCC 11829 and *Propionibacterium acnes* strain C7. *Japan. J. Microbiol.*, **19**, 265–275 (1975).

6. Azuma, I., Sugimura, K., Taniyama, T., Yamawaki, M., Yamamura, Y., Kusumoto, S., Okada, S., and Shiba, T. Adjuvant activity of mycobacterial fractions. Immunological properties of synthetic N-acetylmuramyldipeptides and related compounds. *Infect. Immun.*, **14**, 18–27 (1976).

7. Azuma, I., Sugimura, K., Yamawaki, M., and Yamamura, Y. Mitogenic activity of cell-wall components in mouse spleen cells. *Microbiol. Immunol.*, **21**, 111–115 (1977).

8. Azuma, I., Taniyama, T., Hirao, F., and Yamamura, Y. Antitumor activity of cell-wall skeletons and peptidoglycolipids of mycobacteria and related microorganisms. *Gann*, **65**, 493–505 (1974).

9. Azuma, I., Taniyama, T., Sugimura, K., Aladin, A. A., and Yamamura, Y. Mitogenic activity of the cell walls of mycobacteria, nocardia, corynebacteria, and anaerobic coryneforms. *Japan. J. Microbiol.*, **20**, 263–271 (1976).

10. Azuma, I., Taniyama, T., Yamawaki, M., Sugimura, K., and Yamamura, Y. Adjuvant and antitumor activities of *Nocardia* cell-wall skeletons. *Gann*, **57**, 733–736 (1976).

11. Azuma, I., Yamawaki, M., Yasumoto, K., and Yamamura, Y. Antitumor activity of *Nocardia* cell-wall skeletons in mice, and patients with malignant pleurisy. *Cancer Immunol. Immunother.*, **4**, in press (1978).

12. Brunner, K. T., Mauel, J., Rudolf, H., and Chapuis, B. Studies of allograft immunity in mice. I. Induction, development and *in vitro* assay of cellular immunity. *Immunology*, **18**, 501–515 (1970).

13. Hayata, Y., Obo, K., Ogawa, I., and Taira, O. Immunotherapy for lung cancer cases using BCG or BCG cell-wall skeleton: Primarily intratumoral injections. This volume, pp. 151–160.

14. Hirao, F., Nishikawa, H., Yasaki, S., Ogura, T., Azuma, I., Taniyama, T., Yoshimoto, T., Kishimoto, S., and Yamamura, Y. Effects of oil-attached BCG cell-wall skeleton and thymectomy on the incidence of lung cancer and amyloidosis induced by chemical carcinogens in rabbits. Gann, **69** (No. 4), in press (1978).

15. Igarashi, T., Okada, M., Azuma, I., and Yamamura, Y. Adjuvant activity of N-acetyl-muramyl-L-alanyl-D-isoglutamine and its related compounds on cell-mediated cytotoxicity in syngeneic mice. *Cell. Immunol.*, **34**, 270–278 (1977).

16. Kishimoto, S., Araki, K., and Saito, T. Immunotherapy with BCG or its derivatives in acute myelogenous leukemia. This volume, pp. 189–198.

17. Kitagawa, M., Hamaoka, T., Haba, S., Takatsu, K., and Masaki, H. Selective suppression of T-cells activity in tumor-bearing host and attempt for its improvement. *In* "Host Defence against Cancer and Its Potentiation," ed. by D. Mizuno *et al.*, Japan Scientific Societies Press, Tokyo, pp. 31–42 (1975).

18. Kusumoto, S., Okada, S., Shiba, T., Azuma, I., and Yamamura, Y. Synthesis of 6-O-

mycoloyl-N-acetylmuramyl-L-alanyl-D-isoglutamine with immunoadjuvant activities. *Tetrahedron Lett.*, **47**, 4287–4290 (1976).

19. Meyer, T. J., Ribi, E. E., Azuma, I., and Zbar, B. Biologically active components from mycobacterial cell walls. II. Suppression an regression of strain-2 guinea pig hepatoma. *J. Natl. Cancer Inst.*, **52**, 103–111 (1974).

20. Nakamura, H., Miyoshi, K., Shibata, H., Hayashi, A., Masaoka, T., and Yoshitake, J. Antitumor effect of BCG cell-wall skeleton in acute leukemia. This volume, pp. 217–222.

21. Ogura, T., Azuma, I., Nishikawa, H., Namba, M., Hirao, F., and Yamamura, Y. Effect of oil-attached BCG-cell wall on the kinetics of lymphocytes in tumor-draining node. *Gann*, **66**, 349–354 (1975).

22. Ogura, T., Yoshimoto, T., Nishikawa, H., Sakatani, M., Ito, M., Hirao, F., Azuma, I., and Yamamura, Y. Immunotherapy with BCG cell-wall skeleton in patients with neoplastic pleurisy. This volume, pp. 143–150.

23. Oguro, M., Takagi, T., Majima, H., and Ishiguro, K. Immunochemotherapy of malignant melanoma with BCG-cell-wall skeleton. This volume, pp. 225–230.

24. Ohno, R., Ezaki, K., Kobayashi, M., Takeyama, H., Suzuki, H., Yamada, K., Azuma, I., and Yamamura, Y. Immune response of regional lymph node to BCG cell-wall skeleton and other immunopotentiators. This volume, pp. 109–126.

25. Okuyama, H. and Morikawa, K. Histological study on adjuvanticity of BCG cell-wall: Comparison of adjuvanticity between oil-in-water and water-in-oil forms. This volume, pp. 87–91.

26. Orita, K., Mannami, T., Miwa, H., Ohta, T., Nakahara, T., Konaga, E., and Tanaka, S. Immunotherapy for advanced gastric cancer and colo-rectal cancer using cell-wall skeleton. This volume, pp. 163–171.

27. Sugimura, K., Uemiya, M., Yamawaki, M., Azuma, I., and Yamamura, Y. Macrophage dependency of T-lymphocyte mitogenicity by *Nocardia rubra* cell-wall skeleton. *Microbiol. Immunol.*, **21**, 525–530 (1977).

28. Tanaka, T., Nakagawa, H., Kato, A., Yoshimura, M., Fujita, H., and Kimura, K. Effect of anti-thymocyte serum, anti-macrophage serum, and latex particles on the therapeutic efficacy of BCG or *Corynebacterium liquefaciens* (*Propionibacterium acnes* C7) in syngeneic mice. *Gann*, **68**, 45–52 (1977).

29. Taniyama, T., Azuma, I., Aladin, A. A., and Yamamura, Y. Effect of cell-wall skeleton of *Mycobacterium bovis* BCG on cell-mediated cytotoxicity in tumor-bearing mice. *Gann*, **66**, 705–709 (1976).

30. Taniyama, T., Azuma, I., and Yamamura, Y. Adjuvant activity of mycobacterial fraction. III. Adjuvant effect of cell walls of *Mycobacterium bovis* BCG on cell-mediated cytotoxicity in mice. *Japan. J. Microbiol.*, **19**, 255–264 (1975).

31. Taniyama, T., Watanabe, T., Azuma, I., and Yamamura, Y. Adjuvant activity of mycobacterial fractions. II. *In vitro* adjuvant activity of cell walls of mycobacteria, nocardia and corynebacteria. *Japan. J. Microbiol.*, **18**, 415 (1974).

32. Tokuzen, R., Okabe, M., Nakahara, W., Azuma, I., and Yamamura, Y. Effect of Nocardia and *Mycobaeterium* cell-wall skeletons on autochthonous tumor grafts. *Gann*, **66**, 433–435 (1975).

33. Tokuzen, R., Okabe, M., Nakahara, W., Azuma, I., and Yamamura, Y. Suppression of autochthonous tumors by mixed implantation with *Nocardia rubra* cell-wall skeleton and related bacterial fractions. *Gann*, **69**, 19–24 (1978).

34. Wigzell, H. Quantitative titrations of mouse H-2 antibodies using ^{51}Cr-labeled target cells. *Transplantation*, **3**, 423–431 (1965).

35. Yamada, K., Kawashima, K., Morishima, Y., Esaki, K., Kodera, Y., and Ohno, R. Chemoimmunotherapy of acute myelogenous leukemia in adults with BCG-cell wall skeleton. This volume, pp. 199–209.

36. Yamamura, Y. Immunotherapy of lung cancer with oil-attached cell-wall skeleton of BCG. *In* "Immunotherapy of Cancer: Present Status of Trials in Human Cancer," ed. by W. D. Terry and D. B. Windhorst, Raven Press, New York, pp. 173–179 (1977).

37. Yamamura, Y. Immunotherapy of lung cancer with BCG cell-wall skeleton and related compounds. *In* "Proc. 2nd Int. Congr. Lung Cancer," Raven Press, New York, in press (1978).

38. Yamamura, Y., Azuma, I., Sugimura, K., Yamawaki, M., Uemiya, M., Kusumoto, S., Okada, S., and Shiba, T. Adjuvant activity of 6-O-mycoloyl-N-acetylmuramyl-L-alanyl-D-isoglutamine. *Gann*, **67**, 867–877 (1976).

39. Yamamura, Y., Azuma, I., Sugimura, K., Yamawaki, M., Uemiya, M., Kusumoto, S., Okada, S., and Shiba, T. Immunological and antitumor activities of synthetic 6-O-mycoloyl-N-acetylmuramyldipeptides. *Proc. Japan Acad.*, **53**, 63–66 (1977).

40. Yamamura, Y., Azuma, I., Taniyama, T., Sugimura, K., Hirao, F., Tokuzen, R., Okabe, M., Nakahara, W., Yasumoto, K., and Ohta, M. Immunotherapy of cancer with cell-wall skeleton of *Mycobacterium bovis*-Bacillus Calmette-Guérin: Experimental and clinical results. *Ann. N.Y. Acad. Sci.*, **277**, 209–227 (1976).

41. Yamamura, Y., Ogura, T., Yoshimoto, T., Nishikawa, H., Sakatani, M., Itoh, M., Masuno, T., Namba, M., Yazaki, H., Hirao, F., and Azuma, I. Successful treatment of the patients with malignant pleural effusion with BCG cell-wall skeleton. *Gann*, **67**, 669–677 (1976).

42. Yamamura, Y., Yoshizaki, K., Azuma, I., Yagura, T., and Watanabe, T. Immunotherapy of human malignant melanoma with oil-attached BCG cell-wall skeleton. *Gann*, **66**, 355–363 (1975).

43. Yasumoto, K., Manabe, H., Ohta, M., Nomoto, K., Azuma, I., and Yamamura, Y. Immunotherapy of lung cancer and carcinomatous pleuritis. This volume, pp. 129–141.

44. Yasumoto, K., Manabe, H., Ueno, M., Ohta, M., Ueda, H., Iida, A., Nomoto, K., Azuma, I., and Yamamura, Y. Immunotherapy of human lung cancer with BCG cell-wall skeleton. *Gann*, **67**, 787–795 (1976).

45. Yasumoto, K., Manabe, H., Taniguchi, T., and Nomoto, K. BCG cell-wall skeleton-induced antitumor effect in nude mice. *In* "Proc. 2nd Int. Workshop Nude Mice," ed. by T. Nomura *et al.*, Univ. of Tokyo Press, pp. 533–541 (1977).

46. Yoshimoto, T., Azuma, I., Nishikawa, H., Sakatani, M., Ogura, T., Hirao, F., and Yamamura, Y. Experimental immunotherapy of neoplastic pleural effusion with oil-attached BCG cell-wall skeleton in mice. *Gann*, **67**, 737–740 (1976).

47. Yoshimoto, T., Azuma, I., Sakatani, M., Nishikawa, H., Ogura, T., Hirao, F., and Yamamura, Y. Effect of oil-attached BCG cell-wall skeleton on the induction of pleural fibrosarcoma in mice. *Gann*, **67**, 441–445 (1976).

48. Zbar, B., Ribi, E. E., Meyer, T. J., Azuma, I., and Rapp, H. J. Immunotherapy of cancer: Regression of established intradermal tumors after intralesional injection of mycobacterial cell walls attached to oil droplets. *J. Natl. Cancer Inst.*, **52**, 1571–1577 (1974).

GANN Monograph on Cancer Research 21, 1978

HISTOLOGICAL STUDY ON ADJUVANTICITY OF BCG-CELL WALL: COMPARISON OF ADJUVANTICITY BETWEEN OIL-IN-WATER AND WATER-IN-OIL FORMS

Harue Okuyama and Kazuo Morikawa

*Institute of Immunological Science, Hokkaido University**

BCG-cell wall (CW) adjuvant strongly enhanced both circulating antibody formation and delayed-type hypersensitivity (DTH) when used in the form of water-in-oil (w/o). On the other hand, BCG-CW in the oil-in-water (o/w) form augmented DTH alone, leaving antibody formation at a low level. On histological examination, the injected sites and regional lymph nodes showed remarkable proliferative responses. Differences in the histological changes induced by both adjuvant forms were in quantity and duration rather than in quality. In the o/w groups maximum responses are reached early and decline thereafter, whereas the w/o groups attained a maximum slowly and maintained the high response for a long period. From the immunofluorescence study the appearance and quantity fluctuation of specific antibody-forming cells in both groups paralleled the degree of histological changes and retention. Furthermore, the o/w form of adjuvant developed as high a DTH as the w/o form, but induced only a slight change in the injected sites. Hence, the o/w form is considered to have an advantage as an effective tool for cancer immunotherapy.

Ribi *et al.* (*9*) described a strong adjuvanticity of cell walls isolated from BCG (BCG-CW). Aquired anti-infectious immunity was demonstrated in mice inoculated intravenously with BCG-CW (*1, 10*). Recently BCG has been used effectively in clinical medicine as an immunopotentiating agent against certain cancers. Azuma *et al.* (*3, 8*) found the antitumor effect of cell-wall skeleton (BCG-CWS) purified from physically isolated BCG-CW in animals. In these experiments BCG-CW or -CWS was employed in the form attached to a small amount of mineral oil (o/w). On the contrary, complete adjuvant containing mycobacteria, the most popular agent, has been used in the form of water-in-oil (w/o), namely emulsified in a large amount of oil. Nevertheless, regardless of the difference in the amount of oil between two adjuvants of o/w and w/o, similar adjuvanticity was observed in terms of cellular immunity or delayed-type hypersensitivity (DTH). It is interesting, therefore, to discover whether differences in adjuvanticity exist between the two forms on comparison of immune response, especially as regards morphological changes in the injected sites and regional lymph nodes.

---

* Kita 15, Nishi 7, Kita-ku, Sapporo 060, Japan (奥山春枝, 森川和雄).

Histological Changes in the Regional Lymph Nodes

In the present study sheep erythrocytes (SRBC) or bovine γ-globulin (BGG) was used as the immunogen. When BCG-CW (1 mg) or -CWS (0.5 mg), in the form of o/w or w/o, was introduced into the hind footpad of rabbits, the following proliferating responses in the popliteal lymph nodes were seen, whether or not the immunogen was mixed with adjuvant (Table I): Development of the medullary cords and notable proliferation of pyroninophilic cells therein and in the cortico-medullary junctions, and intensive enlargement of the paracortical areas with proliferation of large pyroninophilic blast cells. These changes reached a peak on day 3 to 6 and then decreased in intensity in the o/w group; in the w/o group maximum changes were observed on day 6 to 10 and maintained thereafter. Many germinal centers developed in the regional lymph nodes of animals receiving immunogen mixed with Freund's incomplete adjuvant (FIA), but the addition of BCG-CW in this form did not provoke germinal center formation beyond that of FIA. From the first stage the lymph node sinuses contained many swollen macrophages, some of which phagocytized oil droplets. After 6 days transformation of cells occurred among reticular cells and macrophages diffusely proliferating around the follicles and in the paracortex. These transformed cells had large, clear cytoplasma and oval, clear nuclei. These cells were identified by electron microscopy as epithelioid cells and took a part in constructing granuloma. Granuloma formation reached a maximum on day 10 to 19 in o/w groups, and after 19 days in w/o groups. Much of the cortex

TABLE I. Histological Changes in Regional Lymph Nodes from Rabbits Immunized with BGG and BCG-CW

After immun.	Germinal center					Pyroninophilic cell									
						Cortico-medullary junction					Medullary cord				
	I	II	III	IV	V	I	II	III	IV	V	I	II	III	IV	V
3 hr	−	±	±	−	−	+	+	±	±	±	±	±	±	−	±
1 day	−	++	+	+	−	++	++	−	−	−	++	++	±	+	+
3 days	+	++	++	++	+	++	+	++	++	++	++	+	++	++	++
6	++	++	+++	++	++	++	+	++	+++	+++	++	++	++	+++	+++
10	+	++	+++	++	++	+	+	++	++	+++	+	++	++	+++	+++
19	+	+	±	++	++	±	±	−	++	++	±	±	±	++	+++

After immun.	Enlargement of paracortex					Pyroninophilic cell in paracortex					Epithelioid cell				
	I	II	III	IV	V	I	II	III	IV	V	I	II	III	IV	V
3 hr	−	±	±	−	−	−	−	±	±	±	−	−	−	−	−
1 day	±	+	−	±	+	+	±	+	+	±	−	−	−	−	−
3 days	+	++	++	+++	++	++	++	++	+++	++	−	−	−	−	−
6	∓	++	+++	+++	+++	+	++	++	+++	++	−	−	+	++	+
10	−	+	++	++	+++	−	+	+	+++	++	−	−	±	+++	++
19	−	−	±	++	+++	−	−	±	++	++	−	−	−	++	+++

Group I: BGG in saline.   II: BGG with oil in o/w form.   III: BGG with FIA in w/o form. IV: BGG with CW in o/w form.   V: BGG with CW in w/o form.

was occupied on occasion by epithelioid granuloma. Langhans giant cells were scattered throughout. BCG-CW produced more severe changes than CWS. Similar changes were observed in guinea pigs inoculated with BCG-CW or BCG-CWS (150 μg) and BGG. These changes have been reported in the lungs of mice given intravenous BCG-CW in o/w (Barclay et al. (5) and Meyer et al. (7)) and in the regional lymph nodes of guinea pigs injected with BCG-CW (Granger et al. (6)). In the present experiment in rabbits, proliferation of pyroninophilic cells in the cortico-medullary junctions and the medullary cords was observed to be maintained, especially in the w/o group. This proliferation correlated with an increment in titer of the serum antibody to BGG and an increase in number of 7S plaque-forming cells (PFC) in the regional lymph nodes of animals sensitized to SRBC. Azuma et al. (2, 4) described a strong augmentation of DTH and antibody production to antigen, when administered together with BCG-CW in the form of w/o. On the other hand BCG-CW in o/w form augmented DTH alone, leaving antibody production at a low level. The o/w group of rabbits in the present study showed a temporal increase in serum antibody level only around day 7. Immunofluorescence study demonstrated that these findings paralleled the production and progress of specific antibody-forming cells in the cortico-medullary junctions and the medullary cords, and further correlated with the transient presence of antigen in the lymph nodes.

The DTH against SRBC or BGG, as stated by Azuma et al. (2, 4), was strongly evoked and maintained in both groups (w/o and o/w), and moreover tuberculin hypersensitivity was produced earlier and more severely in the o/w groups of animals. This process of the reactivity corresponded to the enlargement of the paracortical areas and an early appearance and an intensive proliferation of large pyroninophilic blast cells therein. These findings suggest that, among the morphological changes evoked by BCG-CW adjuvant, the enlargement of paracortical areas and proliferation of large pyroninophilic cells are associated with augmentation of cell-mediated immunity. On the other hand increment of serum antibody formation is related to the intensity of proliferation of pyroninophilic cells in the cortico-medullary junctions and the medullary cords. Accumulation of macrophages and granuloma formation are considered to participate in the two types of immune response at least in the early stage of mobilization and appearance of macrophages, but the function of epithelioid cells transforming from macrophages remains to be elucidated.

Macroscopic and Histological Changes at the Sites of Injection

Abscess formation was observed macroscopically in the injected sites of footpads 3 days after inoculation. In w/o groups the skin became necrotic, softened, and discharged the content. Necrotic foci were surrounded with firm and solid aggregates of granuloma. However, the o/w groups showed neither destruction nor discharge of the abscess. Many polymorphonuclear leukocytes appeared subcutaneously by 3 days and they became concentrated into the center of the abscess. Around them there was accumulation of macrophages loaded with oil droplets, and fibroblastic proliferation occurred. After 10 days the accumulation of cells in this area changed to epithelioid cell granuloma. Lymphocytes and plasma cells were also seen to infiltrate in and around the foci of granuloma. The capacity of o/w adjuvant to produce abscess and granuloma was weak compared to w/o groups which showed persistence of a large abscess and leukocyte infiltration in granuloma even on day 19. Immunofluorescence study indicated antigen retention, due to slow withdrawal from the injected sites, and an especially long duration of antigen deposit in the w/o groups. Specific antibody-producing cells were also demonstrated in the injected sites. Westwater (*11*) presented evidence for the contribution of local antibody formation to the serum antibody level as in regional lymph nodes. It is questionable whether injected adjuvant accelerates the local accumulation of specific antibody-forming cells owing to delayed resorption of antigen, or whether it promotes *in situ* a proliferation of the cell concerned.

Whatever the answer, the fact that cell-mediated immunity alone was strongly elicited in animals by the use of BCG-CW or -CWS in the o/w form will be a convenient way of strengthening antitumor immunity. Clinical safety is also required; the femoral muscle tissue of guinea pigs was chosen as the injected site for a comparative study of the effect of both forms of BCG-CWS (150 μg). The weight of the lymph node was twice normal on day 19 and 28 in the o/w group, and attained about 5 times normal in the w/o group 19 days after. The foci of abscess in the o/w group were small in size, the maximum diameter being 3 mm. Accumulated macrophages and epithelioid cell granuloma in the later stage were morphologically the same. On the other hand, the w/o form caused production of widespread lesions and damage of the neighboring muscle tissues.

CONCLUSION

From this histological study it is considered that the difference of lesions due to the two forms of adjuvants is rather in quantity and duration of changes than in quality. Immunological and immunohistological studies disclosed a distinct difference in serum antibody production without any substantial alteration in the peak of cellular immunity. This disparity is probably due to different mechanisms of stimulation of T and B cells in both immune responses and to the difference in lifespan of the cells concerned. Since BCG-CW or BCG-CWS have the capacity to induce cell-mediated immunity at a high level without obvious tissue damage if used in the form of oil-in-water, they will be utilized as effective tools for cancer immunotherapy.

Acknowledgment
This work was supported by a Grant-in-Aid for Scientific Research from the Ministry of Education, Science and Culture of Japan.

REFERENCES

1. Anacker, R. L., Barclay, W. R., Brehmer, W., Larson, C. L., and Ribi, E. Duration of immunity to tuberculosis in mice vaccinated intravenously with oil-treated cell walls of *Mycobacterium bovis* strain BCG. *J. Immunol.*, **98**, 1265–1273 (1967).
2. Azuma, I., Kanetsuna, F., Taniyama, T., Yamamura, Y., Hori, M., and Tanaka, Y. Adjuvant activity of mycobacterial fractions. I. Purification and *in vivo* adjuvant activity of cell-wall skeletons of *Mycobacterium bovis* BCG, *Nocardia asteroides* 131 and *Corynebacterium diphtheriae* PW8. *Biken J.*, **18**, 1–13 (1975).
3. Azuma, I., Ribi, E. E., Meyer, T. J., and Zbar, B. Biologically active components from

mycobacterial cell walls. I. Isolation and composition of cell-wall skeleton and component P$_3$. *J. Natl. Cancer Inst.*, **52**, 95–101 (1974).

4. Azuma, I., Taniyama, T., Sugimura, K., and Yamamura, Y. Adjuvanticity of mycobacterial cell walls. *Proc. IVth Annu. Meet. Japan. Soc. Immunol.*, **4**, 204–206 (1974) (in Japanese).

5. Barclay, W. R., Anacker, R., Brehmer, W., and Ribi, E. Effect of oil-treated mycobacterial cell walls on the organs of mice. *J. Bacteriol.*, **94**, 1736–1745 (1967).

6. Granger, D. C., Brehmer, W., Yamamoto, K., and Ribi, E. Cutaneous granulomatous response to BCG cell walls with reference to cancer immunotherapy. *Infect. Immun.*, **13**, 543–553 (1976).

7. Meyer, T. J., Ribi, E., and Azuma, I. Biologically active components from mycobacterial cell walls. V. Granuloma formation in mouse lungs and guinea pig skin. *Cell. Immunol.*, **16**, 11–24 (1975).

8. Meyer, T. J., Ribi, E. E., Azuma, I., and Zbar, N. Biologically active components from mycobacterial cell walls. II. Suppression and regulation of strain-2 guinea pig hepatoma. *J. Natl. Cancer Inst.*, **52**, 103–111 (1974).

9. Ribi, E., Larson, C. C., List, R., and Wicht, W. Immunologic significance of the cell wall of *Mycobacteria*. *Proc. Soc. Exp. Biol. Med.*, **29**, 263–265 (1958).

10. Ribi, E., Meyer, T. J., Parker, R., and Brehmer, W. Biologically active components from mycobacterial cell walls. IV. Protection of mice against aerosol infection with virulent *Mycobacterium tuberculosis*. *Cell. Immunol.*, **16**, 1–10 (1975).

11. Westwater, J. O. Antibody formation in a tuberculous lesion at the site of inoculation. *J. Exp. Med.*, **71**, 455–467 (1940).

GANN Monograph on Cancer Research 21, 1978

IMMUNOTHERAPY OF CANCER: THERAPEUTIC EFFICACY OF THE VACCINE CONTAINING ANAEROBIC CORYNEBACTERIUM OR BCG AND TUMOR CELLS IN MICE

Tomiko Tanaka,[*1] Ayako Kato,[*2] Hisayoshi Nakagawa,[*2] Hiroshi Fujita,[*2] and Kiyoji Kimura[*1]

*National Cancer Center[*1] and Tsurumi University,
School of Dental Medicine[*2]*

Cell-mediated antitumor activity of an anaerobic coryneform, *Corynebacterium liquefaciens* ($=Propionibacterium$ *acnes* C7) derived from human bone marrow, was evaluated by intradermal injection of a mixture of it with syngeneic tumor cells, and its therapeutic efficacy was compared with that of the tumor cell-BCG mixtures. (1) When mice given an intradermal inoculation of tumor cells-*P. acnes* (at a 1 mg dose of killed *P. acnes*) vaccine, tumor growth was significantly inhibited at the site of inoculation, but none of the mice developed tumor immunity. (2) The optimal dose of killed *P. acnes* admixed with tumor cells, at a 0.1–0.5 mg dose, was confirmed as optimal for induction of tumor immunity in the present mouse tumor system. (3) For induction of tumor immunity, the use of a vaccine containing killed *P. acnes* and BCG, both with tumor cells, was better than the use of either of them alone. (4) The effect of freshly cultured live *P. acnes* organisms in the vaccine was examined. (5) Treatment with antithymocyte serum completely abolished BCG-mediated tumor suppression but not the killed *P. acnes*-mediated activity. (6) When mice were treated with antimacrophage serum, tumor growth was still highly suppressed and the mice inoculated with tumor cells-*P. acnes* acquired tumor immunity. Similar results were obtained when mice were injected intraperitoneally with latex beads for blocking macrophage function, *i.e.*, the therapeutic efficacy of BCG therapy was abolished by treatment with latex beads in contrast with that of *P. acnes*.

Tumor suppression was not accounted for by death of tumor cells in admixture with *P. acnes* before inoculation within the time-span of an experiment.

Since 1966, anaerobic corynebacteria, like *Corynebacterium parvum*, have been extensively studied experimentally for their antitumor activity. Mostly *C. parvum* was given intraperitoneally (*10, 12, 24, 25, 33*), and major emphasis has been placed on its potent stimulative effect on the host's reticuloendothelial system (*1, 12*), and on the generation of activated macrophages (*8, 19, 20*).

[*1] Tsukiji 5-1-1, Chuo-ku, Tokyo 104, Japan (田中冨子, 木村禧代二).
[*2] Tsurumi 2-1-3, Tsurumi-ku, Yokohama 230, Japan (加藤綾子, 中川久義, 藤田 浩).

This paper deals with *Corynebacterium liquefaciens* which is one of the anaerobic coryneforms inhabiting human bone marrow and which was isolated in the National Cancer Center Hospital in 1965. It was identified as *C. liquefaciens* by Prévôt's classification (*21*) and the category is related to *C. parvum* (*10, 11*). According to survey, the positive incidence of anaerobic corynebacterium in the bone marrow was 73% in healthy adults and 17% in cancer patients, and most of these bacteria were *C. liquefaciens*. The antitumor activity of *C. liquefaciens* in allogeneic and syngeneic mouse tumor systems was reported by Hattori and Mori (*15*) and by ourselves (*17, 30*). In the Eighth Edition of Bergey's Manual (*6*), designation of the anaerobic corynebacterium species was revised as propionibacteria from their physiological and biochemical properties. Therefore, the new designation *Propionibacterium acnes* will be used hereafter, instead of *C. liquefaciens*.

In 1970, Zbar *et al.* (*36–40*) developed an animal model for immunotherapy of cancer, in which intradermal growth of syngeneic guinea pig hepatoma was suppressed if the tumor cells were inoculated with BCG. Following the work of Zbar *et al.*, we have been studying the therapeutic efficacy of the tumor cell-BCG vaccine in syngeneic mice (*28, 29, 31, 32*). In the present work, we demonstrated the use of *P. acnes* (killed or live) in the vaccine instead of BCG, and determined its optimal conditions for tumor suppression at the inoculation site and for induction of systemic tumor immunity. The therapeutic effect of various combinations of *P. acnes* and BCG was also tested. We feel that elucidation of the difference in antitumor mechanism between *P. acnes* and BCG would aid further development of immunotherapy. For this purpose the experiments were undertaken using antithymocyte serum and antimacrophage serum.

In recent years, the chemical and immunological properties of *P. acnes* and other anaerobic coryneforms have been investigated by Azuma *et al.* (*3*) and by Saino *et al.* (*23*).

Mice

Animals used were 8- to 28-week-old Swiss origin inbred mice, SWM/Ms, throughout these experiments. The animals in some experiments were divided into two groups: One group was presensitized with lyophilized BCG (10^7 cells, i.d. or i.p.) or live *P. acnes* C7 (10^7 cells, i.d. or i.p.) 4 to 9 weeks before tumor inoculation; the other group was unsensitized.

Fibrosarcoma was originally induced in mice with a subcutaneous injection of 0.5 mg of 3-methylcholanthrene in olive oil. A mammary tumor that evolved spontaneously in female mice was also used.

A phenol-treated preparation of killed of *P. acnes* C7 was kindly provided by Kowa Co., Ltd. (*23*). This *P. acnes* preparation (20 mg/ml ampule) was washed with Hanks' balanced salt solution (BSS) before use. Freshly cultured organisms used were live *P. acnes* C7 (*30*).

Lyophilized BCG: Mycobacterium bovis, Japan strain (Japan BCG Laboratory, Tokyo), was suspended in saline solution just before use.

Live BCG: Freshly cultured *Mycobacterium bovis*, Japan strain (*30*).

Mouse tumor cells: These were treated with enzymes as described previously (*22, 26*) to make a single cell suspension for intradermal inoculation. A known number of viable tumor cells was inoculated intradermally in the hind quarters of mice. When the tumor cells (or mixture of tumor cells and adjuvant) were injected into mice presensitized with an adjuvant (*P. acnes* or BCG), inoculation was made on the site contralateral to that of presensitization.

Cell-wall fractions of P. acnes and BCG: These were kindly donated by Dr. I. Azuma, Third Department of Internal Medicine, Osaka University Medical School (*3*). Whole cell wall (WCW) or cell-wall skeleton (CWS)-in-oil preparation of BCG was prepared as described elsewhere (*4*), and the product was examined by an optical microscope for the size of droplets (2–20 μm). Since the *P. acnes* fraction does not attach to oil droplets and its antitumor effect was not influenced by the absence of oil droplets (our observation) the fraction was homogenized in Hanks' BSS and used for admixture with tumor cells.

Intradermal tumors in mice were measured weekly as two diameters of the tumor nodule taken at right angles. The square measures were used as the tumor size. Individual growth of the tumor and the dates of death of animals were recorded.

Test for immunity: Animals still alive without any tumor more than 42 to 66 days after the tumor inoculation were challenged intradermally with tumor cells of each line at the site contralateral to the first tumor inoculation. The overall assessment of therapy was based on the rate of tumor-free mice at the time of tumor challenge and induction of tumor immunity after the tumor challenge.

Sera: Rabbit antithymocyte serum, antimacrophage serum, or normal serum, 0.25 ml of each, was injected into the peritoneal cavity of mice 4 or 5 times before and after tumor cell or vaccine inoculation, as indicated in each table. All sera were absorbed with mouse liver or red blood cells as described previously (*30*). The potencies of these absorbed rabbit antithymocyte and antimacrophage sera were titrated by direct cytolysis test against mouse thymocytes and macrophages by serial dilutions of sera and complement (guinea pig serum), respectively. Antithymocyte serum showed 50% cytolysis of thymocytes at about 1:340 dilution, and antimacrophage serum showed 50% cytolysis of macrophages (adherent cells from peritoneal exudate cells) at 1:40 dilution.

Uniform polystyrene particles (diameter, 1.099 μm) were obtained from the Dow Chemical Co., U.S.A. They were suspended in Hanks' BSS in a concentration of 30 mg/0.5 ml just before use, and 0.5 ml of the suspension was injected intraperitoneally 2 hr before tumor inoculation.

Effect of Intradermal Injection of Tumor Cell-P. acnes Vaccine and of Tumor Cell-BCG Vaccine on Tumor Growth and Tumor Immunity in Syngeneic Mice (Experiments 1A and 1B in Table I)

Experiments 1A and 1B were performed to determine the efficacy of tumor cell-*P. acnes* vaccine on tumor suppression and tumor immunity in our mouse tumor system, and compared with that of BCG therapy. Mice sensitized to BCG or unsensitized mice were given intradermal injections of primary and early transplant generation of 3-methylcholanthrene-induced tumor cells mixed with *P. acnes* or BCG in doses indicated in Table I, at room temperature. On the 56th day (1A) or 48th day (1B) after the inoculation, mice free of tumor were challenged with tumor cells of the same line

TABLE I. Effect of Intradermal Injection of Tumor Cell-*P. acnes* C7 (PA-K) and of Tumor Cell-BCG Vaccine on Syngeneic Tumor Growth and Immunity

Exp. No. tumor	Treatment No. of tumor cells+ adjuvant (route)	Presensitized c̄ BCG	Day of tumor challenge No. of tumor-free mice / No. of mice tested on	No. of tumor-free mice / No. of mice challenged
			On day 56	On day 105
1A MCA-fibro-sarcoma[a]	2.5×10^6+PA-K 1 mg (i.d.)	+	7/8	1/7
	2.5×10^6+PA-K 1 mg (i.d.)	−	5/5	0/5
	2.5×10^6+BCG 5×10^7 (i.d.)	+	7/7	3/7
	2.5×10^6+BCG 5×10^7 (i.d.)	−	4/5	0/4
	2.5×10^6 (i.d.), PA-K 1 mg (i.p.)	+	0/8	—
	2.5×10^6 (i.d.)	+	0/7	—
	2.5×10^6 (i.d.)	−	0/5	—
	4.0×10^6 (i.d.) for challenge	+		0/5
		−		0/3
			On day 48	On day 100
1B MCA-fibro-sarcoma[b]	1.2×10^6+PA-K 1 mg (i.d.)	+	5/5	0/5
	1.2×10^6+PA-K 1 mg (i.d.)	−	5/5	0/5
	1.2×10^6+BCG 1.9×10^7 (i.d.)	+	4/5	3/4
	1.2×10^6+BCG 1.9×10^7 (i.d.)	−	2/5	1/2
	1.2×10^6	+	0/5	—
	1.2×10^6	−	0/5	—
	3.0×10^6 for challenge	+		0/4
	3.0×10^6 for challenge	−		0/5

BCG: lyophilized *Mycobacterium bovis*, Japan strain.   *P. acnes*: non-living preparation-Kowa.

[a] Animals: SWS/Ms male 12-week-old mice.   Tumor: 3-methylcholanthrene (MCA)-induced sarcoma, 13 TG, No. 042573 line.   Presensitization: lyophilized BCG (10^7 cells, i.d.) 46 days before tumor inoculation.

[b] Animals: SWM/Ms female, 9- to 12-week-old mice.   Tumor: MCA-induced sarcoma, primary, No. 053174 line.   Presensitization: sensitized with BCG (10^7 cells) 28 days before tumor inoculation.

for assessment of therapeutic efficacy (tumor immunity). As shown by the results presented in Experiment 1, Table I, prior immunization with BCG in both cases of adjuvant is effective for development of systemic tumor immunity (in Exp. 1A, 4/15 *vs.* 0/10, and Exp. 1B, 3/10 *vs.* 1/10) (*26–29*). Intraperitoneal injection of *P. acnes* or BCG did not affect the tumor take of the cells inoculated subsequently, *i.e.*, contact between tumor cells and adjuvant is necessary for optimum efficacy of this therapy (*37*). At a 1 mg dose, *P. acnes* in admixture with tumor cells was effective in inhibiting tumor growth at the site of inoculation but did not affect systemic tumor immunity. In the case of BCG therapy, as we previously reported (*28*), Bartlett *et al.* (*5*) also showed that conditions ideal for tumor suppression were inadequate for the induction of tumor immunity.

Effective Dose of Killed P. acnes in Tumor Cell-P. acnes Vaccine Capable of Inducing Tumor Immunity in Mice (Experiments 2A, 2B, and 2C, Table II)

In this experiment, we tested the optimal dose of killed *P. acnes* in the vaccine required for tumor immunity in our system using three different lines of tumors. The number of tumor cells indicated in Table II were mixed with 0.1–1.0 mg of varied doses of killed *P. acnes* and injected intradermally into mice presensitized with BCG

TABLE II. Effect of Varied Doses of Killed *P. acnes* C7 (PA-K) in the Tumor Cell-PA-K Vaccine on Syngeneic Tumor Growth and Tumor Immunity

Exp. No. tumor	Treatment No. of tumor cells and PA-K	Presensitized c̄ BCG	Day of tumor challenge No. of tumor-free mice — No. of mice tested	No. of tumor-free mice — No. of mice challenged
			On day 66	On day 128
2A MCA-fibro-sarcoma[a]	$2.0 \times 10^6 + 1.0$ mg	—	3/4	0/3
	$2.0 \times 10^6 + 0.5$ mg	—	3/4	1/3
	$2.0 \times 10^6 + 0.1$ mg	—	3/4	0/3
	2.0×10^6	—	0/7	
	3.5×10^6 for challenge			0/6
			On day 44	On day 100
2B MCA-fibro-sarcoma[b]	$8.5 \times 10^5 + 1.0$ mg	—	3/3	0/3
	$8.5 \times 10^5 + 0.5$ mg	+	3/3	3/3
	$8.5 \times 10^5 + 0.5$ mg	—	3/3	3/3
	$8.5 \times 10^5 + 0.1$ mg	—	6/6	3/6
	8.5×10^5	+	0/3	—
	8.5×10^5	—	0/3	—
	10^6 for challenge	—		0/6
			On day 47	On day 96
2C MCA-fibro-sarcoma[c]	$2.4 \times 10^6 + 0.6$ mg	+	5/5	3/5
	$2.4 \times 10^6 + 0.4$ mg	+	5/5	3/5
	$2.4 \times 10^6 + 0.4$ mg	—	4/4	3/4
	$2.4 \times 10^6 + 0.2$ mg	+	5/5	4/5
	$2.4 \times 10^6 + 0.2$ mg	—	4/4	4/4
	$2.4 \times 10^6 + 0.1$ mg	+	5/5	5/5
	$2.4 \times 10^6 + 0.1$ mg	—	4/4	4/4
	2.4×10^6	+	0/5	—
	2.4×10^6	—	0/4	—
	3.2×10^6 for challenge	+		0/4
	3.2×10^6 for challenge	—		0/4

[a] Animal: SWM/Ms male, 9-week-old mice. Tumor: MCA-induced sarcoma, 5 TG, No. 112774 line.

[b] Animal: SWM/Ms male, 8- to 11-week-old mice. Tumor: MCA-induced sarcoma, primary, No. 072275 line. Presensitization: lyophilized BCG (10^7 cells, i.d.) 47 days before tumor inoculation. PA-K: non-living preparation-Kowa.

[c] Animal: SWM/Ms female 10-week-old mice. Tumor: MCA-induced sarcoma, 11 TG, No. 062474 line. Presensitization: lyophilized BCG (10^7 cells, i.d.) 60 days before tumor inoculation.

or unsensitized mice. As shown in Table II, it is apparent that the lower dose of *P. acnes* (0.1–0.5 mg) in the vaccine was better than the higher dose (0.6 and 1 mg) for induction of tumor immunity. One milligram was consistently ineffective on tumor immunity despite its potent local effect, probably due to over-stimulation of the draining node by the higher dose of *P. acnes*. Correlation between the dose of *P. acnes* and its antitumor effect varied depending on the tumor lines used, which differ in their level of antigenicity and growth rates, and on host state such as presensitization or not with BCG.

To test the toxic effect of *P. acnes* on tumor cells, mixtures of *P. acnes* (live or non-living preparation) and tumor cells were incubated *in vitro* and viability of tumor cells

TABLE III. Effect of Tumor Cell-*P. acnes* C7 (PA-K)-BCG Vaccine and of Combination Therapy Using Either Adjuvant on Tumor Growth and Tumor Immunity

Exp. No. tumor	Treatment No. of tumor cells + adjuvant i.d.	Presensitized c̄ BCG (B) or PA-K (P)	Day of tumor challenge No. of tumor-free mice / No. of mice tested	No. of tumor-free mice / No. of mice challenged
			On day 44	On day 62
3A MCA-fibro-sarcoma[a]	8.5×10^5+PA-K 0.5 mg	+ (B)	3/3	3/3
	8.5×10^5+PA-K 0.5 mg	−	3/3	0/3
	8.5×10^5+BCG 10^7	−	6/6	3/6
	8.5×10^5+PA-K 0.5 mg +BCG 10^7	−	7/7	4/7
	8.5×10^5+PA-K 0.25 mg +BCG 5×10^6	−	4/4	3/4
	8.5×10^5	+ (B)	0/3	—
	10^6 for challenge	−	0/3	0/6
			On day 42	On day 73
3B Spontane-ous mammary carcinoma[b]	1.5×10^6+PA-K 0.1 mg	+ (B)	8/8	1/8
	1.5×10^6+PA-K 0.1 mg	−	4/5	0/4
	1.5×10^6+BCG 3.8×10^7	−	3/5	1/3
	1.5×10^6+PA-K 0.1 mg, BCG 10^7 (i.d.)	−	5/5	1/5
	1.5×10^6+BCG 3.8×10^7	+ (P)	3/8	0/3
	1.5×10^6+BCG 3.8×10^7	+ (P, i.p.)	5/10	1/5
	1.5×10^6+BCG 3.8×10^7, PA-K 0.5 mg (i.d.)	−	1/10	0/1
	1.5×10^6+BCG 3.8×10^7, PA-K 0.5 mg (i.p.)	−	2/9	1/2
	1.5×10^6	−	0/5	—
	1.7×10^6 for challenge	−		0/6

BCG : lyophilized *Mycobacterium bovis*, BCG Japan strain. *P. acnes* C7 : Non-living preparation-Kowa.

[a] Animal : SWM/Ms male, 8- to 11-week-old mice. Tumor : MCA-induced sarcoma, primary, No. 07225 line. Presensitized with lyophilized BCG (10^7 cells, i.d.) 47 days before tumor inoculation.

[b] Animal : SWM/Ms female, 10- to 14-week-old mice. Tumor : spontaneous mammay tumor, 2 TG, No. 102275 line. Presensitized with lyophilized BCG (10^7 cells, i.d.) or killed *P. acnes* (0.5 mg, i.d.), 25 days before tumor inoculation.

was measured by the Trypan Blue exclusion test. No significant impairment of tumor cell viability was detected.

Effect of Vaccine Containing P. acnes and BCG Together with Tumor Cells or of Combination Therapy with Vaccine Containing Either Adjuvant and Tumor Cells and Presensitization with Either Adjuvant on Tumor Growth and Tumor Immunity (Experiments 3A and 3B, Table III)

These experiments were conducted to determine which of the single therapy, tumor cell *P. acnes* vaccine or tumor cell-BCG vaccine, combined vaccine (a mixture of tumor cells, *P. acnes*, and BCG), or varied combinations of these two adjuvants, is the most effective for suppression of tumor growth and tumor immunity. This is the first report on treatment of syngeneic tumors in mice with a mixture of tumor cells and two kinds of adjuvant. Its results showed clearly that intradermal inoculation of this mixture of tumor cell-*P. acnes*-BCG was more effective (4/7 and 3/4) than the use of tumor cell-*P. acnes* or tumor cell-BCG mixture alone (0/3 at 0.5 mg of *P. acnes*, 3/6 with BCG) on tumor immunity. It was also found that presensitization of mice with BCG effectively influenced tumor immunity when combined with tumor cell-*P. acnes* vaccine treatment. In contrast, presensitization with *P. acnes* and treatment with tumor cell-BCG vaccine did not alter the effect. Simultaneous injection of *P. acnes* (i.d. or i.p.) with tumor cell-BCG vaccine treatment was also not effective. These data indicate that if an optimal dose of *P. acnes* was used in combination with BCG the therapeutic efficacy of immunotherapy seemed to be synergistic rather than additive. In Experiment 3B the therapeutic efficacy of combination modalities such as either vaccine (tumor cell-*P. acnes* or tumor cell-BCG) treatment in mice presensitized (i.d. or i.p.) with *P. acnes* or BCG was determined. As shown in Table III (3B), its results seemed not to be improved by these combination therapies, but in a group of mice treated with tumor cell-*P. acnes* vaccine and simultaneous injection of BCG at the opposite intradermal site, tumor growth was suppressed significantly (5/5) when compared with those of other groups.

Effect of Live P. acnes and of Live BCG in Mixture with Tumor Cells on Intradermal Syngeneic Tumor Growth and Tumor Immunity (Experiments 4A and 4B, Table IV and Fig. 1)

Experiments 4A and 4B were performed to determine the antitumor activity of live *P. acnes* organisms instead of killed *P. acnes* preparation since this strain of bacteria is present in normal human bone marrow, as mentioned previously (*11, 14*). Mice in Experiment 4B were presensitized with live *P. acnes* organisms. On the 59th day, mice free of tumor were challenged with tumor cells of the same line. Experiment 4A was carried out in almost the same way as Experiment 4B. The results represented in Table IV and Fig. 1 can be summarized as follows: (1) In Experiment 4A, mice presensitized with BCG 6 months ago showed a better effect on this mammary tumor growth when injected with live *P. acnes* compared to that of unsensitized mice (4/5 *vs.* 2/5); development of tumor immunity also was affected (2/4 *vs.* 0/2). (2) In Experiment 4B, tumor cells and live *P. acnes* mixed in a ratio of 1: 0.5 to 1: 50 were all effective for

TABLE IV. Effect of Live *P. acnes* C7 (PA) and of Live BCG in the
Vaccine on Syngeneic Tumor Growth and Tumor Immunity

Exp. No. tumor	Treatment No. of tumor cells+live adj. i.d. (ratio)	Presensitized c̄ BCG (B) or *P. acnes* (P)	Day of tumor challenge No. of tumor-free mice No. of mice tested	No. of tumor-free mice No. of mice challenged
			On day 54	On day 105
4A Spontane- ous mammary carcinoma[a]	1.2×10^6+PA 3.9×10^5 (1:0.3)	+ (B)	4/5	2/4
	1.2×10^6+PA 3.9×10^5 (1:0.3)	−	2/5	0/2
	1.2×10^6	+ (B)	0/5	—
	1.2×10^6	−	0/5	—
	2.5×10^6 for challenge	−		0/5
			On day 59	On day 112
4B MCA-fibro sarcoma[b]	2.5×10^6+PA 1.2×10^8 (1:50)	+ (P)	5/5	4/5
	2.5×10^6+PA 1.2×10^7 (1:5)	+ (P)	5/5	1/5
	2.5×10^6+PA 1.2×10^6 (1:0.5)	+ (P)	5/5	1/5
	2.5×10^6	+ (P)	0/5	—
	3.7×10^6 for challenge	−		0/5

[a] Animal: SWM/Ms female, 10- to 28-week-old mice. Tumor: spontaneous mammary tumor, 7 TG, No. 092074 line. Presensitization: lyophilized BCG (10^7 cells, i.d.) 6 months before tumor inocula-tion.

[b] Animal: SWM/Ms male, 10-week-old mice. Tumor: MCA-induced sarcoma, 8 TG, No. 062474 line. Presensitization: live *P. acnes* C7 (10^7 cells, i.d.) 27 days before tnmor inoculation.

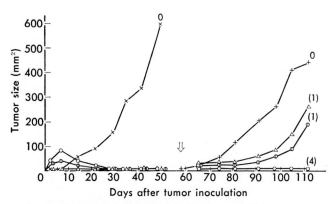

FIG. 1. Suppression of tumor growth and induction of tumor immunity with a mix-ture of tumor cells and live *P. acnes* C7 in mice
　　Animal: SWM/Ms, 10-week-old male mice (Exp. 4B 070775).
　　Tumor: 3-methylcholanthrene (MCA)-induced tumor, 8 TG, No. 062474 line.
　　All mice were presensitized with live *P. acnes* C7 (10^7 cells, i.d.) except the group of control.
　　○ tumor cells (2.5×10^6)+live *P. acnes* (1.2×10^8), av. of 5 mice (4).
　　◉ tumor cells (2.5×10^6)+live *P. acnes* (1.2×10^7), av. of 5 mice (1).
　　△ tumor cells (2.5×10^6)+live *P. acnes* (1.2×10^7), av. of 5 mice (1).
　　× tumor cells (2.5×10^6), av. of 5 mice.
　　+ nonsensitized, challenge control-tumor (3.7×10^6), av. of 5 mice. ⇩ Tumor-free mice received tumor challenge (3.7×10^6 cells, 10th transplant generation of the same tumor) on day 59. Numbers on the graph and in footnote parentheses indicate num-ber of survivors and of mice that acquired tumor immunity, respectively.

tumor suppression and the ratio of 1:50 was the most effective for tumor immunity in mice presensitized with live *P. acnes*. Control mice inoculated with tumor cells alone died of tumor within 61 days. As shown in Fig. 1, there is a clear correlation between the amount of live *P. acnes* and the size of skin reaction or of induction of tumor immunity, as in the case of live BCG (*37*).

Effect of Antithymocyte Serum, Antimacrophage Serum, and Latex Particles on the Antitumor Activity of P. acnes or BCG in Admixture with Tumor Cells in a Syngeneic Mouse System (Experiments 5A and 5B, Table V) (30)

Experiments 5A and 5B were carried out to compare the antitumor mechanisms of *P. acnes* and BCG by treating the mice with antithymocyte serum, antimacrophage serum, or latex particles with a view to clarifying the relative role of different cell populations associated with the antitumor action to *P. acnes* or BCG. The *P. acnes*

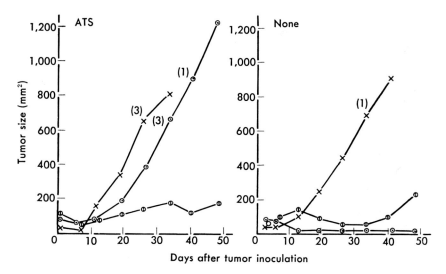

FIG. 2. Effect of antithymocyte serum on the antitumor activity of tumor cell-BCG and tumor cell-*P. acnes* C7 vaccines (Exp. 5A)

Group	Treatment (i.d.) with tumor cells (1.4×10⁸)	No. of mice tested	No. of tumor-free mice on day 48
⊙ ATS	+BCG (CWS-in-oil, 150 μg)	6	0
① ATS	+*P. acnes* (killed preparation, 0.5 mg)	6	2
× ATS	+None	5	0
⊙ None	+BCG (CWS-in-oil, 150 μg)	4	4
① None	+*P. acnes* (killed preparation, 0.5 mg)	4	3
× NS	+None	4	0

Animals: SWM/Ms male mice, 8- to 15-week-old. Tumor: 7 th transplant generation of MCA-induced sarcoma, No. 120574 line. Antithymocyte serum (ATS) or normal serum (NS) was injected (0.25 ml) i.p. on days −2, 0, +2, and +4. Number in parentheses on the graph indicates number of survivors.

used was a killed or non-living preparation and BCG was lyophilized BCG or a non-living preparation (cell wall fractions). Twenty-nine mice were divided into two groups: 17 mice received an intraperitoneal injection of 0.25 ml of antithymocyte serum or normal serum on days -2, 0, $+2$, and $+4$. On day 0, tumor cells alone, tumor cell-*P. acnes* vaccine, or tumor cell-BCG vaccine was inoculated intradermally. The adjuvants used were killed *P. acnes* and BCG-CWS-in-oil preparation, and each of them was mixed with tumor cells. The effect of antithymocyte serum treatment on *P. acnes* and BCG therapy is shown in Fig. 2. Tumor cells injected without *P. acnes* or BCG grew progressively in groups of mice treated with antithymocyte serum, normal or untreated mice, and all died of tumor within 41 days. The effect of antithymocyte serum administration on the antitumor activity of *P. acnes* and BCG was significantly different, as shown in Fig. 2; tumor growth in mice inoculated with the tumor cell-*P. acnes* vaccine was not influenced by treatment with antithymocyte serum, and 2 out of 6 mice showing complete tumor suppression, but not so with the group of mice inoculated with the tumor cell-BCG vaccine. There is convincing evidence that lymphocytes are required for BCG-mediated tumor regression (*9, 13*) but, in the case of killed *P. acnes* therapy, there is evidence that antithymocyte serum treatment does not abrogate the efficacy of *P. acnes*-mediated tumor killing in an allogeneic mouse tumor system (*15*).

Recently, following the work of Mackaness *et al.* (*18*), Yamada and Ohno (*35*) demonstrated cellular responses in popliteal nodes of mice after inoculation of anti-tumor agents in the footpads by measuring ^{3}H-TdR incorporation into DNA, and by determining histological features in responding nodes. Their data indicate that the cells responding to BCG are mainly T cells, and those responding to killed *P. acnes* are probably B cells and macrophages.

With a hope of clarifying more exactly the difference between *P. acnes* and BCG activity, we conducted the next experiment with antimacrophage serum treatment and by intraperitoneal administration of uniform latex particles, which are probably taken up by macrophages and produce selective impairment of macrophage functions (*2, 41*).

TABLE V. Effects of Antithymocyte Serum (ATS), Antimacrophage Serum (AMS), and Latex Particles on the Antitumor Acivity of Tumor Cell-*P. acnes* C7 and Tumor Cell-BCG Vaccine (Exp. 5B)

Treatment (i.d.) with tumor cells (10^6)	No. of tumor-free mice/No. of mice tested on day 35			
	ATS[a]	AMS[a]	Latex[b]	None
+live BCG (1.4×10^7)	0/3	0/3	0/3	3/3
+BCG-CWS-in-oil (100 μg)	0/5			3/3
+live *P. acnes* (5×10^7)	0/3	3/3	3/3	3/3
+*P. acnes*-CWS (100 μg)	1/3			3/3
+none	0/3	0/3	0/3	0/3

Animals: SWM/Ms male mice, 8- to 10-week-old. Tumor: 4th transplant generation of MCA-induced sarcoma, No. 011276 line.

[a] Antisera (0.25 ml) were injected i.p. on days -2, 0, $+5$, and $+7$.

[b] Latex particles (30 mg) were given i.p. 2 hr before the tumor or vaccine inoculation.

The influence of this treatment on the therapecutic effect of each vaccine (*P. acnes* and BCG) was examined.

Forty-eight age-matched mice were divided into 16 groups according to a protocol shown in Table V. Antithymocyte serum or antimacrophage serum was injected intraperitoneally on days -2, 0, $+5$, and $+7$. Tumor cells were mixed with *P. acnes* or BCG, either in living form or a non-living preparation, and inoculated intradermally. The overall assessment of the effect of *P. acnes* or BCG on tumor growth was based on the number of tumor-free animals at the time of tumor challenge (day 35). The adjuvant used was living *P. acnes* or *P. acnes*-CWS preparation, living BCG, or BCG-CWS-in-oil preparation. The results presented in Fig. 3 and Table V can be summarized as follows: (1) The effect of antithymocyte serum on the antitumor activity of living *P. acnes* clearly contrasted with that of non-living *P. acnes*; when mice were

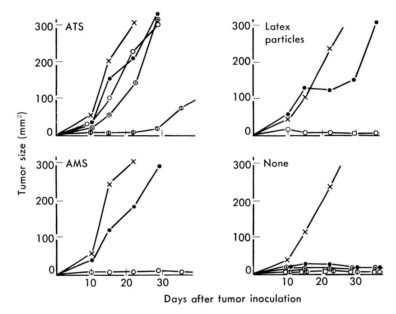

FIG. 3. Effects of antithymocyte serum, antimacrophage serum, and latex particles on the antitumor activity of tumor cell-BCG and tumor cell-*P. acnes* C7 vaccines (Exp. 5B)

Group	Treatment (i.d.) with tumor cells (10^6)
●	+live BCG (1.4×10^7)
⊙	+BCG-CWS-in-oil ($100\ \mu g$)
○	+live *P. acnes* (5×10^7)
⊖	+*P. acnes*-CWS ($100\ \mu g$)
×	+None

Animals: SWM/Ms male mice, 8- to 10-week-old. Tumor: 4 th transplant generation of MCA-induced sarcoma, No. 011276 line. Antisera (0.25 ml) were injected i.p. on days -2, 0, $+5$, and $+7$. Latex particles (30 mg) were given i.p. 2 hr before the tumor or vaccine inoculation.

treated with antithymocyte serum, their response to BCG (both living and non-living) and live *P. acnes* was completely inhibited, but as in Experiment 5A, response to *P. acnes*-CWS was not affected by antithymocyte serum. (2) The effect of antimacrophage serum on the antitumor activity of living BCG and living *P. acnes* was significantly different. When mice were treated with antimacrophage serum, the effect of tumor cell-BCG vaccine against tumor growth was completely suppressed in contrast to that of the tumor cell-*P. acnes* vaccine. Similar results were obtained when mice were injected intraperitoneally with latex beads for blocking macrophage functions. In addition to these experiments, we made a preliminary experiment on latex beads to see whether this treatment abrogates the efficacy to tumor cell-non-living *P. acnes* vaccine or not, and confirmed that the immune response of mice treated with latex beads was not depressed against the tumor cell-non-living *P. acnes* vaccine, 3 out of 4 mice being tumor-free at day 47, in contrast to all 4 mice being tumor-free in normal controls. Tumors grew progressively in both groups of mice, untreated and treated with latex beads, and they all died of tumor. (3) All the normal mice given tumor cell-*P. acnes* (live or CWS) vaccine or tumor cell-BCG (live or CWS-in-oil) vaccine rejected the tumor at the site of inoculation (Fig. 3 and Table V).

There is evidence that intraperitoneal injection of killed *C. parvum*, as in the case of *P. acnes* C7, inhibited syngeneic tumor growth in T cell-deprived mice and it was concluded that the antitumor effect of *C. parvum* depends on macrophage stimulation (7, 24, 34). On the other hand, tumor growth was not inhibited by BCG therapy in T cell-deprived mice (9, 13, 39). Our present results are similar; some additional findings are presented as follows: (1) Antithymocyte serum treatment completely nullified tumor killing mediated by live *P. acnes* but not by the *P. acnes*-CWS preparation. Similarly to tumor cell-live BCG vaccine, the effect of tumor cell-BCG-CWS-in-oil vaccine was also inhibited by antithymocyte serum. It is apparent that a sequence of reactions of cell-mediated immunity to living bacteria is quite different from the reactions produced by the inoculation of non-living bacteria, not only at the reaction site but systemically. Recently, the chemical and immunological properties of *P. acnes* cell wall were reported (3, 23). The different antigenicities of *P. acnes* and BCG might produce different responses in mice treated with antithymocyte serum. (2) When mice were treated with antimacrophage serum or latex particles, the effect of live BCG-mediated tumor killing was completely impaired, in contrast with the effect of tumor suppression mediated by live or non-living *P. acnes*. These results indicate that the antithymocyte serum or antimacrophage serum used reacted with each thymocyte or macrophage specifically, therefore, they reflect the relative roles of different host components which are immunologically committed in the reactions evoked by BCG or *P. acnes*. (3) In the group of normal mice that received tumor cell-*P. acnes* or tumor cell-BCG vaccine, tumor growth was completely suppressed, whereas in control mice inoculated with tumor cells, the tumor grew progressively (Fig. 3).

It should be noted here that the antimacrophage serum we prepared was not completely specific since we have not done absorption studies with lymphocytes; the same applies to antithymocyte serum whose cross reactivity with macrophages was not checked.

The non-specific effect of non-living *P. acnes* has been attributed primarily to stimulation of the reticuloendothelial systems (16, 23), as in the case of *C. parvum* (non-living). The present paper is the first report on a comparative study of macrophage-dependent and lymphocyte-dependent responses in host animals against *P. acnes* and BCG, in both living and non-living preparations. We believe that elucidation of the differences between the antitumor mechanisms of *P. acnes* and BCG is important for the further development of immunotherapy.

Acknowledgment

This work was supported in part by Grants-in-Aid for Cancer Research and for Special Cancer Chemotherapy Program from the Ministry of Health and Welfare, Japan.

REFERENCES

1. Adlam, C. and Scott, M. T. Lympho-reticular stimulatory properties of *Corynebacterium parvum* and related bacteria. *J. Med. Microbiol.*, **6**, 261–274 (1973).
2. Allison, A. C. and Hart, Pd'A. Potentiation by silica of the growth of *Mycobacterium tuberculosis* in macrophage cultures. *Br. J. Exp. Pathol.*, **49**, 465–476 (1968).
3. Azuma, I., Taniyama, T., Sugimura, K., Aladin, A. A., and Yamamura, Y. Chemical and immunological studies on the cell walls of *Propionibacterium acnes* strain C-7 and *Corynebacterium parvum* ATCC 11829. *Japan. J. Microbiol.*, **19**, 265–275 (1975).
4. Azuma, I., Taniyama, T., Hirao, F., and Yamamura, Y. Antitumor activity of cell-wall skeletons and peptidoglycolipids of mycobacteria and related microorganisms in mice and rabbits. *Gann*, **65**, 493–505 (1974).
5. Bartlett, G. L., Purnell, D. M., and Kreider, J. W. BCG inhibition of murine leukemia: Local suppression and systemic tumor immunity require different doses. *Science*, **191**, 299–301 (1976).
6. Bauchanan, R. E. and Gibbons, N. E. "Bergey's Manual of Determinative Bacteriology," 8th ed., Williams & Wilkins Co., Baltimore (1974).
7. Castro, J. E. Antitumor effects of *Corynebacterium parvum* in mice. *Eur. J. Cancer*, **10**, 121–127 (1974).
8. Chaffar, A., Cullen, R. T., Dunbar, N., and Woodruff, M.F.A. Antitumor effect *in vitro* of lymphocytes and macrophages from mice treated with *Corynebacterium parvum*. *Br. J. Cancer*, **29**, 199–205 (1974).
9. Chung, E., Zbar, B., and Rapp, H. J. Tumor regression mediated by *Mycobacterium bovis* (strain BCG)—Effects of isonicotinic acid hydrazide, cortisone acetate and anti-thymocyte serum. *J. Natl. Cancer Inst.*, **51**, 241–250 (1973).
10. Fisher, J. C., Grace, W. R., and Mannick, J. A. The effect of nonspecific immune stimulation with *Corynebacterium parvum* on patterns of tumor growth. *Cancer*, **26**, 1379–1382 (1970).
11. Fujita, H. and Saino, Y. Isolation of anaerobic *Corynebacterium* from human bone marrows and its protective activity against Sarcoma 180. *Kokubyo Gakkai Zasshi*, **38**, 294–299 (1971) (in Japanese).
12. Halpern, B. N., Prevot, A. R., Biozzi, G., Stiffel, C., Mouton, D., Morard, J. C., Bouthillier, Y., and Decreuesfond, C. Stimulation de l'activite phagocytaire du systeme reticuloendothelial provoquee par *Corynebacterium parvum*. *J. Reticuloendothel. Soc.*, **1**, 77–96 (1963).
13. Hanna, M. G., Jr., Snodgrass, M. J., Zbar, B., and Rapp, H. J. Histopathology of tumor regression after intralesional injection of *Mycobacterium bovis*. IV. The development of antitumor and anti-BCG immunity. *J. Natl. Cancer Inst.*, **51**, 897–908 (1973).

14. Hattori, T. and Mori, A. Bacteriological survey of anaerobic corynebacterium in human bone marrow. *Gann*, **64**, 7–14 (1973).

15. Hattori, T. and Mori, A. Antitumor activity of anaerobic *Corynebacterium* isolated from the human bone marrow. *Gann*, **64**, 15–27 (1973).

16. Kato, A. and Fujita, H. Adjuvant effect of *Corynebacterium liquefaciens*. *Gan-to-Kagaku-ryoho*, **3**, 670–676 (1975) (in Japanese).

17. Kato, A., Nakagawa, H., Akimoto, H., Fujita, H., Tanaka, T., and Kimura, K. Antitumor effects of *Corynebacterium liquefaciens*. *Gan-to-Kagakuryoho*, **3**, 677–686 (1976) (in Japanese).

18. Mackaness, G. B., Auclair, D. J., and Lagrange, P. H. Immunopotentiation with BCG. I. Immune response to different strains and preparation. *J. Natl. Cancer Inst.*, **51**, 1655–1667 (1973).

19. Olivotto, M. and Bomford, R. *In vitro* inhibition of tumor cell growth and DNA synthesis by peritoneal and lung macrophages from mice injected with *Corynebacterium parvum*. *Int. J. Cancer*, **13**, 478–488 (1974).

20. O'Neill, G. J., Henderson, D. C., and White, R. G. The role of anaerobic coryneforms on specific and nonspecific immunological reactions. I. Effect on particle clearance and humoral and cell-mediated immunological responses. *Immunology*, **24**, 977–995 (1973).

21. Prévôt, A. "Manual for the Classification of Anaerobic Bacteria," Lea & Febiger, Philadelphia (1966).

22. Rapp, H. J., Churchill, W. H., Jr., Kronman, B. S., Rolley, R. T., Hammond, W. G., and Borsos, T. Antigenicity of a new diethylnitrosamine-induced transplantable guinea pig hepatoma: Pathology and formation of ascites variant. *J. Natl. Cancer Inst.*, **41**, 1–11 (1968).

23. Saino, Y., Eda, J., Nagoya, T., Yoshimura, Y., Yamaguchi, M., and Kobayashi, F. Anaerobic coryneforms isolated from human bone marrow and skin. Chemical, biochemical, and serological studies and some of their biological activities. *Japan. J. Microbiol.*, **20**, 17–25 (1976).

24. Scott, M. T. *Corynebacterium parvum* as an immunotherapeutic anticancer agent. *Semin. Oncol.*, **1**, 367–378 (1974).

25. Smith, S. E. and Scott, M. T. Biological effects of *Corynebacterium parvum*. III. Amplification of resistance and impairment of active immunity to murine tumors. *Br. J. Cancer*, **26**, 361–367, (1972).

26. Tanaka, T. Immunotherapy of cancer: BCG therapy in syngeneic guinea pig. *Igaku-no-Ayumi*, **77**, 599–604 (1971) (in Japanese).

27. Tanaka, T. Effect of intratumor injection of live BCG on 3-methylcholanthrene-induced tumors of primary and early transplantation in mice. *Gann*, **65**, 145–151 (1974).

28. Tanaka, T. and Saito, T. Immunotherapy of cancer: Induction of tumor immunity with a mixture of tumor cell-BCG, and the effect of intratumor injection of BCG and of nonliving BCG preparation. *Gann*, **66**, 631–640 (1975).

29. Tanaka, T. and Sasaki, N. Effect of immunotherapy, chemotherapy, and surgery on tumor immunity in mice. *Gann*, **65**, 395–402 (1974).

30. Tanaka, T., Nakagawa, H., Kato, A., Yoshimura, M., Fujita, H., and Kimura, K. Effect of anti-thymocyte serum, anti-macrophage serum, and latex particles on the therapeutic efficacy of BCG or *Corynebacterium liquefaciens* (*Propionibacterium acnes* C7) in syngeneic mice. *Gann*, **68**, 45–52 (1977).

31. Tanaka, T. and Tokunaga, T. Suppression of tumor growth and induction of specific tumor immunity by intradermal inoculation of a mixture of living tumor cells and live *Mycobacterium bovis* in syngeneic mice. *Gann*, **62**, 433–434 (1971).

32. Tokunaga, T., Kataoka, T., Nakamura, R. M., Yamamoti, S., and Tanaka, T. Tumor immunity induced by BCG-tumor cell mixtures in syngeneic mice. *Japan. J. Med. Sci. Biol.*, **26**, 71–85 (1973).

33. Woodruff, M.F.A. and Boak, J. L. Inhibitory effect of injection of *Corynebacterium parvum* on the growth of tumor transplants in syngeneic host. *Br. J. Cancer*, **20**, 345–355 (1966).

34. Woodruff, M.F.A., Dunbar, N., and Chaffar, A. The growth of tumors in T cell-deprived mice and their response to treatment with *Corynebacterium parvum*. *Proc. Roy. Soc. London, Ser. B*, **184**, 97–102 (1973).

35. Yamada, K. and Ohno, R. Comparison of the immunological potentiating effect of several antitumor agents in germ-free and nude mice. *Igaku-no-Ayumi*, **96**, 263–270 (1976) (in Japanese).

36. Zbar, B., Bernstein, I., Bartlett, G. L., and Rapp, H. J. Immunotherapy of cancer: Regression of intradermal tumors and prevention of growth of lymph node metastases after intralesional injection of living *Mycobacterium bovis*. *J. Natl. Cancer Inst.*, **49**, 119–130 (1972).

37. Zbar, B., Bernstein, I., and Rapp, H. J. Suppression of tumor growth at the site of injection of living Bacillus Calmette-Guerin. *J. Natl. Cancer Inst.*, **46**, 831–839 (1971).

38. Zbar, B., Bernstein, I., Tanaka, T., and Rapp, H. J. Tumor immunity produced by the intradermal inoculation of living tumor cells and living *Mycobacterium bovis* (strain BCG). *Science*, **170**, 1217–1218 (1970).

39. Zbar, B. and Rapp, H. J. Immunotherapy of guinea pig cancer with BCG. *Cancer*, **34**, 1532–1540 (1974).

40. Zbar, B. and Tanaka, T. Immunotherapy of cancer: Regression of tumors after intralesional injection of living *Mycobacterium bovis*. *Science*, **172**, 271–273 (1971).

41. Zisman, B., Hirsch, M. S., and Allison, A. C. Selective effects of anti-macrophage serum, silica and anti-lymphocyte serum on pathogenesis of herpes virus infection of young adult mice. *J. Immunol.*, **104**, 1155–1159 (1970).

GANN Monograph on Cancer Research 21, 1978

IMMUNE RESPONSE OF REGIONAL LYMPH NODE TO BCG CELL-WALL SKELETON AND OTHER IMMUNOPOTENTIATORS

Ryuzo Ohno,[*1] Kohji Ezaki,[*1] Masahide Kobayashi,[*1] Hideo Takeyama,[*1] Hisamitsu Suzuki,[*1] Kazumasa Yamada,[*1] Ichiro Azuma,[*2] and Yuichi Yamamura[*2]

*First Department of Internal Medicine, Nagoya University School of Medicine,[*1] and Third Department of Internal Medicine, Osaka University Medical School[*2]*

Quantitative and morphological aspects of the cellular response provoked by BCG cell-wall skeleton (BCG-CWS), *Nocardia rubra*-CWS, *Propionibacterium acnes*-CWS, *P. acnes* C7-whole cells, D-CMI, PS-K, and OK-432 were studied in the regional lymphoid tissues, by comparing the responses in normal mice with those in T cell-deficient nude mice, in order to investigate the modes of action of these immunopotentiators. The immunological effects of the immunopotentiators were found to be not unidirectional but they exert their effects on all of the 3 lines of immunocompetent cells; T cells, B cells, and macrophage-histiocytes. However, BCG-CWS exerts its effect mainly on T cells and evoked lymphoblast proliferation in the paracortical area. *P. acnes* C7, both whole cells and CWS, mainly evoked strong macrophage-histiocyte proliferation. *N. rubra*-CWS, D-CMI, and PS-K seemed to work on both T cells and macrophage-histiocytes, and OK-432 on both T cells and B cells. Adjuvant activities and also antitumor actions of these immunopotentiators are probably dependent on the cell lines which these agents mainly stimulate.

Immunotherapy with living cells of *Mycobacterium bovis* strain BCG has been shown to be effective in malignant melanoma, acute leukemia and other malignancies (3, 4). So far BCG has been most widely used as a nonspecific immunostimulator in immunotherapy of human cancer. When live BCG cells are applied, however, there are several disadvantages for practical use. Serious side effects including disseminated BCG infection and granulomatous hepatitis have been reported (14). Therefore the use of non-living subcomponents of BCG has been studied to avoid these disadvantages. Azuma *et al.* (1) have purified cell-wall skeleton of BCG, a fraction with adjuvant and antitumor activity. Successful clinical applications of the fraction have been reported for malignant melanoma by Yamamura *et al.* (18) and for lung cancer by Yasumoto *et al.* (19).

[*1] Tsurumai-cho 65, Showa-ku, Nagoya 466, Japan (大野竜三, 江崎幸治, 小林政英, 竹山英夫, 鈴木久三, 山田一正).
[*2] Fukushima 1-1-50, Fukushima-ku, Osaka 553, Japan (東 市郎, 山村雄一).

Besides BCG and its cell-wall skeleton, methanol extraction residue of BCG (*17*), *Corynebacterium parvum* (*5*) and Levamizole (*12*) have been applied clinically for cancer with some effectiveness. In Japan, protein-bound polysaccharide preparation from *Basidiomycetes* (PS-K), Su strain of *Streptococcus haemolyticus* (OK-432), and *Propionibacterium acnes* C7 have also been tested for human malignancy with some effects (*6, 7*).

Azuma *et al.* (*2*) showed that not only cell-wall skeleton of BCG but cell-wall skeletons prepared from *Mycobacterium kansasii*, *Mycobacterium tuberculosis* H37Rv, *Nocardia rubra*, *Nocardia asteroides*, *Corynebacterium diphtheriae*, and *P. acnes* possessed suppressive activities on experimental tumor growth. Azuma *et al.* (*2*) also found that peptidoglycolipids (D-CMI and D-CMI-A) of *M. tuberculosis* Aoyama B was effective for the suppression of tumor growth in syngeneic mice.

In an attempt to investigate the modes of action of cell-wall skeleton of BCG and other immunopotentiators with antitumor activity, we studied quantitative and morphological aspects of the cellular response provoked by these agents in the regional lymphoid tissues, by comparing the responses in normal mice with those in T cell-deficient nude mice.

Immunopotentiators Tested

The following 7 immunopotentiators which had been developed in Japan and shown to possess antitumor activity at least against experimental tumors were tested.

1) Cell-wall skeleton of *M. bovis* strain BCG (BCG-CWS) (*2*).
2) Cell-wall skeleton of *N. rubra* (*N. rubra*-CWS) (*2*).
3) Chloroform-methanol insoluble peptidoglycolipids from the so-called "wax D" fraction of *M. tuberculosis* Aoyama B strain (D-CMI) (*2*).
4) Phenol-treated cells of *P. acnes* C7 (*P. acnes*-whole cells) (*13*).
5) Cell-wall skeleton of *P. acnes* C7 (*P. acnes*-CWS) (*2*).
6) Protein-bound polysaccharide preparation extracted from *Coriolus versicolor* (PS-K) (*15*).
7) Penicillin G treated *Streptococcus haemolyticus* Su strain (OK-432) (*10*).

BCG-CWS, *N. rubra*-CWS, and D-CMI were prepared in the form of oil-in-water as described previously (*2*). Other agents were dissolved or suspended in sterile saline.

Experimental Animals and Measurements of Immunological Responses of Regional Lymphoid Tissues

Male and female germ-free ICR mice (ICR-GF) (CLEA Japan Inc.) and male Balb/c mice from a specific pathogen-free colony (Balb/c-SPF) (Shizuoka Exp. Animal Coop.) were used as normal mice. Male and female Balb/c-nu/nu mice were used as T cell-deficient mice. All the mice were maintained in an infection-free environment and fed a sterile and vitamin-supplemented diet in a sterile isolator (Trexler type, Nihon CLEA Japan Inc.). All experiments were performed in sterile condition. As emphasized by Old *et al.* (*11*), the need for these precautions is very great in such studies.

The extent of cellular proliferation in response to BCG-CWS and other immunopotentiators was measured in the popliteal lymph nodes of mice which were injected with the agents in their hind footpads. To measure and express the relative rate of cell division in responding nodes, ^{3}H-thymidine (^{3}H-TdR) was incorporated into DNA. Groups of mice were inoculated in hind footpads with 0.05 ml of a suspension of an appropriate concentration of the immunopotentiators. At intervals thereafter, 3 mice from each group received intravenous injection of 20 μCi ^{3}H-TdR (10 Ci/mmol, New England Nuclear). Forty-five minutes later, the popliteal nodes were excised anp minced thoroughly. Each node was extracted twice with cold 5% trichloroacetic acid. The precipitate was then dissolved in Sluene (Packard Instruments) and transferred to a counting vial to which 10 ml of toluene containing 0.5% PPO and 0.01% POPOP was added. The incorporated radioactivity was counted in a liquid scintillation counter (LS-335, Beckman Instruments) and expressed as counts per minute (cpm) per node.

To examine the morphological changes in the responding nodes, the nodes were stained with hematoxylin-eosin and also with methyl green-pyronin. Histoautoradiogram was prepared to clarify the localization of ^{3}H-TdR incorporating cells. The node was also examined by electron microscopy to confirm the exact nature of the proliferating cells.

Adjuvant Effect of BCG-CWS and Other Immunopotentiators in Regional Lymph Nodes

In order to confirm the adjuvant activities of 7 immunopotentiators in the regional lymphoid tissues, augmentation of plaque-forming cell (PFC) production in the popliteal lymph nodes was examined. Fourteen days after the injection of the immunopotentiators into hind footpads, 10^8 sheep red blood cells (SRBC) were administered into the same footpads. Direct PFC in the popliteal nodes were assayed 4 days later according to Cunningham's method with a slight modification (9). As shown in Table I, all of the 7 immunopotentiators tested were found to augment the PFC production in the nodes. Thus it was ascertained that all these agents worked as adjuvants for the immune response in the regional lymph nodes.

TABLE I. PFC in the Popliteal Lymph Nodes of Balb/c-SPF Mice Immunized with SRBC into the Hind Footpads

Agent given	Dose	PFC per	
		10^6 cells	Node
None	—	272	1,461 (1.0)[a]
BCG-CWS	100 μg	325	7,808 (5.3)
N. rubra-CWS	100 μg	551	10,375 (7.1)
P. acnes-whole cells	100 μg	428	11,618 (7.9)
P. acnes-CWS	100 μg	515	9,904 (6.8)
D-CMI	100 μg	485	15,441 (10.5)
PS-K	5 mg	662	8,774 (6.0)
OK-432	0.5 KE	756	9,214 (6.5)

[a] Stimulation ratios.

Time Course and Histologic Features of Immune Response to Immunopotentiators

After the footpad injection of the same amount of oil droplets or saline as used for the preparation of immunopotentiators, no significant changes in lymph node morphology and no increase of ³H-TdR incorporation were observed in both the normal and the nude mice (Photos 1, 2, and 3). After the footpad injection of the immunopotentiators, significant enlargement and morphological changes were noted in the draining nodes as follows.

1) BCG-CWS

Figure 1 (a) shows the TdR incorporation into DNA by the popliteal lymph nodes of ICR-GF mice, which were injected with 100 or 50 μg of BCG-CWS into the hind footpads. The incorporation was maximum at day 14 and was relatively well sustained at day 21. Figure 1 (b) shows the incorporation in Balb/c-nu/nu mice. The magnitude of the response in the nude mice was far less than that in the normal mice.

Histologic features of the popliteal nodes are schematically illustrated in Fig. 2. In the normal mice, the observed lymph node enlargement was mainly due to hyperplasia of the paracortical area (Photo 5) and increased numbers of pyroninophilic blast cells were located in this region (Photo 4). These cells were identified as lymphoblasts by electron microscopy (Photo 9). ³H-TdR-labeled cells were mainly located in the paracortical area in the histoautoradiogram. The formation of a few germinal centers in the cortex was noted together with the accumulation of plasma cells in the medullary cord. In the nude mice, lymph node enlargement was minimum and no cell proliferation was observed in the paracortical area. A few germinal centers in the cortex with the accumulation of plasma cells in the medullary cord were observed.

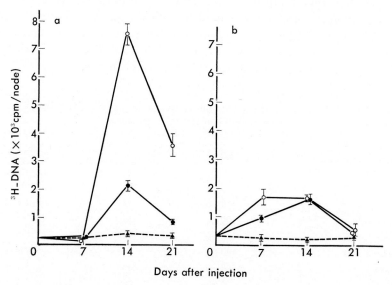

FIG. 1.　³H-TdR incorporation into DNA by the popliteal lymph nodes of ICR-GF mice (a) and Balb/c-nu/nu mice (b) after 100 or 50 μg of BCG-CWS into the hind footpads

○ BCG-CWS, 100 μg;　● BCG-CWS, 50 μg;　▲ control.

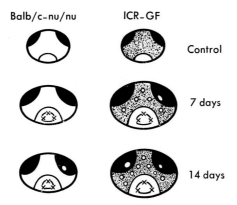

FIG. 2. Histologic features of the popliteal lymph nodes after BCG-CWS injection into the hind footpads

○ pyroninophilic blasts; × plasmablasts, plasma cells.

2) *N. rubra*-CWS

Figure 3 (a) shows the TdR incorporation into DNA by the popliteal lymph nodes of Balb/c-SPF mice after the footpad injection of 100 or 20 μg of *N. rubra*-CWS. Marked TdR incorporation was observed at days 14 and 21. In the nodes of Balb/c-nu/nu mice, only a little incorporation was seen at day 21 (Fig. 3 (b)). Histologic features are schematically illustrated in Fig. 4. Enlargement of the draining nodes was significant in the normal mice but it was minimum in the nude mice. In the normal mice, lymphoblast proliferation in the paracortical area was the prominent feature. In addition to this, granuloma formation was observed spreading from the medulla

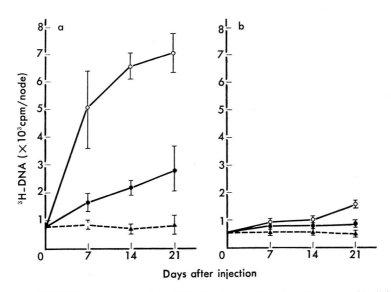

FIG. 3. ³H-TdR incorporation into DNA by the popliteal lymph nodes of Balb/c-SPF mice (a) and Balb/c-nu/nu mice (b) after 100 or 20 μg of *N. rubra*-CWS into the hind footpads.

○ *N. rubra*-CWS, 100 μg; ● *N. rubra*-CWS, 20 μg; ▲ control.

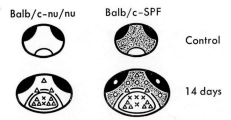

FIG. 4. Histologic features of the popliteal lymph nodes after *N. rubra*-CWS injection into the hind footpads
      ○ pyroninophilic blasts; × plasmablasts, plasma cells; △ granuloma.

to the cortex (Photo 6). The cells in the granuloma were identified as histiocytes by electron microscopy (Photo 10). In the nude mice granuloma formation was the main feature. Formation of germinal centers in the cortex and accumulation of plasma cells in the medullary cords were observed both in the normal and the nude mice.

3) *P. acnes-whole cells*

Figure 5 (a) shows the TdR incorporation into DNA by the popliteal lymph nodes of ICR-GF mice after 250 or 125 μg of *P. acnes*-whole cells. High and distinct incorporation was observed at days 7 and 14. Also in Balb/c-nu/nu mice high incorporation was noted (Fig. 5 (b)). Marked enlargement of lymph nodes was noted in both the normal and the nude mice. The main histological feature was the extensive granuloma formation spreading from the medulla to the cortex (Fig. 6) in both kinds of mice. The cells were identified as histiocytes by electron microscopy and ^{3}H-TdR-labeled cells were mainly observed in the area of the granuloma formation (Photo 7).

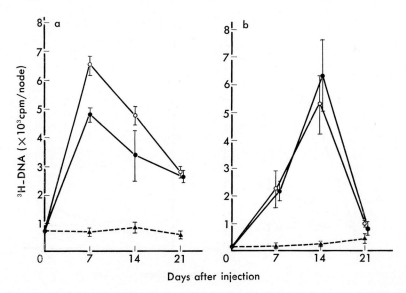

FIG. 5. ^{3}H-TdR incorporation into DNA by the popliteal lymph nodes of ICR-GF mice (a) and Balb/c-nu/nu mice (b) after 250 and 125 μg of *P. acnes*-whole cells into the hind footpads
      ○ *P. acnes*-whole cells, 250 μg; ● *P. acnes*-whole cells, 125 μg; ▲ control.

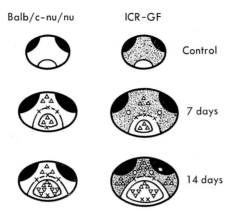

FIG. 6. Histologic features of the popliteal lymph nodes after *P. acnes*-whole cell injection into the hind footpads

○ pyroninophilic blasts; × plasmablasts, plasma cells; △ granuloma.

4) *P. acnes-CWS*

Figure 7 (a) shows the TdR incorporation into DNA by the popliteal lymph nodes of Balb/c-SPF mice after 250 or 50 μg of *P. acnes*-CWS. High and distinct incorporation was observed at days 7 and 14. Also in Balb/c-nu/nu mice high incorporation was noted (Fig. 7(b)). The time course and the magnitude of the incorporation revealed the same tendency as those in *P. acnes*-whole cells. Also the degree of lymph node enlargement and the histologic features were almost the same as in the case of

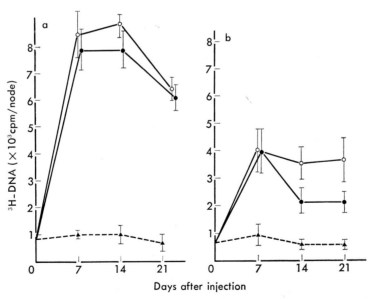

FIG. 7. ³H-TdR incorporation into DNA by the popliteal lymph nodes of Balb/c-SPF mice (a) and Balb/c-nu/nu mice (b) after 250 or 50 μg of *P. acnes*-CWS into the hind footpads

○ *P. acnes*-CWS, 250 μg; ● *P. acnes*-CWS, 50 μg; ▲ control.

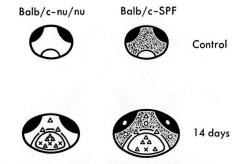

FIG. 8.   Histologic features of the popliteal lymph nodes after *P. acnes*-CWS injection into the hind footpads

○ pyroninophilic blasts;   × plasmablasts, plasma cells;   △ granuloma.

P. acnes-whole cells (Photo 8, Fig. 8). The main histologic feature was the extensive granuloma formation both in the normal and the nude mice. Proliferation of lymphoblasts in the paracortical area of the normal mice, however, was more prominent by *P. acnes*-CWS than in *P. acnes*-whole cells.

5)   *D-CMI*

Figure 9 (a) shows the TdR incorporation into DNA by the popliteal lymph nodes of Balb/c-SPF mice after 100 or 20 μg of D-CMI. This agent produced the highest incorporation of ³H-TdR among the 7 immunopotentiators tested. The incorporation at day 14 was 19,000 cpm/node. There was also a considerable incorporation

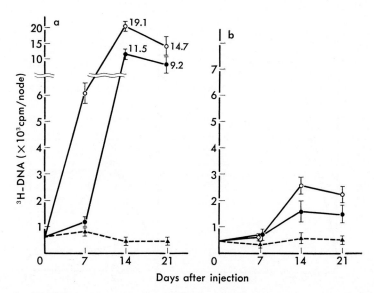

FIG. 9.   ³H-TdR incorporation into DNA by the popliteal lymph nodes of Balb/c-SPF mice (a) and Balb/c-nu/nu mice (b) after 100 or 20 μg of D-CMI into the hind footpads

○ D-CMI, 100 μg;   ● D-CMI, 20 μg;   ▲ control.

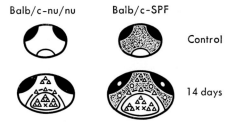

Balb/c-nu/nu   Balb/c-SPF

Control

14 days

Fig. 10.   Histologic features of the popliteal lymph nodes after D-CMI injection into the hind footpads
    ○ pyroninophilic blasts;   × plasmablasts, plasma cells;   △ granuloma.

in the nude mice (2,400 cpm at day 14) as shown in Fig. 9 (b). Incorporation in the latter, however, was only 13% of the former. Therefore, the cellular response provoked by D-CMI was much higher in the normal mice. Histologic features are schematically illustrated in Fig. 10. Marked enlargement of lymph nodes was seen in the normal mice, and also in the nude mice to a lesser degree. In the normal mice, proliferation of lymphoblasts in the paracortical area was marked. Granuloma formation and accumulation of plasma cells were also observed in the medulla. In the nude mice, only granuloma formation and accumulation of plasma cells were noted.

6)   PS-K

Figure 11 shows the TdR incorporation into the regional lymph nodes of ICR-GF mice and Balb/c-nu/nu mice after 5 or 2.5 mg of PS-K. A considerable increase of the incorporation was observed in the normal mice, but no increase was noted in the nude mice. Mild enlargement of the nodes was noted in the normal mice, and histologically, proliferation of lymphoblasts in the paracortical area and granuloma formation in the medulla were observed (Fig. 12). In the nude mice, enlargement of the nodes was minimal, but granuloma formation spreading from the medulla to the cortex was present.

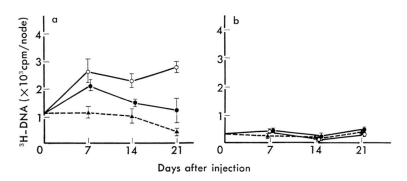

Fig. 11. ^{3}H-TdR incorporation into DNA by the popliteal lymph nodes of ICR-GF mice (a) and Balb/c-nu/nu mice (b) after 5 or 2.5 mg of PS-K into the hind footpads
    ○ PS-K, 5 mg;   ● PS-K, 2.5 mg;   ▲ control.

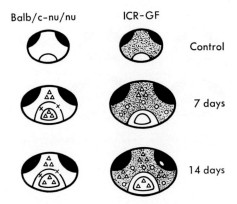

FIG. 12. Histologic features of the popliteal lymph nodes after PS-K injection into the hind footpads

○ pyroninophilic blasts; × plasmablasts, plasma cells; △ granuloma.

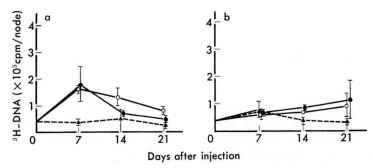

FIG. 13. ³H-TdR incorporation into DNA by the popliteal lymph nodes of ICR-GF mice (a) and Balb/c-nu/nu mice (b) after 0.5 or 0.25 KE of OK-432 into the hind footpads

○ OK-432, 0.5 KE; ● OK-432, 0.25 KE; ▲ control.

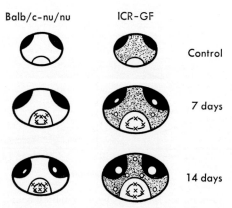

FIG. 14. Histologic features of the popliteal lymph nodes after OK-432 injection into the hind footpads

○ pyroninophilic blasts; × plasmablasts, plasma cells.

7)   OK-432

Figure 13 shows the TdR incorporation in the regional lymph nodes of ICR-GF mice and Balb/c-nu/nu mice after 0.5 or 0.25 KE* of OK-432. Both in the normal and the nude mice, a slight increase of the incorporation was observed. Enlargement of the lymph nodes was mild, and histologically, formation of germinal centers in the cortex and accumulation of plasma cells in the medulla were noted in both kinds of mice. Proliferation of lymphoblasts in the paracortical area was also seen in normal mice.

Macrophage Colony-forming Cells in the Regional Lymph Nodes

In order to investigate whether the histiocytes, consisting of granulomas in the immunopotentiator-treated lymph nodes, are derived only from outside sources such as bone marrow, or they multiply and proliferate also in the lymph nodes, macrophage colony-forming cells in the regional lymph nodes were assayed according to the method of Van Furth (16) with a slight modification.

Five days after the injections of the immunopotentiators in the hind footpads of Balb/c-SPF mice, 1 to 10×10^5 cells of the popliteal lymph nodes were cultured in 0.5 ml of Eagle's minimal essential medium (MEM) supplemented with 10% fetal calf serum and 20% conditioned medium in a Lab-Tek tissue culture chamber/slide (Lab-Tek Products) in a humidified incubator with 5% CO_2 in air at 37°. The conditioned medium was the supernatant culture fluid of L cell in Eagle's MEM.

TABLE II.   Macrophage Colony Assay in the Popliteal Lymph
Nodes of Balb/c-SPF Mice

Agent injected into hind footpads	Macrophage colony
None (control)	—
P. acnes-whole cells	⧪⧪⧪
P. acnes-CWS	⧪⧪⧪
D-CMI	$+ \sim +\!+$
PS-K	$+ \sim +\!+$
N. rubra-CWS	+
BCG-CWS	+
OK-432	+

From day 3 to day 6 of the culture period, the supernatant culture fluid was discarded and the cultures were washed with Eagle's MEM to remove the cells which had not firmly attached to the glass. At day 3 the glass adherent cells were degenerating macrophages, as seen in Photo 11. At day 4 and later, colonies of glass adherent cells were observed (Photos 12 and 13). They were confirmed as macrophages by their vigorous phagocytic activities. Observation of cells in mitosis as shown in Photo 12 confirmed the self-proliferating ability of colony-forming cells.

In the popliteal lymph nodes of untreated Balb/c-SPF, there were no macrophage colony-forming cells in this experimental system (Table II). In the draining nodes of

* 1 KE = 100 μg cells.

mice treated with immunopotentiators, macrophage colony-forming cells appeared. Both in *P. acnes*-whole cells- and *P. acnes*-CWS-treated nodes, numerous macrophage colony-forming cells were observed. The number of colonies was almost impossible to count owing to confluence of the colonies in our experimental system. In D-CMI- and PS-K-treated mice, several macrophage colonies per 10^6 lymph node cells appeared. In BCG-CWS, *N. rubra*-CWS- or OK-432-treated mice, only a few colonies per 10^6 cells were observed. Not only the number of colonies but also that of the cells in each colony were exceedingly greater in the nodes of *P. acnes*-whole cells- or *P. acnes*-CWS-treated mice than those in the nodes treated with other immunopotentiators. Thus both *P. acnes*-whole cells and *P. acnes*-CWS induced not only the massive migration of a large number of histiocytes or their precursors into the draining nodes but provoked definite proliferation of these cells in the nodes.

COMMENT

The immunological responses evoked by the 7 immunopotentiators in the regional lymphoid tissues of the normal mice and T cell-deficient nude mice were different. Figure 15 summarizes the highest ^{3}H-TdR incorporation into DNA by the popliteal lymph nodes of both the normal and the nude mice, after the injection of each immunopotentiator. BCG-CWS, *N. rubra*-CWS, and D-CMI produced much more intense reaction in the normal mice than in the nude mice since the TdR incorporations were much higher in the former. Thus BCG-CWS, *N. rubra*-CWS, and D-CMI seem to stimulate T cells or at least evoke immunological effects by way of T cells. On the other hand, both *P. acnes*-whole cells and *P. acnes*-CWS stimulated the lymphoid tissues of the normal and nude mice almost equally. There was no remarkable difference in TdR incorporation between the two sets of mice. In *P. acnes*-whole cells

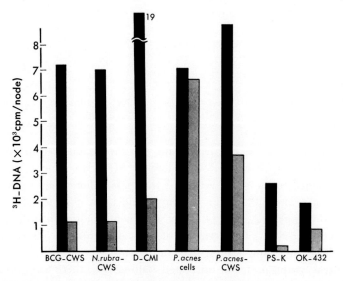

FIG. 15.   Summary of the highest ^{3}H-TdR incorporation into DNA by the popliteal lymph nodes after the injection of each immunopotentiator
■ Balb/c-SPF or ICR-GF;   ▨ Balb/c-nu/nu.

TABLE III. Summary of Histologic Features of the Popliteal Lymph Nodes

Agent injected into footpads	Lymphoblast in paracortical area	Macrophage-histiocytes	Plasma cells in medulla
BCG-CWS	++	±	+
N. rubra-CWS	+	+	+
D-CMI	+ ~ ++	++	+
P. acnes-whole cells	±	+++	+
P. acnes-CWS	+	+++	+
PS-K	+	+ ~ ++	+
OK-432	+	±	++

there was almost no difference. In *P. acnes*-CWS, however, the nodes of the normal mice incorporated more ^{3}H-TdR than those of the nude mice. This could be explained by the histological observation that in the paracortical area of the nodes of *P. acnes*-CWS-treated mice, there was a notably increased number of lymphoblasts compared to the same area in *P. acnes*-whole cell-treated mice. At any rate it is of great interest that CWS of *P. acnes* evoked almost the same immunological effects as the whole cells. The increase of ^{3}H-TdR incorporation by PS-K- and OK-432-treated nodes was significant but not remarkable. In PS-K-treated nodes the incorporation was higher in the normal mice; in OK-432 the incorporation was also observed in the nude mice.

Table III summarizes histologic features of the draining nodes evoked by the 7 immunopotentiators. These 7 seem to be of 4 types according to the observations. Characteristic of the first type is the proliferation of lymphoblasts in the paracortical area that dominates the histological changes, as seen in BCG-CWS. The blasts are pyroninophilic and are most likely T cells, since in the T cell-deficient nude mice no such lymphoproliferative response was observed. The dominant feature of the second type is the proliferation of macrophage-histiocytes. *P. acnes*-whole cells and *P. acnes*-CWS belong to this type. The third type possesses the characteristics of the first and second type. The proliferation of both lymphoblasts and macrophage-histiocytes is observed in this type, as seen in *N. rubra*-CWS, D-CMI, and PS-K. OK-432 belongs to the fourth type, in which the accumulation of plasma cells in the medullary cord is observed in addition to that of lymphoblasts in the paracortical area. In each of the 4 types, however, the 3 lines of immunocompetent cells, lymphoblasts in the paracortical area, plasma cells in the medullary cord, and macrophage-histiocytes spreading from the medulla to the cortex, are found to proliferate in the draining nodes although the degree of proliferation differs substantially. Thus the immunological effects of the 7 immunopotentiators are not unidirectional but they exert their effects on all of the 3 immunocompetent cell lines.

From the above-mentioned observations, BCG-CWS exerts its effect mainly on T cells, and *P. acnes*, both whole cells and CWS, mainly evokes strong macrophage-histiocyte proliferation. *N. rubra*-CWS, D-CMI, and PS-K seem to work on both T cells and macrophage-histiocytes, and OK-432 on both T cells and B cells. As seen in our study adjuvant activities and antitumor actions of these immunopotentiators are probably dependent on the cell lines which these agents mainly stimulate.

It is of great interest that cell-wall skeletons of each of the 3 microorganisms showed characteristic immunological effects. The cell-wall skeletons of BCG showed a similar effect on the regional lymph nodes as the whole cells of BCG. The time course of the response and the histologic features of the nodes after injection of BCG whole cells are very similar to our observations on the nodes of BCG-CWS-treated mice according to the report of Mackaness *et al.* (*8*). The cell-wall skeletons of *P. acnes* also showed a very similar effects as the whole cells of this bacterium. A slight difference was that the cell-wall skeletons induced more lymphoblast proliferation in the paracortical area of normal mice, while the whole cells caused higher ^{3}H-TdR incorporation in the nodes of nude mice. In the case of BCG preparations, Mackaness *et al.* (*8*) reported that soluble antigenic materials in lyophilized commercial BCG preparations produced germinal center formation in the cortex and massive accumulation of plasma cells in the medullary cord. If it may be assumed that this is applicable to the *P. acnes* preparations, the phenol-killed whole cells may contain these antigenic materials, thus inducing more plasma cell proliferation both in normal and nude mice than the cell-wall skeletons, the more purified active component presumably lacking these antigenic materials.

Knowing the characteristics of these immunopotentiators, one should try the clinical application of not only single but multiple combination therapy with these agents against human cancer in the future.

Acknowledgment

We wish to thank Dr. Norio Hirabayashi, Dr. Mikio Shamoto, and Dr. Takashi Yokochi for their helpful suggestions and discussions, and Miss Sayoko Sugiura for her excellent technical assistance.

REFERENCES

1. Azuma, I., Ribi, E. E., Meyer, T., and Zbar, B. Biologically active components from mycobacterial cell walls. I. Isolation and composition of cell wall skeleton and component P$_3$. *J. Natl. Cancer Inst.*, **52**, 95–101 (1974).
2. Azuma, I., Taniyama, T., Hirao, F., and Yamamura, Y. Antitumor activity of cell-wall skeletons and peptidoglycolipids of mycobacteria and related microorganisms in mice and rabbits. *Gann*, **65**, 493–505, (1974).
3. Gutterman, J. U., Mavligid, G. M., Reed, R. C., and Hersh, E. M. Immunotherapy of human cancer. *Semin. Oncol.*, **1**, 409–423, (1974).
4. Hersh, E. M., Gutterman, J. U., Mavligid, G. M., Reed, R. C., and Richman, S. P. BCG vaccine and its derivatives. Potential, practical consideration and precautions in human cancer immunotherapy. *J. Am. Med. Assoc.*, **235**, 646–650 (1976).
5. Israel, L. Immunochemotherapy with *Corynebacterium parvum* in disseminated cancer. *Ann. N.Y. Acad. Sci.*, **277**, 241–251 (1976).
6. Ito, I. and Mitomi, T. Clinical and experimental study of protein-bound polysaccharide, PS-K. *Igaku-no-Ayumi*, **91**, 511–515 (1974) (in Japanese).
7. Kimura, I., Ohnoshi, T., Yasuhara, S., Sugiyama, M., Urabe, Y., Fujii, M., and Machida, K. Immunotherapy in human lung cancer using the streptococcal agent OK-432. *Cancer*, **27**, 2201–2203 (1976).
8. Mackaness, G. B., Auclair, D. J., and Lagrange, P. H. Immunopotentiation with BCG. I. Immune response to different strains and preparations. *J. Natl. Cancer Inst.*, **51**, 1655–1667 (1973).

9. Ohno, R., Yokomaku, S., Wakayama, K., Imai, K., and Yamada, K. Effect of protein-bound polysaccharide preparation, PS-K, on the immune response of mice to sheep red blood cells. *Gann*, **67**, 97–99 (1976).

10. Okamoto, H., Shoin, S., Koshimura, S., and Shimizu, R. Studies on the anticancer and streptolysin-S forming abilities of hemolytic streptococci. *Japan. J. Microbiol.*, **11**, 323–326 (1967).

11. Old, L. J., Benaceraf, B., Clarke, D. A., Carswell, E. A., and Stockert, E. The role of the reticuloendothelial system in the host reaction to neoplasia. *Cancer Res.*, **21**, 1281–1300 (1961).

12. Rojas, A. F., Mickiewicz, E., Feierstein, J. N., Glait, H., and Olivari, A. J. Levamizole in advanced human breast cancer. *Lancet*, **1**, 211–215 (1976).

13. Sasao, T., Niimoto, M., Yamagata, S., and Hattori, T. Effect of anaerobic Corynebacterium on anti-tumor activity of the tumor bearing mice. *Gan-to-Kagakuryoho*, **2**, 35–43 (1975) (in Japanese).

14. Sparks, F. C. Hazards and complications of BCG immunotherapy. *Med. Clin. North Am.*, **60**, 499–509 (1976).

15. Tsukagoshi, S. and Ohashi, F. Protein-bound polysaccharide preparation, PS-K, effective against mouse sarcoma-180 and rat ascites hepatoma AH-13 by oral use. *Gann*, **65**, 557–558 (1974).

16. Van Furth, R., Hirsh, J. G., and Fedorko, M. E. Morphology and peroxidase cytochemistry of mouse promonocytes, monocytes and macrophages. *J. Exp. Med.*, **132**, 794–805 (1970).

17. Weiss, D. W. MER and other mycobacterial fractions in immunotherapy of cancer. *Med. Clin. North Am.*, **60**, 473–497 (1976).

18. Yamamura, Y., Yoshizaki, K., Azuma, I., Yagura, T., and Watanabe, T. Immunotherapy of human malignant melanoma with oil-attached BCG cell-wall skeleton. *Gann*, **66**, 335–363 (1975).

19. Yasumoto, K., Manabe, H., Ueno, M., Ohta, M., Ueda, H., Iida, A., Nomoto, K., Azuma, I., and Yamamura, Y. Immunotherapy of human lung cancer with BCG cell-wall skeleton. *Gann*, **67**, 787–795 (1976).

EXPLANATION OF PHOTOS

PHOTO 1.   Popliteal lymph node of ICR-GF mice. Hematoxylin-Eosin stain (H-E).

PHOTO 2.   Popliteal lymph node of Balb/c-SPG mice. H-E.

PHOTO 3.   Popliteal lymph node of Balb/c-nu/nu mice. H-E.

PHOTO 4.   Pyroninophilic blast cells in the paracortical area of the popliteal lymph node of BCG-CWS-treated ICR-GF mice. Methyl green-pyronin stain.

PHOTO 5.   Popliteal lymph node of BCG-CWS-treated ICR-GF mice. H-E.

PHOTO 6.   Popliteal lymph node of *N. rubra*-CW-Streated Balb/c-SPF mice. H-E.

PHOTO 7.   Histoautoradiogram showing ^{3}H-TdR-labeled cells in the area of the granuloma formation in the popliteal lymph node of *P. acnes*-whole cells-treated ICR-GF mice.

PHOTO 8.   Popliteal lymph node of *P. acnes*-CWS treated Balb/c-SPF mice. H-E.

PHOTO 9.   Lymphoblasts in the paracortical area of the popliteal lymph node of BCG-CWS-treated ICR-GF mice.

PHOTO 10.   Histiocytes in the medulla of the popliteal lymph node of *N. rubra*-CWS-treated Balb/c-SPF mice.

PHOTO 11.   Glass adherent cells at day 3 of the culture.

PHOTO 12.   Glass adherent macrophage colony appearing at day 4. Note the cells in mitosis.

PHOTO 13.   Fully developed glass adherent macrophage colony at day 6 of the culture.

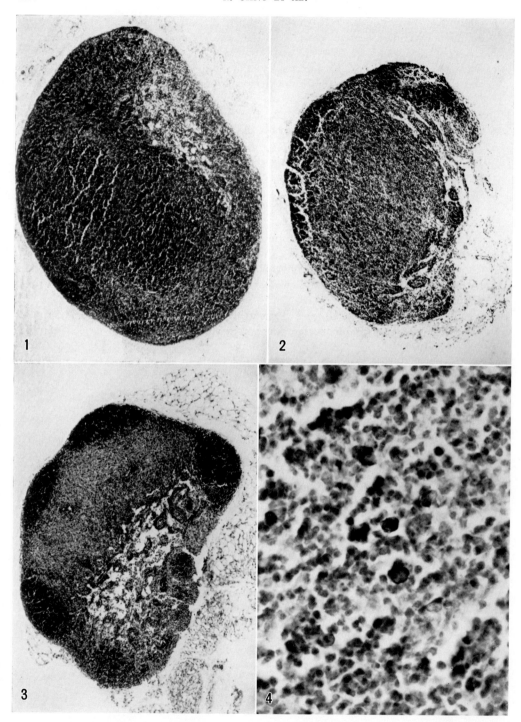

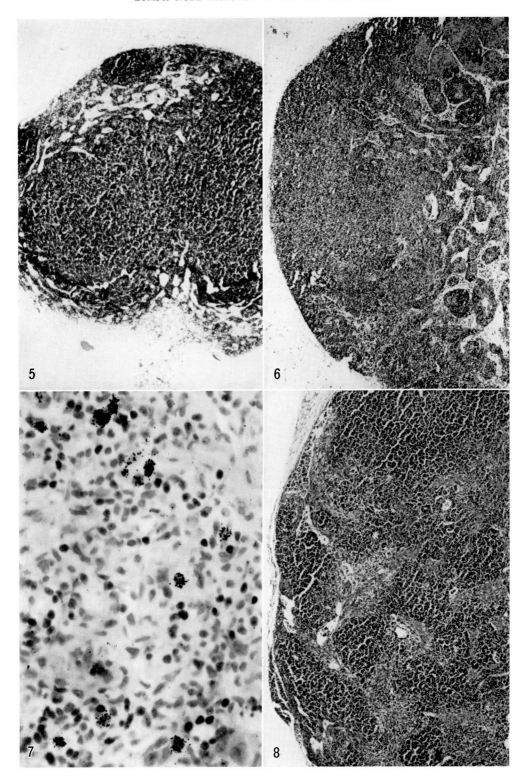

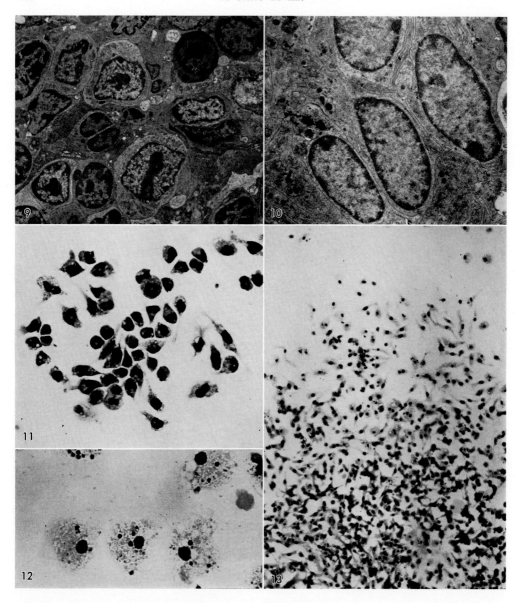

CLINICAL TRIALS. I. IMMUNOTHERAPY OF LUNG CANCER AND MALIGNANT PLEURITIS

GANN Monograph on Cancer Research 21, 1978

IMMUNOTHERAPY OF LUNG CANCER AND CARCINOMATOUS PLEURITIS

Kosei Yasumoto,[*1] Hideo Manabe,[*1] Mitsuo Ohta,[*1] Kikuo Nomoto,[*2] Ichiro Azuma,[*3] and Yuichi Yamamura[*3]

*Department of Chest Surgery, Kyushu Cancer Center,[*1] Laboratory for Immunology, Cancer Research Institute, Faculty of Medicine, Kyushu University,[*2] and Third Department of Internal Medicine, Osaka University Medical School[*3]*

Immunotherapy with BCG cell-wall skeleton (BCG-CWS) was applied to lung cancer patients after the usual modalities of treatments. Effectiveness of immunotherapy was determined by prolongation of survival, augmentation or restoration of lymphocyte responses, and pathological findings suggesting host resistance.

1) Lymphocyte responsiveness in lung cancer patients was depressed with an advance of the clinical stage before the start of treatment, when assessed by *in vivo* skin test to purified protein derivative, *in vitro* lymphocyte response to phytohemagglutinin, and *in vitro* lymphocyte cytotoxicity against allogeneic cells of a cultured lung cancer line.

2) Such lymphocyte responses were restored or augmented in many of the patients after BCG-CWS immunotherapy.

3) Prolongation of survival period was revealed after BCG-CWS treatment in each clinical stage of lung cancer. However, complete cure of lung cancer was expected only in stage I.

4) *In vitro* lymphocyte responses which were assessed 4 months after the start of BCG-CWS treatment was correlated well with the prognosis of patients.

5) Pathological examinations of autopsied cases suggested that BCG-CWS augmented not only anticancer resistance but also resistance against microorganisms.

6) Intrapleural injection of BCG-CWS was effective in controlling the pleural effusion and prolonging the survival period of patients with carcinomatous pleuritis. The tentative results on intrapleural administration of cell-wall skeleton of *Nocardia rubra* suggest that it has a stronger potentiality in augmentation of antitumor resistance than BCG-CWS.

Immunological responses have proved to contribute to the resistance against a variety of experimental tumors in autochthonous or syngeneic hosts. Elimination of tumor cells in such cases may be attributable to a cytotoxic effect of killer T cells,

---

[*1] Notame 595, Minami-ku, Fukuoka 815, Japan (安元公正, 真鍋英夫, 大田満夫).
[*2] Maidashi 3-1-1, Higashi-ku, Fukuoka 812, Japan (野本亀久雄).
[*3] Fukushima 1-1-50, Fukushima-ku, Osaka 553, Japan (東 市郎, 山村雄一).

cytotoxic or cytostatic effects of activated macrophages, or antibody-dependent cell-mediated cytotoxicity, at least with respect to epithelial tumors. Immunological mechanisms have been expected to be involved specifically or nonspecifically also in human cancer, since antigen-specific or nonspecific lymphocyte responsiveness as demonstrated by delayed skin reactions (6) or *in vitro* proliferative response to plant lectins (10, 11, 16) has been confirmed to be depressed in the late stage of various kinds of malignant tumor. Thus, many assay systems have been applied to monitor lymphocyte responsiveness to tumor-specific antigens in cancer patients. Mixed lymphocyte-tumor cell culture (20, 39), *in vitro* proliferative response to extracted tumor antigens (33), and cytotoxicity test against tumor cells (28, 29, 41) have been attempted for such a purpose. Nonetheless, the contribution of specific immune responses to the resistance against human cancer appears to be far from being defined clearly. Therefore, the establishment of reliable assay systems may be required to monitor immunological status at various stages of cancers or during the therapy in antigen-specific or nonspecific terms.

A variety of immunopotentiators have been proposed for immunotherapy of human cancer on the basis of the results obtained with experimental tumors. Experimental trials for immunotherapy were performed extensively after the successful treatment of line 10 hepatoma with BCG in syngeneic guinea pigs by Zbar *et al.* (43, 44). The success in BCG immunotherapy for human malignant melanoma by Morton *et al.* (23, 24) has promoted clinical trials for a variety of human tumors. Although live BCG is used most commonly in clinical fields, such a treatment is accompanied by severe side effects including liver damage, anaphylactic reaction, and septicemia (13, 26, 32, 34, 35). Yamamura and his co-workers have found that BCG cell-wall skeleton (BCG-CWS) attached to oil droplets is as active as live BCG in the suppression of growth of a syngeneic guinea pig tumor and gave a low incidence of toxic side effects (2, 22, 38, 40).

Oil-attached BCG-CWS has been applied to the immunotherapy of lung cancer patients in Kyushu Cancer Center; their immunological status has been observed (42). In this communication, effects of BCG-CWS immunotherapy on the survival period of lung cancer patients, various kinds of lymphocyte responsiveness, and pathological reactions will be summarized on the basis of 3-year results. The effect of such a therapy was most striking in those cases with carcinomatous pleuritis. Results of a tentative application of cell-wall skeleton of *Nocardia rubra* (N-CWS) to the therapy of carcinomatous pleuritis will also be presented briefly.

Immunological Status of Patients with Lung Cancer

It is important to assess the immunological responsiveness of patients with lung cancer before immunotherapy. Lymphocyte responsiveness was estimated by assessment of *in vivo* delayed hypersensitivity reaction to purified protein derivative (PPD), lymphocyte proliferative response to phytohemagglutinin (PHA), and lymphocyte cytotoxic activity against cultured allogeneic lung cancer cells. The ratios of positive skin reaction to PPD in normal healthy controls, in patients at stages I and II, and in those at stages III and IV of lung cancer were 87, 80, and 58%, respectively. In other words, the ratio of negative reactions increased with an advance of the clinical stage.

Presence of such a correlation has been shown by some other investigators (*1, 14*), but not accepted by others (*7, 17*). Lymphocyte response to PHA was examined by the method of ^{3}H-TdR incorporation. Lymphocytes were separated from the peripheral blood of patients by the Conray-Ficoll method (*5*). Average values of ^{3}H-TdR incorporation were $5,900\pm140$ in healthy persons and $3,900\pm1,270$ in patients with benign lung diseases. The values at stages I and II, stage III, and stage IV of lung cancer were $4,300\pm1,960$, $1,400\pm790$, and 700 ± 360, respectively. The responsiveness to PHA declined with an advance of the clinical stage. Han and Takita (*10*) reported also that the PHA response was markedly impaired in most lung cancer patients at late stages, compared to those with resectable lung cancer.

Our third assay system to monitor the immunological status of patients with lung cancer was lymphocyte cytotoxicity against allogeneic lung cancer cells of an established line. The method was mentioned in detail elsewhere (*41*). The cytotoxic activity of lymphocytes was $32\pm7\%$ in healthy persons, while those in patients in stage I, stage II, stage III, and stage IV of lung cancer were 50 ± 18, 45 ± 13, 40 ± 13, and $23\pm18\%$, respectively. The cytotoxic activities declined with advance of the clinical stage of lung cancer. The decline in such a reactivity with the progression of tumors was also observed by Pierce *et al.* (*30*) and by Takasugi *et al.* (*37*). Therefore, this microcytotoxicity assay appears to be useful in the estimation of immunological status of lung cancer patients, although the meaning of such an assay system is not understood clearly and the concept of a non-specific cytotoxic effect is supported by many investigators (*3, 12, 36*). Patients with lung cancer possess impaired reactivities in PPD skin reaction, PHA response, and lymphocyte cytotoxicity before the start of treatment.

Protocol for BCG-CWS Immunotherapy of Lung Cancer

Immunotherapy has been expected to augment resistance against cancer and to restore the depressed capacity of lymphocytes to mediate cellular immune response. We have chosen BCG-CWS as the standard immunopotentiator.

Before the start of BCG-CWS immunotherapy, all patients were subjected to the usual modalities of anticancer treatment, *i.e.*, surgical resection of tumor, radiotherapy, and/or anticancer chemotherapy, except for some of the patients with carcinomatous pleuritis. After the completion of the usual modalities of treatments, the patients were classified into the following 5 groups: Tumor-resected cases (Group 1), the cases who were subjected to surgery but whose tumors could not be resected (Group 2), the cases carrying palpable surface metastatic tumors (Group 3), the cases with pleural effusion (Group 4), and the miscellaneous cases (Group 5). Procedures for BCG-CWS administration were varied according to this classification, as shown in Table I.

The clinical effect of BCG-CWS in each stage of lung cancer was assessed by comparing the survival time to that of historic control patients who did not receive BCG-CWS treatment. Although the controls were historic, the average age, ratio of males, and histological variations at each stage were almost the same between controls and cases treated with BCG-CWS, as shown in Table II. In order to observe the effects of BCG-CWS treatment on lymphocyte responsiveness, PPD skin test, lymphocyte proliferative response to PHA, and lymphocyte cytotoxicity against allogeneic

TABLE I. Protocol for Immunotherapy of Lung Cancer Patients
with Oil-attached BCG-CWS

Group No.	Clinical stages[a] of patients	Patients treated	Protocols for immunotherapy	
1	I, II, III	Resected cases	1st:	Irradiated autologous tumor cells 1×10^8 mixed with BCG-CWS 300 μg, intradermally at 7-10 days after resection
			2nd:[b]	BCG-CWS 200 μg, intradermally
2	III	Cases subjected to exploratory thoracotomy	1st:	BCG-CWS 300 μg, intralesional injection at the time of surgery
			2nd:	BCG-CWS 200 μg, intradermally
3	IV	Cases with surface metastatic tumor	1st:	BCG-CWS 300 μg, intralesional injection
			2nd:	BCG-CWS 200 μg, intradermal or intralesional injection
4	III, IV	Cases with pleural effusion	1st:	BCG-CWS 300 μg, intrapleural injection
			2nd:	BCG-CWS 200 μg, intradermal or intrapleural injection
5	I, II, III, IV	Miscellaneous cases	1st:	BCG-CWS 300 μg, intradermally
			2nd:	BCG-CWS 200 μg, intradermally

[a] According to the clinical staging of lung cancer in the Japanese Lung Cancer Society.
[b] From the second time of the injection, 200 μg of BCG-CWS was injected every 2 weeks for 30 weeks and every 4 weeks thereafter.

TABLE II. Histological Classification of Lung Cancer in the Present Study

Histological classification	No. of patients in each clinical stage							
	Stage I		Stage II		Stage III		Stage IV	
	Control	BCG-CWS treated	Control	BCG-CWS treated	Control	BCG-CWS treated	Control	BCG-CWS treated
Adenocarcinoma	11	4	11	3	25	29	21	24
Squamous cell	4	4	11	9	35	23	8	6
Small cell	0	1	1	2	2	6	6	3
Large cell	0	1	3	0	7	3	6	3
Adenoacanthoma	0	0	0	1	2	3	2	1
Alveolar cell	1	0	0	0	1	0	0	0
Unknown	0	0	0	1	0	0	0	0
Total	16	11	26	16	72	64	43	37

cultured cells of lung cancer were assessed. Additionally, pathological examinations were made to evaluate the effectiveness of BCG-CWS treatment in 24 autopsied patients.

Evaluation of the Clinical Effect of BCG-CWS Treatment

The survivals of 128 patients who were treate withd BCG-CWS were compared with those of 157 patients who were not treated with BCG-CWS (control) at each clinical stage of lung cancer. Observation period reached over 30 months in some cases after the start of BCG-CWS treatment. The survival rate of the patients in each stage was determined by the life table method.

In stage I, the survival rate at 30 months was 79% in control patients, while that of BCG-CWS treated cases was 100%. None of the 11 patients treated with BCG-CWS has died within 30 months of the observation period. However, one patient had a metastatic focus in the brain and is now receiving radiotherapy (Fig. 1). The survival rates of control and BCG-CWS treated patients in stage II were 35 and 42% at 30 months, respectively. Their median survival periods were 21 and 25.6 months, respectively, in control and BCG-CWS treated cases (Fig. 2). The survival rates of control and BCG-CWS treated patients in stage III were 7 and 25% at 27 months, respectively.

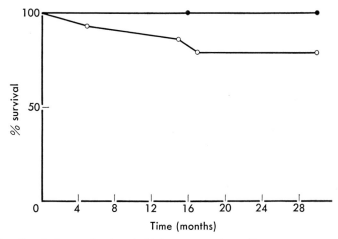

FIG. 1. Survival rate of patients with lung cancer (stage I)
○ patients who did not receive BCG-CWS (16 cases); ● patients treated with BCG-CWS (11 cases).

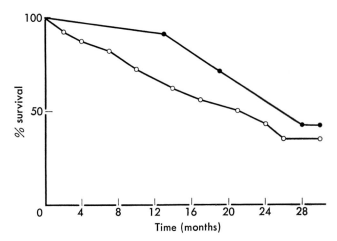

FIG. 2. Survival rate of patients with lung cancer (stage II)
○ patients who did not receive BCG-CWS (26 cases); ● patients treated with BCG-CWS (16 cases).

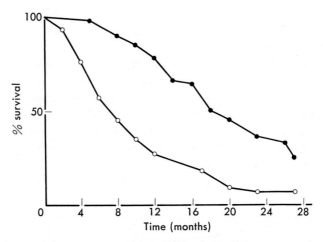

FIG. 3.　Survival rate of patients with lung cancer (stage III)
○ patients who did not receive BCG-CWS (72 cases);　● patients treated with BCG-CWS (64 cases).

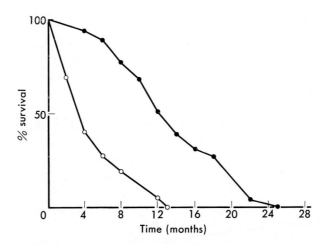

FIG. 4.　Survival rate of patients with lung cancer (stage IV)
○ patients who did not receive BCG-CWS (43 cases);　● patients treated with BCG-CWS (37 cases).

Their median survival periods were 7.2 and 18 months, respectively, in control and BCG-CWS treated cases (Fig. 3). Median survival periods of patients at stage IV were 3.4 and 12.2 months, respectively, in control and BCG-CWS treated cases. None of the patients at stage IV survived over 13 and 25 months, respectively, in control and in BCG-CWS treated cases (Fig. 4).

Thus, the BCG-CWS immunotherapy of lung cancer appears to prolong survival period, although complete cure may be expected only in stage I cases, whose number of residual tumor cells after surgical resection are expected to be small. McKneally et al. (21) reported that the intrapleural inoculation of BCG was effective in patients with stage I lung cancer, but not in patients with more advanced lung cancer, when the effects were judged by the prolongation of their survival periods. Oldham *et al.* (*27*) also reported that immunotherapy with BCG was not effective in advanced lung cancer under their randomized study. Many investigators agree that the success of cancer immunotherapy can be expected in patients with limited tumor burdens (*19, 25, 27, 31*). However, BCG-CWS immunotherapy was effective also in advanced cases at stages III and IV. This discrepancy may be ascribed to the differences of immuno-stimulants (live BCG and BCG-CWS) or of immunotherapy protocols. Although the results presented here were not based on a randomized study, the effect of BCG-CWS immunotherapy was also supported by immunological tests and pathological findings.

Immunological Monitoring during Immunotherapy

Lymphocyte responsiveness has to be estimated as accurately as possible in order to follow the clinical courses after immunotherapy and to obtain a final conclusion as to its effectiveness. Therefore, delayed skin reaction to PPD, proliferative response of peripheral blood lymphocytes to PHA, and *in vitro* lymphocyte cytotoxicity to an allogeneic cultured cell line of lung cancer were assessed. Lymphocyte activity assessed by these 3 methods was depressed especially in advanced cases before the start of the treatment. The ratio of positive reactions in the PPD skin test increased from 16 to 24 weeks after the start of BCG-CWS immunotherapy (*42*). Although the patients with negative PPD skin reactions after BCG-CWS immunotherapy appeared to have a rel-atively poor prognosis, the positive reactions did not necessarily anticipate good prog-noses. This fact is supported by many investigators using live BCG (*8, 9, 27*). The lymphocyte proliferative response to PHA increased to the normal range during BCG-CWS treatment in the majority of patients as compared to the depressed response before the start of treatment. The augmented response was correlated with good prog-nosis of the patients (*42*). Lieberman *et al.* (*18*) and Gross *et al.* (*9*) also reported that high values of PHA response were predictive of the efficacy of BCG immunotherapy. As lymphocyte response to PHA reflects nonspecific activity of T lymphocytes, BCG-CWS, and BCG are presumed to augment the T cell function generally.

In the microcytotoxicity assays against allogeneic target cells of lung cancer, the cytotoxic activities of lymphocytes were augmented during the course of BCG-CWS treatments. The maximum cytotoxic activity was obtained around 4 months after the start of BCG-CWS treatment. The cytotoxic values obtained at 4 months or later cor-related with the prognosis of the patients (*42*). Berkelhammer *et al.* (*4*) reported that cytotoxic activities of lymphocytes against melanoma cells and bladder carcinoma cells were augmented during the course of BCG treatment of malignant melanoma patients. In their study, correlation between the augmentation of such cytotoxic activities and the clinical course of the disease was equivocal. Such a result may be ascribed to the fact that the last point of their assessment was 10 weeks after the start of BCG im-munotherapy. In our study also, cytotoxic values during the first 4 months of BCG-CWS immunotherapy did not correlate with the clinical course of patients.

The meaning of microcytotoxicity assays is controversial. Most investigators, in-cluding ourselves, presume that the main mechanism of this assay is nonspecific. Exact mechanisms of this assay system remain to be defined in terms of populations of effector cells, target cells, and technical factors. Still, the microcytotoxicity assay appears to be useful for anticipating the prognosis of patients and estimating the efficacy of BCG-CWS immunotherapy of lung cancer.

Pathological Findings after BCG-CWS Treatment

The third method for estimating the effectiveness of immunotherapy against cancer is pathological examination. Such histological findings as lymphocyte infiltration into the cancer tissue, macrophage infiltration, and fibrous tissue formation around the cancer tissue may be ascribed to the effect of immunotherapy.

Hematogenous and lymphatic metastases were compared between the 24 autopsied patients who had received BCG-CWS treatment and the 46 autopsied patients who had not received such a treatment. Some characteristic histological findings in patients treated with BCG-CWS will be presented. As shown in Table III, organs involved in hematogenous metastasis were examined macroscopically. Seven or more organs were involved in 11 out of 46 control cases (24%). On the other hand, only one patient given BCG-CWS treatment (4%) had such a high degree of hematogenous metastases. Any organ was not involved in hematogenous metastasis in 11 cases of controls (24%) and one case of BCG-CWS treated (4%). The main cause of death of these patients appeared to be infectious diseases such as bronchopneumonia. Therefore, BCG-CWS treatment may augment not only the resistance against cancer but also against microorganisms. There was no significant difference in lymph node metastases between controls and BCG-CWS treated patients (Table IV).

In some autopsied cases who received BCG-CWS treatment, histological findings indicated the effectiveness of such a treatment. In one case who received intratumoral

TABLE III.   Degree of Hematogenous Metastases in Autopsied
Cases With Lung Cancer

No. of organs involved	Control		BCG-CWS	
	No. of cases	%	No. of cases	%
0	11	23.9	1	4.2
1	3	6.5	3	12.5
2	6	13.0	5	20.8
3	4	8.7	3	12.5
4	7	15.2	4	16.7
5	2	4.3	4	16.7
6	2	4.3	3	12.5
7	4	8.7	0	0
8	3	6.5	0	0
9	1	2.2	1	4.2
10	2	4.3	0	0
11	0	0	0	0
12	0	0	0	0
13	1	2.2	1	0
Total	46	100.0	24	100.0

TABLE IV. Degree of Lymph Node Metastases in Autopsied Cases with Lung Cancer

Metastatic spread	Control		BCG-CWS	
	No. of cases	%	No. of cases	%
None	4	8.7	0	0
Intrathoracic	19	41.3	9	37.5
Cervical or retroperitoneal	20	43.4	14	58.3
Axillary or inguinal	3	6.5	1	4.2
Total	46	100	24	100

BCG-CWS injection at the time of exploratory thoracotomy, followed by intradermal injection of BCG-CWS biweekly, marked lymphoid cell and giant cell infiltrations into the cancer tissue were found. Other parts of the primary lesion in this case showed formation of several fibrous nodules. Cancer tissue was included in one nodule, but not in others. Such findings were reported by Lieberman et al. (18) and by Khalil et al. (15) in patients with malignant melanoma injected intratumorally with live BCG.

Immunotherapy of Carcinomatous Pleuritis

We will illustrate an intrapleural administration of BCG-CWS against carcinomatous pleuritis from our 5 methods of BCG-CWS administration. Generally, carcinomatous pleuritis occurs in the terminal stage of various kind of malignancies; it rapidly leads to patient death. Various procedures have been attempted to control pleural effusions but these have failed to prolong survival. Most of the procedures were directed only to local management of pleural effusion thereby perhaps explaining the failures.

As reported previously (42), direct injections of BCG-CWS into the pleural space of patients with carcinomatous pleuritis due to lung cancer are effective in controlling pleural effusion and in prolonging the survival period. Table V demonstrates results of the longer observation of the same patients as reported in this paper. The mean survival period of 7 patients at stage III was 7 months when they were not subjected to BCG-CWS treatment (control). The mean survival time of 6 patients at stage III was 16 months when they received BCG-CWS administration. This prolongation of the survival period was statistically significant. In stage IV, the mean survival periods were 5 and 7 months, respectively, in controls and BCG-CWS treated patients. Although 2 months' survival prolongation was obtained, such an extent was not statistically significant. Tumor cells disappeared from the exudate in approximately 70% of patients after this type of treatment. Immunological or non-immunological activities of lymphocytes were restored in many of these cases to the normal ranges when assessed by PPD skin test, PHA response, and microcytotoxicity test. Nevertheless, almost all patients died from cancer after their prolonged survival period. In order to achieve more effective immunotherapy, combination with anticancer chemotherapy must be tried.

The N-CWS was reported to have a higher potentiality to exert antitumor effects than BCG-CWS in some experimental tumors (2). Therefore, we have applied intrapleural administration of N-CWS to the treatment of carcinomatous pleuritis. Oil-

TABLE V. Effect of BCG-CWS on Patients with Carcinomatous Pleuritis

Group	Patients			Stage	Histological classification[a]	Survival period (months)	Status
	Name	Sex	Age (years)				
Controls	S.I.	M	77	III	Large cell	13	Dead
	K.H.	M	79	III	Adeno	9	Dead
	S.F.	M	49	III	Adeno	9	Dead
	K. K.	M	70	III	Adeno	6	Dead
	S. K.	M	63	III	Adeno	4	Dead
	Y. M.	M	68	III	Squamous	4	Dead
	Y. I.	M	75	III	Squamous	3	Dead
	N. H.	M	32	IV	Adeno	8	Dead
	Y. K.	M	63	IV	Large cell	7	Dead
	S. K.	F	39	IV	Adeno	6	Dead
	M. K.	M	50	IV	Adeno	5	Dead
	H. N.	M	51	IV	Adeno	4	Dead
	A. I.	M	50	IV	Adeno	4	Dead
	T. N.	F	54	IV	Adeno	3	Dead
	T. K.	F	75	IV	Squamous	3	Dead
	T. M.	F	66	IV	Adeno	1	Dead
Cases treated with BCG-CWS	M. M.	F	38	III	Adeno	27	Dead
	S. N.	F	64	III	Adeno	23	Alive
	K. I.	M	49	III	Adeno	18	Dead
	M. O.	F	61	III	Adeno	11	Dead
	H. F.	F	62	III	Adeno	9	Dead
	Y. N.	M	62	III	Adeno	7	Dead
	M. K.	F	56	IV	Adeno	12	Dead
	I. Y.	M	64	IV	Adeno	8	Dead
	A. K.	M	64	IV	Adeno	8	Dead
	I. K.	M	52	IV	Adeno	7	Dead
	K. Y.	F	52	IV	Adeno	5	Dead
	T. S.	F	36	IV	Adeno	5	Dead
	T. S.	M	58	IV	Squamous	4	Dead

[a] Large cell, large cell carcinoma ; adeno, adenocarcinoma ; squamous, squamous cell carcinoma.

attached N-CWS was prepared for clinical use in the same manner as BCG-CWS (42). Three hundred μg of N-CWS was injected into the pleural cavity every 2 weeks. Since the maximal observation time of patients subjected to N-CWS immunotherapy is 9 months at this time, we will present only cytological changes in the pleural effusion as local effects. As demonstrated in Table VI, 6 of 7 patients given N-CWS immuno-therapy showed disappearance of malignant cells from their pleural effusion after 2 to 5 times of administration of 300 μg of N-CWS. As the malignant cells disappeared, the exudation of pleural effusion was reduced in volume. Types of cells accumulating in the pleural effusion altered during the courses of N-CWS administration. In the initial phase of N-CWS treatment (1 to 3 days after the first administration of N-CWS), the accumulating cells were mainly neutrophils. Following this phase, lymphocytes

TABLE VI. Analysis of Patients Receiving Intrapleural Injection of N-CWS

Patient	Sex	Age	Primary lesion	Histological classification	Detection of tumor cells in pleural effusion	
					Before treatment	After treatment
M. H.	M	66	Lung	Adenocarcinoma	Positive	Converted to negative after 2 times injection
Y. Y.	M	53	Lung	Adenocarcinoma	Positive	Converted to negative after single injection
S. M.	M	62	Lung	Adenocarcinoma	Positive	Converted to negative after single injection
T. A.	M	38	Unknown	Adenocarcinoma	Positive	Converted to negative after 3 times injection
M. I.	M	38	Unknown	Adenocarcinoma	Positive	Converted to negative after 3 times injection
M. In.	M	42	Unknown	Adenocarcinoma	Positive	Converted to negative after 5 times injection
K. O.	M	64	Unknown	Adenocarcinoma	Positive	Died after 4 times injection

and histiocytes became predominant in the effusion by 7 to 14 days from the start of N-CWS treatment. The predominance of lymphocytes and histiocytes was sustained as long as the malignant cells existed in the effusion. The predominant lymphocyte reactions during concomitant existence of malignant cells may suggest the contribution of tumor-specific immunological mechanisms for elimination of malignant cells. After the disappearance of malignant cells from the effusion, neutrophils became predominant again. These neutrophils may act only as scavenger cells to remove dead malignant cells.

REFERENCES

1. Anthony, H. M., Templeman, G. H., Madsen, K. E., and Mason, M. K. The prognostic significance of DHS skin tests in patients with carcinoma of bronchus. *Cancer*, **34**, 1901–1905 (1974).
2. Azuma, I., Taniyama, T., Hirao, F., and Yamamura, Y. Antitumor activity of cell-wall skeletons and peptidoglycolipids of mycobacteria and related microorganisms in mice and rabbits. *Gann*, **65**, 493–505 (1974).
3. Baldwin, R. W. *In vitro* assays of cell-mediated immunity to human solid tumors: Problems of quantitation, specificity, and interpretation. *J. Natl. Cancer Inst.*, **55**, 745–748 (1975).
4. Berkelhammer, J., Mastrangelo, M. J., Laucius, J. F., Bodurtha, A. J., and Prehn, R. T. Sequential *in vitro* reactivity of lymphocytes from melanoma patients receiving immunotherapy compared with the reactivity of lymphocytes from healthy donors. *Int. J. Cancer*, **16**, 571–578 (1975).
5. Böyum, A. Isolation of mononuclear cells and granulocytes from human blood. *Scand. J. Clin. Lab. Invest.*, **21** (Suppl. 97), 9–50 (1968).
6. Eilber, F. R. and Morton, D. L. Impaired immunologic reactivity and recurrence following cancer surgery. *Cancer*, **25**, 362–367 (1970).
7. Golub, S. H., O'Connell, T. X., and Morton, D. L. Correlation of *in vivo* and *in vitro* assays of immunocompetence in cancer patients. *Cancer Res.*, **34**, 1833–1837 (1974).

8. Golub, S. H., Forsythe, A. B., and Morton, D. L. Sequential examination of lymphocyte proliferative capacity in patients with malignant melanoma receiving BCG immunotherapy. *Int. J. Cancer*, **19**, 18–26 (1977).

9. Gross, N. J. and Quartey, A.C.E. Monitoring of immunologic status of patients receiving BCG therapy for malignant disease. *Cancer*, **37**, 2183–2193 (1976).

10. Han, T. and Takita, H. Immunologic impairment in bronchogenic carcinoma: A study of lymphocyte response to phytohemagglutinin. *Cancer*, **30**, 616–620 (1972).

11. Han, T. and Takita, H. Impaired lymphocyte response to allogeneic cultured lymphoid cells in patients with lung cancer. *New Engl. J. Med.*, **186**, 605–606 (1972).

12. Herberman, R. B. and Oldham, R. K. Problems associated with study of cell-mediated immunity to human tumors by microcytotoxicity assays. *J. Natl. Cancer Inst.*, **55**, 749–753 (1975).

13. Hunt, J. S., Silverstein, M. J., and Sparks, F. C. Granulomatous hepatitis—A complication of BCG immunotherapy. *Lancet*, **ii**, 820–821 (1973).

14. Israel, L. Cell-mediated immunity in lung cancer patients: Data, problems, and propositions. *Cancer Chemother. Rep.*, **4**, 279–281 (1973).

15. Khalil, A., Rappaport, H., and Misset, J. L. Kinetics of histologic changes in human melanoma after local immunotherapy with BCG. *Cancer Immunol. Immunother.*, **1**, 193–196 (1976).

16. Krant, M. J., Manskopf, G., Bradrup, C. S., and Madoff, M. A. Immunologic alterations in bronchogenic cancer. *Cancer*, **21**, 623–631 (1968).

17. Lee, Y. N., Sparks, F. C., Eilber, F. R., and Morton, D. L. Delayed cutaneous hypersensitivity and peripheral lymphocyte counts in patients with advanced cancer. *Cancer*, **35**, 748–755 (1975).

18. Lieberman, R., Wybran, J., and Epstein, W. The immunologic and histopathologic changes of BCG-mediated tumor regression in patients with malignant melanoma. *Cancer*, **35**, 756–777 (1975).

19. Mathé, G., Pouillart, P., Schwarzenberg, L., Amiel, J. L., Schneider, M., Hayat, M., DeVassal, F., Jasmin, C., Rosenfeld, C., Weiner, R., and Rappaport, H. Attempt at immunotherapy of 100 acute lymphoid leukemia patients: Some factors influencing results. *Natl. Cancer Inst. Monogr.*, **35**, 361–374 (1972).

20. Mavligit, G. M., Hersh, E. M., and McBride, C. M. Lymphocyte blastogenic response to autochthonous viable and nonviable human tumor cells. *J. Natl. Cancer Inst.*, **51**, 337–343 (1973).

21. McKneally, M. F., Maver, C., Kausel, H. W., and Alley, R. D. Regional immunotherapy with intrapleural BCG for lung cancer. *J. Thorac. Cardiovasc. Surg.*, **72**, 333–338 (1976).

22. Meyer, T. J., Ribi, E., Azuma, I., and Zbar, B. Biologically active components from mycobacterial cell walls. II. Suppression and regression of strain-2 guinea pig hepatoma. *J. Natl. Cancer Inst.*, **52**, 103–111 (1974).

23. Morton, D. L., Holmes, E. C., Eilber, F. R., and Wood, W. C. Immunological aspects of neoplasia: A rational basis for immunotherapy. *Ann. Intern. Med.*, **74**, 587–604 (1971).

24. Morton, D. L. Immunotherapy of human melanoma and sarcomas. *Natl. Cancer Inst. Monogr.*, **35**, 375–378 (1972).

25. Morton, D. L. Immunotherapy of cancer: Present status and future potential. *Cancer*, **30**, 1647–1655 (1972).

26. O'Brien, T. F. and Galdabini, J. J. Case records of the Massachusetts General Hospital. *New Engl. J. Med.*, **293**, 443–448 (1975).

27. Oldham, R. K., Weese, J. L., Herberman, R. B., Perlin, E., Mills, M., Heims, W., Blom, J., Green, D., Reid, J., Bellinger, S., Law, I., McCoy, J. L., Dean, J. H., Cannon,

G. B., and Djeu, J. Immunological monitoring and immunotherapy in carcinoma of the lung. *Int. J. Cancer*, **18**, 739–749 (1976).

28. O'Toole, C., Perlmann, P., Unsgaard, B., Moberger, G., and Edsmyr, F. Cellular immunity to human urinary bladder carcinoma. I. Correlation to clinical stage and radiotherapy. *Int. J. Cancer*, **10**, 77–91 (1972).

29. O'Toole, C., Perlmann, P., Unsgaard, B., Almgard, L. E., Johansson, B., Moberger, G., and Edsmyr, F. Cellular immunity to human urinary bladder carcinoma. II. Effect of surgery and preoperative irradiation. *Int. J. Cancer*, **10**, 92–98 (1972).

30. Pierce, G. E. and DeVald, B. Microcytotoxicity assays of tumor immunity in patients with bronchogenic carcinoma correlated well with clinical status. *Cancer Res.*, **35**, 3577–3584 (1975).

31. Powles, R. L., Crowther, D., Bateman, C.J.T., Beard, M.E.J., McElwain, T. J., Russell, J., Lister, T. A., Whitehouse, J.M.A., Wrigley, P.F.M., Pike, M., Alexander, P., and Fairley, G. H. Immunotherapy for acute myelogenous leukaemia. *Br. J. Cancer*, **28**, 365–376 (1973).

32. Rosenberg, E. B., Kanner, S. P., and Schwartzman, R. J. Systemic infection following BCG therapy. *Arch. Intern. Med.*, **134**, 769–773 (1974).

33. Roth, J. A., Holmes, E. C., Boddie, A. W., and Morton, D. L. Lymphocyte responses of lung cancer patients to tumor-associated antigen measured by leucine incorporation. *J. Thorac. Cardiovasc. Surg.*, **70**, 613–618 (1975).

34. Schwarzenberg, L., Simmler, M. C., and Pico, J. L. Toxicology and possible adverse effect of BCG. *Cancer Immunol. Immunother.*, **1**, 69–76 (1976).

35. Sparks, F. C., Silverstein, M. J., Hunt, J. S., Haskell, C. M., Pilch, Y. H., and Morton, D. L. Complications of BCG immunotherapy in patients with cancer. *New Engl. J. Med.*, **289**, 827–830 (1973).

36. Takasugi, M., Mickey, M. R., and Terasaki, P. I. Studies on specificity of cell-mediated immunity to human tumors. *J. Natl. Cancer Inst.*, **53**, 1527–1538 (1974).

37. Takasugi, M., Ramseyer, A., and Takasugi, J. Decline of natural nonselective cell-mediated cytotoxicity in patients with tumor progression. *Cancer Res.*, **37**, 413–418 (1977).

38. Taniyama, T., Azuma, I., Aladin, A. A., and Yamamura, Y. Effect of cell-wall skeleton of *Mycobacterium bovis* BCG on cell-mediated cytotoxicity in tumor-bearing mice. *Gann*, **66**, 705–709 (1975).

39. Watkins, E. W., Ovata, Y., Anderson, L. L., Watkins, E. III., and Waters, M. F. Activation of host lymphocytes cultured with cancer cells treated with neuraminidase. *Nature New Biol.*, **231**, 83–85 (1971).

40. Yamamura, Y., Yoshizaki, K., Azuma, I., Yagura, T., and Watanabe, T. Immunotherapy of human malignant melanoma with oil-attached BCG cell-wall skeleton. *Gann*, **66**, 355–363 (1975).

41. Yasumoto, K., Ohta, M., and Nomoto, K. Cytotoxic activity of lymphocytes to bronchogenic carcinoma cells in patients with lung cancer. *Gann*, **67**, 505–511 (1976).

42. Yasumoto, K., Manabe, H., Ueno, M., Ohta, M., Ueda, H., Iida, A., Nomoto, K., Azuma, I., and Yamamura, Y. Immunotherapy of human lung cancer with BCG cell-wall skeleton. *Gann*, **67**, 787–795 (1976).

43. Zbar, B. and Tanaka, T. Immunotherapy of cancer—Regression of tumors after intralesional injection of living *Mycobacterium bovis*. *Science*, **172**, 271–273 (1971).

44. Zbar, B. Tumor regression mediated by *Mycobacterium bovis* (strain BCG). *Natl. Cancer Inst. Monogr.*, **35**, 341–344 (1972).

IMMUNOTHERAPY WITH BCG CELL-WALL SKELETON IN PATIENTS WITH NEOPLASTIC PLEURISY

Takeshi Ogura, Takahiko Yoshimoto, Hideki Nishikawa,
Mitsunori Sakatani, Masami Ito, Fumio Hirao,
Ichiro Azuma, and Yuichi Yamamura

*Third Department of Internal Medicine,
Osaka University Medical School**

Oil-attached cell-wall skeleton of *Mycobacterium bovis* BCG (BCG-CWS) was used in the treatment of neoplastic pleurisy in 5 cancer patients. Intrapleural injections of BCG-CWS combined with preceding anticancer chemotherapy resulted in eradication of both tumor cells and effusion in the affected pleural cavity. These effects were maintained successfully in 4 patients by monthly intradermal injections of the agent. The patients with a good response to the treatment appeared to survive well-conditioned. The possible mechanisms responsible for these therapeutic effects were discussed in relation to the host's immune response and an inflammatory reaction leading to obliteration of the pleural space.

Neoplastic pleurisy is a common complication of malignant disease and is still one of the most serious problems in the management of a patient with cancer.

A potent suppressive effect of oil-attached BCG cell-wall skeleton (BCG-CWS) in human tumors as well as in animal tumors has been reported (*6–12*). In recent preliminary studies in 2 patients with neoplastic pleurisy, it was demonstrated that BCG-CWS, particularly when injected into the affected pleural cavity, had a therapeutic effect on both disappearance of tumor cells in the neoplastic effusion and prevention of accumulation of the effusion (*10*).

The purpose of this report is to detail the patients with treatment of neoplastic pleurisy, with special emphasis on the use of intrapleural injections of BCG-CWS.

Patients and Method of Treatment

1) Patients

The subject consisted of 5 patients including 2 patients reported preliminarily (*10*), entered recently for 2 years into the Osaka University Hospital, Third Departmenf of Internal Medicine. All the patients had the clinical characteristics of lung cancer and cytological proof of neoplastic effusion. Details of the patients are summarized in Table I.

---
* Fukushima 1-1-50, Fukushima-ku, Osaka 553, Japan (小倉 剛, 吉本崇彦, 西川秀樹, 坂谷光則, 伊藤正己, 平尾文男, 東 市郎, 山村雄一).

TABLE I. Patients Studied

Patient No.	Sex	Age (yr)	Histological type	Clinical stage[a]	Initial therapy[b]
1[c]	M	67	Anaplastic carcinoma (small)	IV	CQ+5-FU (i.v.) (×6) Linac (3,000R)
2[c]	F	44	Adenocarcinoma	III	MMC (i.p.) (×4) MTX (i.p.) (×5)
3	M	74	Adenocarcinoma	III	MMC (i.p.) (×4) Linac (3,600R)
4	M	48	Adenocarcinoma	III	MMC (i.p.) (×2)
5	M	48	Anaplastic carcinoma (large)	IV	MMC (i.p.) (×3) Linac (3,000R)

[a] According to the Clinical Staging of Lung Cancer in the Japanese Lung Cancer Society.

[b] CQ, carbazilquinone; 5-FU, 5-fluorouracil; MMC, mitomycin C; MTX, methotrexate; i.v., intravenously; i.p., intrapleurally.

[c] These patients were preliminarily reported.

2) Oil-attached BCG-CWS

Oil-attached BCG-CWS was prepared by the same method as described previously (10–12).

3) Treatment procedure

All the patients were given antineoplastic agents as initial therapy before treatment with BCG-CWS, intravenously in the first case and intrapleurally in the other cases, as indicated in Table I. Three patients (cases 1, 3, and 5) were supplemented with irradiation therapy for either vena cava superior syndrome or atelectasis due to intrabronchial tumor growth.

After aspiration of pleural fluid as completely as possible, 100 or 200 μg of oil-attached BCG-CWS suspended in 10 ml saline was injected into the pleural cavity as induction therapy. In the second case, the injection dose was reduced to 50 μg because she showed a strong skin reaction for both purified protein derivative (PPD) and 10 μg of BCG-CWS. The treatment was applied more than twice at various intervals according to response to the treatment and clinical condition of the patient. When prevention of reaccumulation of the effusion was attained by intrapleural injections, the patient was referred to maintenance therapy in which 100 μg of BCG-CWS was injected monthly into the skin at the bilateral upper arms to shoulders.

Clinical Result

1) Clinical response to induction therapy with intrapleural injection of BCG-CWS

In all the patients, induction therapy with BCG-CWS led to disappearance of malignant cells in the effusion which could not be eradicated by the preceding chemotherapy. In 3 cases clusterings of mononuclear cells around such a malignant cell were

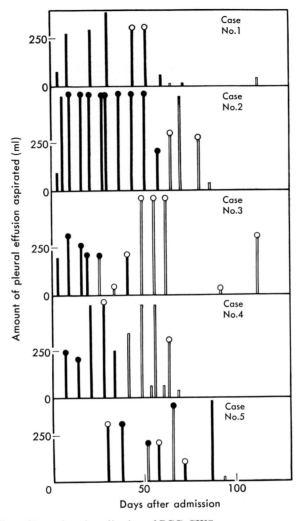

FIG. 1. Effect of intrapleural application of BCG-CWS
    Amount of the effusion aspirated with each thoracentesis is represented by vertical bar (■ tumor cell positive; □ tumor cell negative). Closed and open round symbols at top of the bar represent individual intrapleural application of anticancer drug and BCG-CWS, respectively. The agent was injected immediately after the thoracentesis.

found, as shown in Photos 1 and 2. Other changes in cellular distribution in the effusion before and during the therapy are summarized in Fig. 1. Except for eosinophilia induced by intrapleural chemotherapy, neutrophilia was the most distinct response in the effusion.

    Intrapleural injection of BCG-CWS also resulted in a remarkable decrease of pleural effusion as shown in Fig. 2. In 3 patients pleural effusion was increased transiently on chest roentgenogram taken a few days after the first injection of BCG-CWS. The effusions aspirated thereafter became slightly blooded but turned gradually yellowish and serous.

    In laboratory findings elevations of erythrocyte sedimentation rate (ESR), CRP-

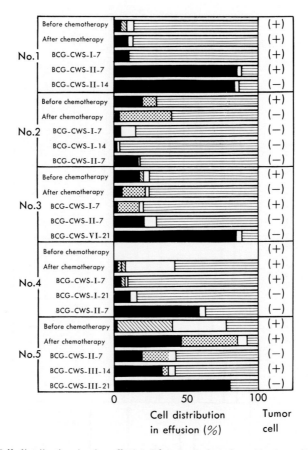

Fig. 2. Cell distribution in the effusion after intrapleural application of BCG-CWS
    In case 1 chemotherapy was given intravenously.
    Roman numerals, No. of intrapleural BCG-CWS applications; arabic numerals,
days after intrapleural BCG-CWS application. ■ neutrophil; ▦ eosinophil;
▨ mesothelial cell; ☐ histiocyte; ☰ lymphocyte.

positivity, and content of plasma fibrinogen were observed. Leucocytosis in the peripheral blood was also remarkable but not always related to lymphocytosis or monocy-
tosis.

The main complaints with intrapleural injection of BCG-CWS were discomfort,
mild to moderate fever, and local pain. These, however, were not serious and were
controlled with care.

2) *Clinical changes during maintenance therapy*
    Prevention of reaccumulation of pleural effusion during the maintenance therapy
was so complete that no patients needed to receive further thoracentesis as well as
anticancer chemotherapy. This made it possible for 3 patients to be out of hospital for
a long time as shown in Table II. The period from final therapeutic thoracentesis to
either death or to May 1, 1977, in each patient is indicated as remission duration of the
effusions (Table II).

TABLE II. Effect of Treatment with BCG-CWS

Patient No.	Dose of BCG-CWS (i.p. injection) (μg × times)	Reaction	Remission (month)	Survival after admission (month)
1	100 × 2	Local pain Fever	20[a] (dead)	23 (5 — 15 — 3) in- out- in- patient patient patient
2	50 × 2	Local pain Fever Nausea (mild)	21[b] (alive)	23 (5 —— 18) in- out- patient patient
3	200 × 7	Nil	3[b] (alive)	7 (in-patient)
4	200 × 1 50 × 1	Local pain	8[b] (alive)	10 (2 —— 8) in- out- patient patient
5	50 × 1 200 × 2	Discomfort	1[a] (dead)	4 (in-patient)

[a] No recurrence of effusion until death due to systemic spreading of the disease.
[b] No recurrence of effusion after final i.p. administration of BCG-CWS.

Skin test with PPD was positive in all the patients before initial chemotherapy and the reactivity was augmented during the maintenance therapy in 3 cases. No negative conversion was observed. In one case positive conversion of skin test with dinitrochlorobenzene was observed. During the maintenance therapy patients had few complaints. The skin ulceration induced by intracutaneous injections was fairly small.

3) Pathological study in an autopsied patient

Postmortem examination was performed on the first case. Characteristic was an extreme thickening and firm fibrous adhesion of the pleurae (Photo 3). The original pleural space remained localized in the lower lateral portion of the right hemithorax and contained a very small amount of serous, yellowish effusion. This change was limited only to the pleural cavity given BCG-CWS. Other metastatic involvements were found in the liver, ribs, and spinal bones. On microscopic examination malignant cells were scattered or clustered in thickened pleurae and infiltration of mononuclear cells, such as lymphocytes, was not apparent. In some areas adjacent to the primary pulmonary tumor, however, lymphocyte infiltration was found. The pleural effusion was scarce and contained no malignant cells on cytological examination.

DISCUSSION

The use of BCG-CWS in the treatment of neoplastic pleural effusion was originally based on its suppressive effect on tumor growth by potentiating an immunological response at various levels (7, 9, 11, 12). It has been generally accepted that immunotherapy with an immunopotentiating agent is most effective when the agent is administered at the tumor site. Accordingly, intrapleural injection of BCG-CWS appears to be optimum in lung cancer patients with neoplastic pleurisy.

In the present study, neoplastic cells still present in the effusion escaping from the initial attack with chemotherapy were completely eradicated after intrapleural administration of BCG-CWS. Although no direct evidence for the effect could be demonstrated, mononuclear cells rosette-forming with a tumor cell were found in the effusion after BCG-CWS administration and may be responsible for the effect as suggested by Sulitzeanu (6).

Another important therapeutic effect was reduction of the pleural effusion. Although the pathogenesis involved in the production of the effusion in neoplastic pleurisy is often complicated, tumor cell seeding, lymphatic and venous obstruction are most important locally. Production of a fibrous union between the affected pleurae resulting in obliteration of the pleural space has been considered to be the most effective reaction (1–4).

BCG-CWS, when injected into the pleural cavity, appears also to induce an inflammatory reaction at the pleural surfaces with resulting adhesive fibrosis, as presented by subjective symptoms, elevated value of CRP and ESR, increased plasma fibrinogen, and marked by thickened pleurae at autopsy. From this view, it is suggested that success with BCG-CWS is due to potentiated immune response and partly to the local inflammatory reaction.

Maintenance therapy not only kept the patients out of hospital for a long time but also restricted application of the antineoplastic drugs and palliative thoracentesis. This also contributed indirectly to keeping the patients' immune response from declining. Thus, in the treatment of neoplastic pleurisy BCG-CWS seems to be equal to or more successful than other agents reported previously (1–5), and merits further usage in cancer patients having a recurrent metastatic pleurisy.

REFERENCES

1. Anderson, C. B., Philpott, G. W., and Ferguson, T. B. The treatment of malignant pleural effusions. *Cancer*, **33**, 916–922 (1974).
2. Borja, E. R. and Pugh, R. P. Single-dose quinacrine (Atabrine) and thoracotomy in the control of pleural effusions in patients with neoplastic diseases. *Cancer*, **31**, 899–902 (1973).
3. Hickman, J. A. and Jones, M. C. Treatment of neoplastic pleural effusions with local instillations of quinacrine (mepacrine) hydrochloride. *Thorax*, **25**, 226–229 (1970).
4. Jones, G. R. Treatment of recurrent malignant pleural effusion by iodized talc pleurodesis. *Thorax*, **24**, 69–73 (1969).
5. Martini, N., Bains, M. S., and Beattie, E. J., Jr. Indication for pleurectomy in malignant effusion. *Cancer*, **35**, 734–738 (1975).
6. Sulitzeanu, D., Gorsky, Y., Paglish, S., and Weiss, D. Morphological evidence suggestive of host-tumor cell interactions *in vivo* in human cancer patients. *J. Natl. Cancer Inst.*, **52**, 603–604 (1974).
7. Taniyama, T., Azuma, I., Aladin, A. A., and Yamamura, Y. Effect of cell-wall skeleton of *Mycobacterium bovis* BCG on cell-mediated cytotoxicity in tumor-bearing mice. *Gann*, **66**, 705–709 (1975).
8. Yamamura, Y., Azuma, I., Taniyama, T., Ribi, E., and Zbar, B. Suppression of tumor growth and regression of established tumor in mice with oil-attached mycobacterial fractions. *Gann*, **65**, 179–181 (1974).

9. Yamamura, Y., Yoshizaki, K., Azuma, I., Yagura, T., and Watanabe, T. Immuno-therapy of human malignant melanoma with oil-attached BCG cell-wall skeleton. *Gann*, **66**, 355–363 (1975).
10. Yamamura, Y., Ogura, T., Yoshimoto, T., Nishikawa, H., Sakatani, M., Itoh, M., Masuno, T., Namba, M., Yazaki, H., Hirao, F., and Azuma, I. Successful treatment of the patients with malignant pleural effusion with BCG cell-wall skeleton. *Gann*, **67**, 669–667 (1976).
11. Yamamura, Y., Azuma, I., Taniyama, T., Sugimura, K., Hirao, F., Tokuzen, R., Okabe, M., Nakahara, W., Yasumoto, K., and Ohta, M. Immunotherapy of cancer with cell-wall skeleton of *Mycobacterium bovis* Bacillus Calmette-Guerin: Experimental and clinical results. *Ann. N.Y. Acad. Sci.*, **277**, 209–226 (1976).
12. Yasumoto, K., Manabe, H., Ueno, M., Ohta, M., Ueda, H., Iida, A., Nomoto, K., Azuma, I., and Yamamura, Y. Immunotherapy of human lung cancer with BCG cell-wall skeleton. *Gann*, **67**, 787–795 (1976).
13. Yoshimoto, T., Azuma, I., Nishikawa, H., Sakatani, M., Ogura, T., Hirao, F., and Yamamura, Y. Experimental immunotherapy of neoplastic pleural effusion with oil-attached BCG cell-wall skeleton in mice. *Gann*, **67**, 737–740 (1976).

EXPLANATION OF PHOTOS

PHOTO 1. Mononuclear cells rosette-forming with tumor cells in the effusion in case 1 (7 days after 2nd intrapleural application of BCG-CWS). May-Giemsa stain. ×1,000.

PHOTO 2. Similar rosette formation in case 5 (2 weeks after 2nd intrapleural application of BCG-CWS). May-Giemsa stain. ×1,000.

PHOTO 3. Gross appearance of the dorsal cut surface of the lungs. Note the thickening and adhesion of pleurae. Original pleural space is localized in lower lateral part. Primary tumor is indicated with arrow.

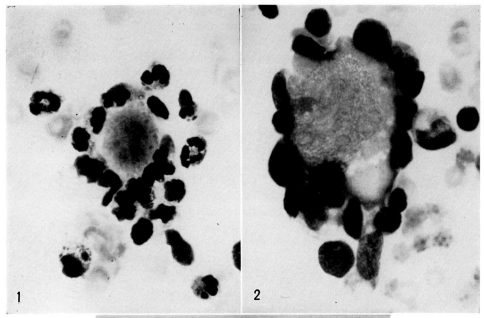

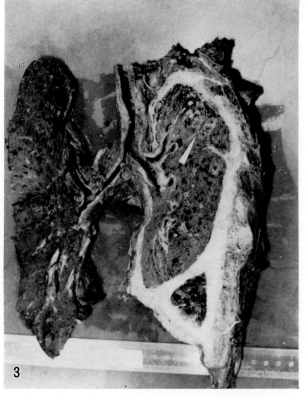

IMMUNOTHERAPY FOR LUNG CANCER CASES USING BCG OR BCG CELL-WALL SKELETON: INTRATUMORAL INJECTIONS

Yoshihiro Hayata, Kenkichi Ohbo, Ippei Ogawa, and Osamu Taira

*Department of Surgery, Tokyo Medical College**

BCG or BCG cell-wall skeleton (BCG-CWS) was used to treat a total of 135 lung cancer cases. Of these, intratumoral injection was given in 52 cases, consisting of 32 cases of transbronchofiberscopic injection by means of a specially-developed needle, 6 percutaneous injections, 6 under thoracotomy and 8 cases of injection to metastatic skin lesions. The regional efficacy was examined in terms of tumor disappearance or regression or opening of the bronchus. It was found that cases which received intratumoral injection of BCG-CWS compared favorably with cases injected with mitomycin C (MMC). There was also a significant difference in histological changes between the BCG-CWS group and the MMC group. Remarkable tumor regression was obtained in 40% of cases treated with intratumoral injections of BCG-CWS percutaneously or under thoracotomy. Adenocarcinoma cases responded best to both types of therapy. It was suggested that combined therapy is necessary with BCG or BCG-CWS in order to obtain optimum results.

Intratumoral injection of BCG has been employed as a regional or general treatment for melanoma by Morton et al. (8) and others, and its regional efficacy is well known. However, there are few reports extant on the subject of regional BCG or BCG-cell-wall skeleton (BCG-CWS) therapy. Since October 1974, the authors have been administering BCG intradermally in lung cancer cases treated at Tokyo Medical College Hospital, and since February 1976 they have been administering BCG-CWS intradermally, intratumorally, intralymphatically, or intrapleurally.

Patients and Methods of Immunotherapy

Between October 1974 and March 1977, 135 lung cancer patients were treated with BCG or BCG-CWS. All received intradermal inoculations; 52 cases received intratumoral injections, 11 cases received intrapleural injections, and one case was injected intralymphatically. Of the 52 cases in which the tumor was injected directly, 32 cases were injected by means of a needle which the authors had developed for that specific purpose. Six cases of peripheral tumors received percutaneous injections and 6 cases of intrapulmonary tumor or metastatic lymph nodes were injected under thoracotomy, 3 of which underwent open lung irradiation of the primary or metastatic

* Nishishinjuku 6-7-1, Shinjuku-ku, Tokyo 160, Japan (早田義博, 於保健吉, 小川一平, 平良 修).

lesion, doses varying from 2,000 to 3,000 R, using a Betatron or linear accelerator X-ray. Eight cases of metastatic skin lesions were also injected.

BCG was only given intradermally, and the direct intratumoral injection of BCG-CWS was of varying dosages; transbronchofiberscopic injections, 3–21 times per case, of 200 μg doses, percutaneous injections of 500 μg BCG-CWS were given 1–3 times, while injection under thoracotomy consisted of a single massive dose of 1,000–3,000 μg.

Histologically the 32 cases injected transbronchofiberscopically consisted of 11 cases of squamous cell carcinoma, 12 adenocarcinoma, 8 small cell carcinoma, and one large cell carcinoma. All were stage III cases and all were treated with intradermal inoculations of BCG-CWS and received 3 or more transbronchofiberscopic injections, while undergoing combined treatment with chemotherapy and/or irradiation.

Immune response changes following BCG-CWS injections were examined by T cell population (7) and blast formation of lymphocytes by phytohemagglutinin (PHA) (13).

The control group consisted of 25 cases of central type lung cancer receiving either irradiation therapy or multicombined chemotherapy with irradiation, and 3 cases received 2 or 3 transbronchofiberscopic intratumoral injections of 2 mg mitomycin C (MMC). These cases served as a basis for comparing and evaluating bronchofiberscopic and histological findings. The former group of 25 cases consisted of 11 squamous cell carcinoma cases, 8 adenocarcinoma, and 6 small cell carcinoma cases.

Clinical Effect with Immunotherapy

1) Immune response changes following transbronchofiberscopic BCG-CWS injections
Comparison of T cell population changes following intradermally injected BCG or BCG-CWS and transbronchofiberscopically injected BCG-CWS showed increasing

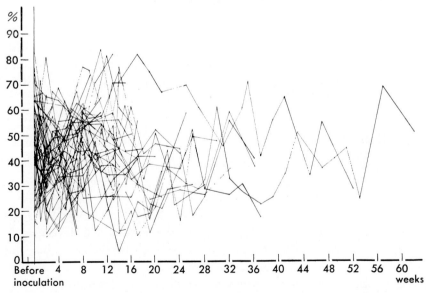

FIG. 1.   Changes in T cell population after BCG-CWS inoculation in stage III lung cancer cases

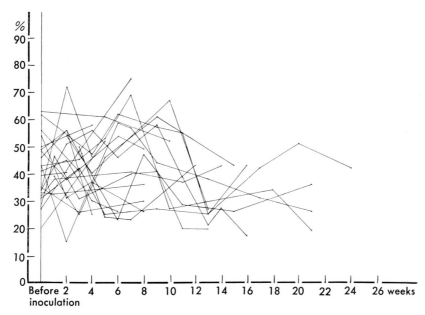

FIG. 2. Changes in T cell population after transbronchofiberscopic injection of BCG-CWS

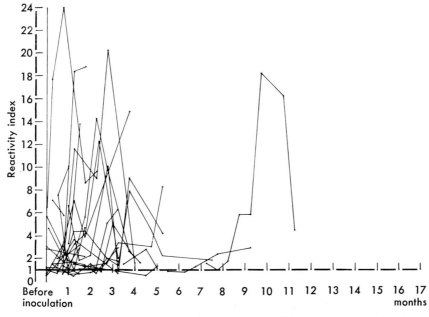

FIG. 3. Changes in blast formation to PHA of stage III lung cancer cases after inoculation with BCG or BCG-CWS

immune response in some cases, although between the two groups there was no significant difference (Figs. 1 and 2). This was reflected by the blast formation of lymphocytes by PHA (Figs. 3 and 4).

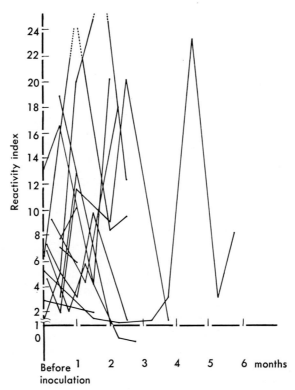

FIG. 4. Changes in blast formation to PHA after transbronchofiberscopic intratumoral injection of BCG-CWS

2) Changes in bronchofiberscopic findings and histology after injection of BCG-CWS

Figure 5 shows a case in which the left upper lobe bronchus displayed a decrease in redness, swelling, and dilatation of the vessels one week after injection of 200 μg BCG-CWS. No significant changes were observed after one case received an injection

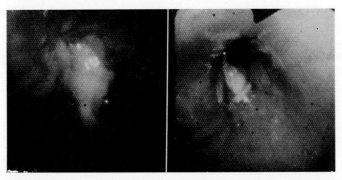

FIG. 5. Bronchofiberscopic findings before and after intratumoral BCG-CWS injection in a case of squamous cell carcinoma

The photograph on the left shows an infiltrative tumor and obstruction of the left upper lobe bronchus. In the photograph on the right, which was taken after weekly injections of 200 μg BCG-CWS, significant opening of the lumen can be observed.

of 2 mg MMC (Fig. 6). Comparison of histological findings at the injection site of a case receiving 3 injections of 200 μg BCG-CWS was made with a case receiving the same number of 2 mg MMC injections (Figs. 7 and 8). Remarkable degeneration of

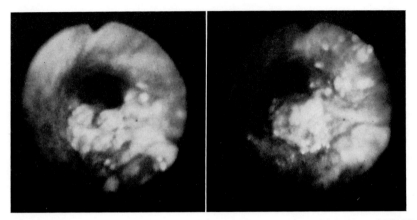

FIG. 6. Bronchofiberscopic findings before and after intratumoral injection of MMC
The infiltrating tumor situated in the right truncus intermedius seen in the photograph on the left was a low-differentiated squamous cell carcinoma, and, as seen on the right, 3 weekly injections of 2 mg MMC did not result in any significant difference.

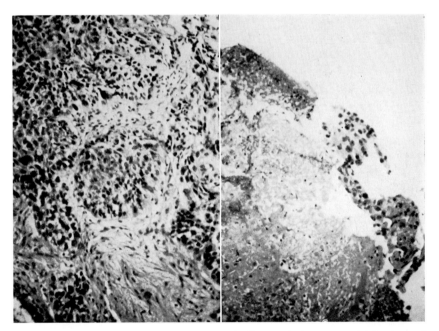

FIG. 7. Histologic changes after transbronchofiberscopic intratumoral injections of BCG-CWS
Features of low-differentiated squamous cell carcinoma can be seen on the left, and on the right, after 3 weekly injections of 200 μg BCG-CWS, necrosis of tumor nests and degeneration of tumor cells can be seen. Hematoxylin-eosin stain (H-E). ×100.

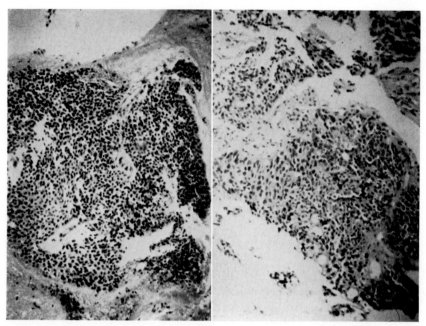

FIG. 8.   On the right, features of low-differentiated squamous cell carcinoma before 3 weekly injections of 2 mg MMC
    No significant differences can be seen after the treatment in the photograph on the left. H-E. ×100.

tumor cells was recognized in the BCG-CWS case, but no significant degeneration was seen in the mitomycin case (Figs. 7 and 8).

Table I delineates the changes as seen bronchofiberscopically within 3 weeks after 3 transbronchofiberscopic injections of BCG-CWS. Tumor regression was observed in 37.5% of cases and moderate opening of the bronchial lumen in 28.1%, but no case of total tumor disappearance or complete opening of the bronchial lumen was seen. The same cases were then treated with chemotherapy and/or irradiation after 3 or 4 more injections of BCG-CWS, and, subsequent to the combined therapy, disappearance of the tumor was noted in 18.7% of cases and complete opening of the bronchus in

TABLE I.   Changes of Bronchofiberscopic Findings in Stage III Lung Cancer Cases Injected Transbronchofiberscopically with BCG-CWS (Feb. 1975–March 1977)

Histological type	Tumor changes			Changes in bronchial lumen		
	Disap-pearance	Regression	Un-changed	Signifi-cantly opened	Moder-ately opened	Un-changed
Squamous cell carcinoma	0	4	7	0	4	7
Adenocarcinoma	0	4	8	0	3	9
Small cell carcinoma	0	4	4	0	2	6
Large cell carcinoma	0	0	1	0	0	1
Total	0	12	20	0	9	23

TABLE II. Changes of Bronchofiberscopic Findings of Cases Receiving
Transbronchofiberscopic Intratumoral BCG-CWS Injection and
Combined Therapy (Stage III Cases) (Feb. 1975–March 1977)

Histological type	Tumor changes			Changes in bronchial lumen		
	Disap-pearance	Regression	Un-changed	Signifi-cantly opened	Moder-ately opened	Un-changed
Squamous cell carcinoma	0	7	4	2	5	4
Adenocarcinoma	1	2	8	3	2	6
Small cell carcinoma	4	3	2	5	1	3
Large cell carcinoma	0	0	1	0	0	1
Total	5	12	15	10	8	14

TABLE III. Changes of Bronchofiberscopic Findings in Cases Receiving Irradiation and
Chemotherapy (Stage III, Non-resected Cases) (Sept. 1974–April 1976)

Histological type	Tumor changes			Changes in bronchial lumen		
	Disap-pearance	Regression	Un-changed	Signifi-cantly opened	Moder-ately opened	Un-changed
Squamous cell carcinoma	1	7	3	3	5	3
Adenocarcinoma	0	2	6	1	0	7
Small cell carcinoma	1	4	1	2	3	1
Total	2	13	10	6	8	11

31.2% (Table II). Better results were observed in adenocarcinoma and small cell carcinoma cases. Cases receiving irradiation or irradiation plus chemotherapy, but without BCG-CWS, did not exhibit as high a rate of improvement of bronchial findings as the BCG-CWS therapy group (Table III).

3) Percutaneous intratumoral BCG-CWS injection and injection under thoracotomy
Figure 9 shows a case of adenocarcinoma in which tumor decreased markedly after 2 percutaneous injections of 500 μg BCG-CWS. Of 6 percutaneously injected tumor cases, a remarkable decrease was observed in 3, and in 6 cases injected with BCG-CWS under thoracotomy tumor shadows disappeared in 3. However, with the exception of the single case shown in Fig. 9, all these cases were treated with chemotherapy and/or irradiation following BCG-CWS injection.

4) Survival of cases injected with BCG or BCG-CWS
Immunotherapy using BCG or BCG-CWS was performed in most cases of lung cancer treated recently at Tokyo Medical College. In stage I cases no non-surgical therapy was given, while in stage II cases combined therapy with BCG or BCG-CWS was given following resection. Sufficient time has not yet elapsed since the commencement of this type of therapy to permit any definitive discussion of the extent of its effect on survival.

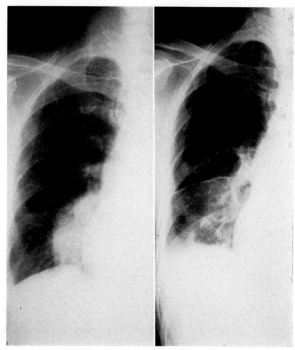

FIG. 9. Chest X-rays before (right) and after (left) percutaneous BCG-CWS
intratumoral injections
   The tumor shadow decreased significantly after 2 injections of 500 μg BCG-CWS.

FURTHER COMMENTS

There are many reports concerning regional efficacy and changes in immun reponse
as a result of BCG injections for melanoma (1–4, 8, 9) and the relationship between
immune response and tumor remission has also been examined. Experiments on tumor-
bearing mice (10, 11, 14) have also shown the regional and general effects of BCG.
Exceedingly few reports exist on BCG immunotherapy for lung cancer, although some
promising results were obtained by BCG or BCG-CWS inoculation in lung cancer
cases by Yasumoto (12, 13) and by intrapleural injection by McKneally (5, 6).

   Of a total of 135 cases treated with BCG or BCG-CWS, the primary tumor was
injected with BCG-CWS transbronchofiberscopically, percutaneously, or under thoracotomy in 44 cases. Observation of T-cell population changes, blast formation, and
purified protein derivative response revealed increases in immune response following
the intratumoral injection of BCG-CWS and also in intradermally inoculated cases.
No serious complications were experienced.

   In terms of regional effects, total disappearance of the tumor or complete opening
of the bronchial lumen was not observed in cases treated by intratumoral injection of
BCG-CWS alone, but such results were obtained when injection of BCG-CWS was
combined with chemotherapy and/or irradiation. Cases which did not receive BCG-
CWS treatment did not display such a high rate of tumor disappearance or opening
of the bronchial lumen. Furthermore, cases treated by intratumoral injection of BCG-

CWS percutaneously or under thoracotomy showed a higher rate of tumor shadow disappearance and/or decrease than cases which received no BCG treatment, and better results were obtained even in central type adenocarcinoma cases. However, these cases also received combined therapy, which indicates that better results can be obtained when intratumoral BCG-CWS is combined with irradiation or irradiation plus chemotherapy; this agrees with McKneally's results (5, 6).

Thus, intratumoral BCG-CWS injections are effective regional lung cancer treatment, and the transbronchofiberscopic injection seems to be safe, which brings a greater range of cases within the applicable range of this therapy.

Acknowledgment

The authors express their sincere gratitude for the cooperation of Drs. Yamamura and Azuma of Osaka University in extracting and providing the BCG-CWS without which this study would not have been possible.

This study was partly aided by a Grant-in-Aid for Cancer Research from the Ministry of Health and Welfare, Japan, and the Tokyo Medical College Hospital Cancer Center, which are gratefully acknowledged.

REFERENCES

1. Baker, M. A. and Taub, R. N. Immunotherapy of human cancer. *Progr. Allergy*, **17**, 227–299 (1973).
2. Grant, R. M., Mackie, R., Cochran, A. J., Murray, E. A., Hoyle, D., and Ross, C. Results of administering B.C.G. to patients with melanoma. *Lancet*, **i**, 1096–1100 (1974).
3. Gutterman, J. U., Mavligit, G., McBride, C., Frei, E., Freireich, E. J., and Hersh, E. M. Active immunotherapy with B.C.G. for recurrent malignant melanoma. *Lancet*, **i**, 1208–1212 (1973).
4. Mastrangelo, M. J., Sulit, H. L., Prehn, L., Bornstein, R. S., Yarbro, J. W., and Prehn, R. T. Intralesional BCG in the treatment of metastatic malignant melanoma. *Cancer*, **37**, 684–692 (1976).
5. McKneally, M. F., Maver, C., and Kausel, H. W. Regional immunotherapy of lung cancer with intrapleural B.C.G. *Lancet*, **i**, 377–379 (1976).
6. McKneally, M. F., Maver, C., Kausel, H. W., and Alley, R. D. Regional immunotherapy with intrapleural BCG for lung cancer. *J. Thorac. Cardiovasc. Surg.*, **72**, 333–338 (1976).
7. Mitchell, M. S., Kirkpatrick, D., Mokyr, M. B., and Gery, I. On the mode of action of BCG. *Nature*, **243**, 216–218 (1973).
8. Morton, D. L., Eilber, F. R., Malmgren, R. A., and Wood, W. C. Immunological factors which influence response to immunotherapy in malignant melanoma. *Surgery*, **68**, 158–164 (1970).
9. Nathanson, L. Regression of intradermal malignant melanoma after intralesional injection of *Mycobacterium bovis* strain BCG. *Cancer Chemother. Rep.*, **56**, 659–666 (1973).
10. Smith, H. G., Bast, R. C., Jr., Zbar, B., and Rapp, H. J. Eradication of microscopic lymph node metastases after injection of living BCG adjacent to the primary tumor. *J. Natl. Cancer Inst.*, **55**, 1345–1352 (1975).
11. Tanaka, T. and Saito, T. Immunotherapy of cancer: Induction of tumor immunity with a mixture of tumor cell-BCG, and the effect of intratumor injection of BCG and of non-living BCG preparation. *Gann*, **66**, 631–640 (1975).

12. Yasumoto, K., Ohta, M., and Nomoto, K. Cytotoxic activity of lymphocytes to bronchogenic carcinoma cells in patients with lung cancer. *Gann*, **67**, 505–511 (1976).

13. Yasumoto, K., Manabe, H., Ueno, M., Ohta, M., Ueda, H., Iida, A., Nomoto, K., Azuma, I., and Yamamura, Y. Immunotherapy of human lung cancer with BCG cell-wall skeleton. *Gann*, **67**, 787–795 (1976).

14. Yamamura, Y., Azuma, I., and Taniyama, T. Immunotherapy of cancer with BCG. *Saishin Igaku*, **30**, 51–55 (1975) (in Japanese).

CLINICAL TRIALS. II.
IMMUNOTHERAPY OF
GASTROINTESTINAL CANCERS

IMMUNOTHERAPY FOR ADVANCED GASTRIC CANCER AND COLO-RECTAL CANCER USING BCG CELL-WALL SKELETON

Kunzo Orita, Tetsuya Mannami, Hiroaki Miwa, Tamotsu Ohta, Harutsugu Nakahara, Eiji Konaga, and Sanae Tanaka

Department of Surgery, Okayama University Medical School*

Postoperative immunotherapy is being conducted in cases of advanced gastric cancer, stages III and IV, and cases of colo-rectal cancer B and C by Dukes' classification in whom the main tumor at least has been extirpated. The series has been divided into three groups: (1) Those who received 0.1–1 mg BCG plus autochthonous tumor cells, intradermally (i.d.), (2) those who received 200 μg of oil-attached BCG cell-wall skeleton (BCG-CWS) i.d., and (3) those who received an intratumor injection of 500 μg of oil-attached BCG-CWS once before operation at endoscopy and again after operation. There have been no adverse effects in any of these groups. The greatest prolongation of life has occurred in the second group. The postoperative change in the blast formation rate of peripheral blood lymphocytes to phytohemagglutinin reflects the effect of immunotherapy relatively well.

In Europe and North America, there seems to have been little study on cell-mediated immunity in relation to digestive tract cancer, especially on that which is most prevalent in Japan, gastric cancer. In particular, there has been no report as yet on the use of immunotherapy in gastric cancer. Similarly, the study of colo-rectal cancer (prevalent in Europeans and Americans) is far behind that of melanoma and leukemia, even though digestive tract cancer generally does not differ immunologically from any other solid cancer. Gastric cancers (20, 22) and colo-rectal cancers (2, 10) possess tumor antigens that are not found in normal tissues, so that the possibility that the host can mobilize its cell-mediated immunity against a tumor by the aid of lymphocytes is gradually being recognized. With the widely-used BCG as an immunopotentiator, immunotherapy for gastric cancer and colo-rectal cancer is now being attempted.

Staging of Gastric Cancer and Colo-rectal Cancer

The clinical stage of gastric cancer was evaluated macroscopically at operation, according to the rules of the Japanese Research Society for Gastric Cancer (12). This staging is based on a combination of four factors: Serosal invasion (S_0–S_3); peritoneal dissemination (P_0–P_3); lymph node metastasis (N_0–N_4); and hepatic metastasis (H_0–H_3); and is divided into stages I, II, III, and IV. The staging of colo-rectal cancer was

---

* Shikatacho 2-5-1, Okayama 700, Japan (折田薫三, 万波徹也, 三輪恕昭, 太田 保, 中原東亜, 小長英二, 田中早苗).

carried out according to Dukes' classification. For the present study of immunotherapy, cases in stages III and IV gastric cancer and colo-rectal cancer of Dukes' B and C classification were selected.

Immunological Parameters

Until a tumor reaches a certain size, the lymphocytes of the host usually have antitumor activity (*19*). T and B lymphocytes undergo immune reactions to tumor antigens through the mediation of macrophages. There are 4 kinds of activated T cells: Effector (cytotoxic) T cells that aggregate on tumor cells to destroy them or to inhibit their proliferation; delayed hypersensitivity initiation T cells that produce lymphokines when they come in contact with tumor antigens; helper T cells that augment the activity of B cells; and suppressor T cells that inhibit the activity of B cells and T cells (*5*). The humoral antibody produced by B cells against tumor antigen acts in two ways. One is lymphocyte-dependent antibody that has an antitumor activity (*9*), and the other is an antibody that combines with soluble tumor antigens to form the so-called blocking factor, which inhibits the activity of activated T cells (*11*). On the other hand, there are many substances in the serum of a cancer patient that impede the activity of T cells nonspecifically. In advanced cancer, a fall in the nonspecific activity of T cells often occurs (*23*).

On the dasis of the above observations, certain parameters of cell-mediated immunity, including macrophage migration inhibitory factor (MIF) by George and Vaughan's method (*6*) was measured, and in colo-rectal cancer, the activity of effector T cells and blocking factor using a P cell line derived from colon cancer cells (*17*) as target cells by Takasugi and Klein's method (*25*) was tested. As parameters of nonspecific cell-mediated immunity, purified protein derivative (PPD) skin tests were performed, the blast formation rate of lymphocytes to phytohemagglutinin (PHA) was estimated from the appearance rate of large and intermediate lymphocytes after 3 days' culture (*21*), and the rate of rosette formation with sheep erythrocytes of T lymphocytes was calculated by Tachibana and Ishikawa's method (*26*). Such tests were conducted throughout the course before and after operation, using peripheral blood lymphocytes.

Postoperative Immunotherapy against Gastric Cancer and Colo-rectal Cancer

Even since Mathé's report (*13*) that the remission induced by chemotherapy of acute lymphoblastic leukemia in infants can be maintained for a longer period of time by the administration of BCG in a large dose, BCG has come to be used as an important immunopotentiator. Gutterman *et al.* (*8*) obtained favorable results in cases of melanoma with extensive metastasis where the tumors could not be removed completely, by giving postoperative chemotherapy combined with BCG administration. It seems that a cancer patient can be cured permanently if the tumor mass is reduced to a minimum by some method and immunotherapy is then conducted.

1) Immunotherapy against gastric cancer using BCG and autochthonous tumor cells
The following immunotherapy protocol was used from November 1973 to November 1975. Free tumor cells are isolated from 0.5 g of resected tumor tissue, treated with

TABLE I. Gastric Cancer Patients Receiving More than 3 i.d. Injections
of BCG+Autochthonous Tumor Cells (Protocol-73)

Case No.	Age (yr.)	Sex	Stage	Preoperative		Follow-up (months)
				PPD	MIF	
1	75	M	III	−	+	37, alive
2	64	M	III	+	−	13, died of other disease
3	69	M	III	+	+	28, alive
4	69	M	III	−	+	20, alive
5	46	F	IV	±	+	10, died of tumor
6	63	F	IV	−	−	39, alive
7	70	M	IV	+	+	9, died of tumor
8	57	M	IV	−	+	10, died of tumor
9	60	F	IV	±	+	16, died of other disease
10	67	F	IV		+	7, died of tumor
11	57	F	IV	−	−	21, alive

12.5 mg/ml of mitomycin C for 30 min, mixed with 0.1–1 mg of BCG, and the mixture
is injected intradermally (i.d.) into the exterior side of the upper arm on the 1st or
2nd postoperative day. The remaining tumor cells are stored in a liquid nitrogen
bomb, and depending on size of the tumor, the immunization is repeated in the 2nd,
4th, and 8th postoperative weeks. As anticancer agents, 40 mg mitomycin C is given
within one postoperative month and 250 mg of 5-fluorouracil (5-FU) is injected twice
a week intravenously (i.v.) to a total of 10 g. In addition, depending on the individual,
oral administration of 6 g/day PSK (a protein bound polysaccharide from a basidiomycetes) is given on consecutive days. Table I shows data on 11 cases of advanced
gastric cancer receiving more than 3 injections of BCG+autochthonous tumor cells.
Case No. 6 is of P_1 whose MIF became positive after operation, but who is now surviving 37 months after operation. Case No. 9 is a case of $S_2P_3H_0N_3$ in the terminal stage
showing cancer dissemination throughout the entire peritoneal cavity at operation, but
the MIF for 6 months after operation was weakly positive, while the T cell rate and
the blast formation rate to PHA tended to rise. The MIF disappeared in the 10th
postoperative month and the T cell rate as well as blast formation rate to PHA tended
to decrease, so that the case was given only a further 2 mg BCG, MIF again increased
and, at a laparotomy for ileus, the peritoneal dissemination observed at the first operation had practically disappeared.

2) *Immunotherapy against gastric cancer with BCG-CWS*

Cell-wall skeleton of *Mycobacterium bovis* BCG (BCG-CWS) produced by Yama-
mura-Azuma is said to have fewer side-effects than BCG, its chemical profile is uniform and it has a far stronger immunopotentiating activity than BCG (*15, 27*). We have
been using i.d. injections of BCG-CWS together with chemotherapy since December
1975. Following Azuma's method (*1*) 200 μg of oil-attached BCG-CWS is given i.d.
on the exterior side of the upper arm. Oil-attached BCG-CWS is injected once a week
for 4 postoperative weeks, once every two weeks from the 4th to the 12th postoperative
week, once a month from the 12th week to 6 months, and once every 3 months from 6

TABLE II. Gastric Cancer Patients Receiving i.d. 200 μg
of Oil-attached BCG-CWS (Protocol-75)

Case No.	Age (yr.)	Sex	Stage	Preoperative				Follow-up (months)
				PPD	PHA (%)	T cell (%)	MIF	
1	54	M	III	+		48.1	−	16, alive
2	48	F	III	+	65.5	44.1	−	16, alive
3	51	M	III	++	8.8	64.6	−	14, alive
4	63	M	III	++		63.9		9, alive
5	60	M	IV	+		42.7	−	16, alive
6	38	M	IV	+	54.0		+	15, died of tumor
7	49	F	IV	++		29.2	−	9, died of tumor
8	58	M	IV	−	56.3	58.6	−	7, died of tumor
9	59	M	IV	++	39.3	62.0	−	12, alive
10	33	F	IV	++	62.3	43.6	+	12, alive
11	65	M	IV	−	53.0	68.3	−	12, alive

to 24 months. Table II shows results of 11 cases of advanced gastric cancer who received BCG-CWS.

*3) Immunotherapy with preoperative intratumor injection of BCG-CWS plus the 2nd
protocol*

There have been many reports since Morton (*18*) first described the shrinkage of
tumor mass following intratumor injection of BCG. Under endoscopic view, 500 μg
of oil-attached BCG-CWS is injected into the tumor in several different places 7–10
days before operation. After operation according to the 2nd protocol described above,
BCG-CWS is injected periodically in combination with chemotherapy. As illustrated
in Table III, terminal stage cases were specially selected, and intratumor injections
were instituted. In cases responding positively to PPD skin tests, redness and swelling
similar to the PPD skin test occurred at the site of intratumor injection. When such

TABLE III. Gastric Cancer Patients Receiving Both Preoperative Intratumor Injection
of 500 μg Oil-attached BCG-CWS and i.d. Injection BCG-CWS (Protocol-75)

Case No.	Age (yr.)	Sex	Stage	Preoperative					Follow-up (months)
				PPD	DNCB	MIF	PHA (%)	T cell (%)	
1	58	M	IV (H_1P_3)	−	++	−	56.3	58.6	7, died
2	50	M	IV (S_3)	++	++		30.6		14, alive
3	67	M	IV ($H_2P_3N_4S_3$)	±	−		25.3		7, died
4	72	M	IV (N_4S_3)	+		−	21.2	47.3	5, died of other disease
5	51	M	IV (N_4)	++	−	−	8.8	76.3	15, alive
6[a]	19	M	IV ($P_3N_4S_3$)	+	++		61.6	33.5	7, died
7[a]	31	M	IV (P_3S_3)	+	−		65.3		3, died

[a] 6, 7: No surgery.

spots are observed under the microscope, marked round cell infiltration, Langhan's giant cells, and the destruction of tumor cells can be seen. Regional lymph nodes are also markedly swollen.

4) Immunotherapy against colo-rectal cancer with BCG or BCG-CWS

In the 1st protocol of 1973, BCG+autochthonous tumor cells were given to 3 cases, and in the 2nd protocol, oil-attached BCG-CWS was given to 5 cases (Table IV). The number of cases used so far is small and we have not yet made any randomization of cases, hence it is impossible to determine the effects of immunotherapy in these cases. All cases of stage III gastric cancer, whether given BCG or oil-attached BCG-CWS, are surviving at present. The results for stage IV gastric cancer cases are shown in Fig. 1. The non-immunotherapy group of 22 cases since 1973 was taken as

TABLE IV. Colo-rectal Cancer Patients Receiving BCG or BCG-CWS

Case No.	Age (yr.)	Sex	Disease	Stage (Dukes)	Preoperative				Follow-up (months)
					PPD	PHA	T cell	MIF	
Protocol-73[a]									
1	58	M	Rectal cancer	C	+	45.6	52.3	+	31, died
2	67	M	Rectal cancer	B	+	33.0	40.7	−	4, died of other disease
3	60	F	Rectal cancer	C	+	55.3	53.1	+	
4	70	M	Rectal cancer	C	−	49.2	61.2	−	32, alive
Protocol-75[b]									
1	74	M	Rectal cancer	C	±	28.6		−	7, died
2	64	F	Colon cancer	C	±	11.0	54.8	−	16, alive
3	45	M	Rectal cancer	B	−	14.8		−	14, alive
4	35	M	Rectal cancer	C	−	28.0	14.0	+	5, alive
5	71	M	Rectal cancer	C	++	32.3	24.2	+	3, alive

[a] Cases in protocol-73 receiving more than 3 i.d. injections of BCG + autochthonous tumor cells.
[b] Cases in protocol-75 periodically receiving i.d. 200 μg of oil-attached BCG-CWS.

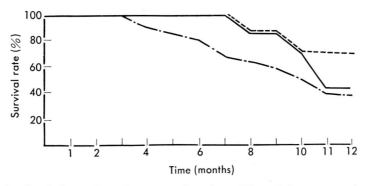

FIG. 1. Survival rate of gastric cancer patients (stage IV) receiving postoperative immunotherapy
—— protocol-73 (BCG); - - - - protocol-75 (BCG-CWS); —·— control (non-immunotherapy).

the control. In the group with BCG administered by the 1st protocol of 1973, 100% of the cases survived for 6 postoperative months but by 12 months, the survival rate was about the same as that of the control group. In the group injected with BCG-CWS by the 2nd protocol of 1975, all cases survived 6 months, 4/6 cases (70%) survived 12 months, and 2/4 cases were still surviving 16 months after operation. In those receiving an intratumor injection of BCG-CWS before operation and i.d. injection of BCG-CWS after operation, there was hardly any difference from the control group. Two cases whose preoperative PPD skin test was intermediately positive were still surviving 14 and 15 months after operation.

In a series of 35 cases consisting of gastric cancer, hepatoma, pancreatic cancer, and colon cancer that terminated in either simple laparotomy or palliative operation, Falk *et al.* (4) injected 2 mg BCG into the peritoneal cavity, followed by oral administration of 120 mg BCG, 5-FU, and cyclophosphamide every week for 8 weeks. They reported that BCG administration was most effective in cases of colon cancer. The average survival period of 19 cases was 13.2 months, with the survival period of liver-metastatic cases being 12.8 months. In 177 cases not receiving BCG, the survival period was 5 months or less. Mavligit *et al.* (14) divided 58 cases of colon cancer of Dukes' C classification who underwent the definitive operation into two groups: One group of immunotherapy with only BCG, and the other group of immunochemotherapy with BCG and 5-FU from about the 4th to the 8th postoperative week. Both groups were followed for 21 months. Viable organisms of BCG of the Pasteur strain in a dose of 6×10^8 cells were administered by scarification once a week for 3 months, and thereafter, once every 2 weeks. 5-FU was administered 5 days a week in a dose of 100 mg/m² and this was repeated once every 4 weeks. With BCG administration alone, recurrence occurred in 5/26 cases and death in 2/26 cases. In the BCG+5-FU group, recurrence was seen in 2/32 cases and there were no deaths. The diagnosis of recurrence was derived from carcinoembryonic antigen (CEA) values.

Changes in Immunological Parameters during Immunotherapy

In general, when immunotherapy with BCG is effective, not only the PPD skin reaction but also the nonspecific and specific immunological capacities are elevated. In advanced cancer patients with low preoperative immunity where a curative operation was performed and the postoperative course was favorable, immunity can gradually be restored even without immunotherapy (24). Eilber and Morton (3) administered a strong dose of BCG after sufficient extirpation of melanoma and sarcoma, and repeatedly tested DNCB skin reaction. For melanoma, those with positive DNCB reactions before operation totalled 65 cases, of whom 41 showed a reinforced postoperative reaction. Thirty-seven of these 41 cases (90%) continued to have a favorable course without recurrence. The 7 cases whose DNCB reaction turned negative all had recurrences. Gross and Libiol (7) administered Tice strain BCG to 14 cases of lung cancer and 12 cases of melanoma. In all cases, the tumors had been eradicated by surgery or irradiation. They stated that in the cases without recurrence and having a smooth course, intradermal reactions against 6 recall antigens such as PPD, histoplasma and streptokinase-streptodornase (SK-SD) were elevated, and especially that the blast formation of peripheral blood lymphocytes to PHA correlated closely with the prognosis.

Minton (*16*) also observed a rise in PPD skin reaction and MIF after injection of a mixture of BCG and mumps virus into the metastatic foci of melanoma.

With i.d. injection of BCG+autochthonous tumor cells according to our 1973 protocol, cases in whom the PPD skin reaction turned positive 4 weeks after operation totaled 3/12 cases. In the group undergoing operation only, this occurred in 8/45 cases. Follow-up of the MIF of peripheral blood lymphocytes in the immunotherapy group suggests that MIF remains positive for a long time. MIF turned negative about the same time as a recurrence or aggravation was confirmed clinically. In the gastric cancer patients who received i.d. injections of oil-attached BCG-CWS according to our 1975 protocol, there was no definite trend obvious in the immunological parameters, but there was a rapid rise in the blast formation rate to PHA by the 2nd and 3rd post-operative months. Even prior to death the rate continued at a high level. The difference in protocol between 1973 and 1975 was reflected in the changes in immunological

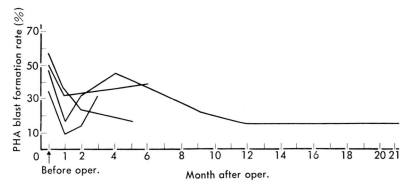

FIG. 2.   PHA blast formation rate in colo-rectal cancer patients receiving BCG (i.d.) (protocol-73)

   In those cases given BCG+autochthonous tumor cells, the PHA blast formation rate decreased rapidly in the first postoperative month.

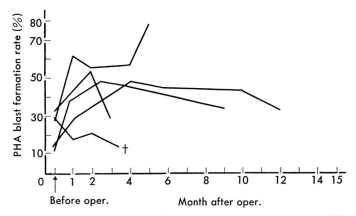

FIG. 3.   PHA blast formation rate in colo-rectal cancer patients receiving BCG-CWS (i.d.) (protocol-75)

   In those cases given oil-attached BCG-CWS, the PHA blast formation rate was somewhat elevated in the first postoperative month.

parameters and was particularly marked in the colo-rectal cancer group. With the 1973 protocol, the PHA blast formation rate decreased rapidly during the first postoperative month, whereas in the group who received oil-attached BCG-CWS, there was no fall in the blast formation rate (Figs. 2 and 3). A rate of over 40% was maintained in cases having a favorable course. The percentage of T cells was high in most of the cases one month after operation. During the first 2–3 months after operation, the MIF level in the immunotherapy group tended to be maintained at a higher level than in the non-immunotherapy group. The oil-attached BCG-CWS group had a stronger MIF after operation than the BCG+autochthonous tumor cell-treated group.

In colo-rectal cancer patients, we are conducting studies on the cytotoxic activity of peripheral blood lymphocytes and blocking factor in serum. So far, these indicate a tendency for the blocking factor to disappear early in cases who are given oil-attached BCG-CWS.

Based on these results, we have instituted postoperative immunotherapy using BCG or BCG-CWS. It is, however, not yet possible to draw conclusions because the number of cases is small and the period of our observations is short. Nonetheless, immunotherapy can be used for gastric and colo-rectal cancer, and even with advanced digestive tract cancer. Provided that immunotherapy follows a surgical operation aimed at leaving a minimal tumor tissue residue, recurrence after operation can be prevented.

REFERENCES

1. Azuma, I., Ribi, E. E., Meyer, T. J., and Zbar, B. Biologically active components from mycobacterial cell walls. 1. Isolation and composition of cell-wall skeleton and component P_3. *J. Natl. Cancer Inst.*, **52**, 95–101 (1974).
2. Baldwin, R. W., Embleton, M. J., Jones, J.S.P., and Langman, M.J.S. Cell-mediated and humoral immune reaction to human tumors. *Int. J. Cancer*, **12**, 73–83 (1973).
3. Eilber, F. R. and Morton, D. L. Sequential evaluation of general immune competence in cancer patients. Correlation with clinical course. *Cancer*, **35**, 660–665 (1975).
4. Falk, R. E., McGregor, A. S., Landi, S., Ambus, U., and Langer, B. Immunostimulation with intraperitoneally administered Bacille Calmette-Guérin for advanced malignant tumors of the gastrointestinal tract. *Surg. Gynecol. Obstet.*, **142**, 363–368 (1976).
5. Fujimoto, S., Green, M. I., and Sehon, A. H. Regulation of the immune response to tumor antigens. II. The nature of immunosuppressor cells in tumor-bearing hosts. *J. Immunol.*, **116**, 800–806 (1976).
6. George, M. and Vaughan, J. H. *In vitro* cell migration as a model for delayed hypersensitivity. *Proc. Soc. Exp. Biol. Med.*, **111**, 514–521 (1962).
7. Gross, N. J. and Libiol, E.Q.A. Monitoring of immunologic status of patients receiving BCG therapy for malignant disease. *Cancer*, **37**, 2183–2193 (1976).
8. Gutterman, J. U., Mavligit, G. M., Gottlieb, J. A., Burges, M. A., McBride, C. M., Einhorn, L., Freireich, E. J., and Hersh, E. M. Chemoimmunotherapy of disseminated malignant melanoma with dimethyl triazeno imidazole carboxamide and Bacillus Calmette-Guerin. *N. Engl. J. Med.*, **291**, 592–597 (1974).
9. Hakala, T. R. and Lange, P. H. Serum induced lymphoid cell-mediated cytotoxicity to human transitional cell carcinomas of the genitourinary tract. *Science*, **184**, 795–797 (1974).
10. Hellström, I., Hellström, K. E., and Sheppard, T. H. Cell-mediated immunity against

antigens common to human colonic carcinomas and fetal gut epithelium. *Int. J. Cancer*, **6**, 346–351 (1970).

11. Hellström, I., Sjögren, H. O., Warner, G. A., and Hellström, K. E. Blocking of cell-mediated tumor immunity by sera from patients with growing neoplasms. *Int. J. Cancer*, **7**, 226–237 (1971).

12. Japanese Research Society for Gastric Cancer. The general rules for the gastric cancer study in surgery. *Japan. J. Surg.*, **3**, 61–71 (1973).

13. Mathé, G., Amiel, J. L., Schwarzenberg, L., Schneider, M., Cattan, A., Schlumberger, J. R., Hayat, M., and Vassal, F. Active immunotherapy for acute lymphobalstic leukemia. *Lancet*, **i**, 697–699 (1969).

14. Mavligit, G. M., Gutterman, J. U., Burgess, M. A., Khankhanian, N., Seibert, G. B., Speer, J. E., Reed, R. C., Jubert, A. V., Martin, R. C., McBride, C. M., Copeland, E. M., Gehan, E., and Hersh, E. M. Adjuvant immunotherapy and chemoimmunotherapy in colo-rectal cancer of the Dukes' C classification. Preliminary clinical results. *Cancer*, **36**, 2421–2427 (1975).

15. Mayer, T. J., Ribi, E. E., Azuma, I., and Zbar, B. Biologically active components from mycobacterial cell walls. II. Suppression and regression of strain-2 guinea pig hepatoma. *J. Natl. Cancer Inst.*, **52**, 103–111 (1974).

16. Minton, J. P. Mumps virus and BCG vaccine in metastatic melanoma. *Arch. Surg.*, **106**, 503–506 (1973).

17. Moore, G. E. and Koike, A. Growth of human tumor cells *in vitro* and *in vivo*. *Cancer*, **17**, 11–20 (1964).

18. Morton, D. L. Immunological factors which influence response to immunotherapy in malignant melanoma. *Surgery*, **68**, 158–164 (1970).

19. Orita, K. Reaction of lymphoid cells on target cells *in vitro*. *Acta Haematol. Japon.*, **31**, 697–709 (1968).

20. Orita, K., Kobayashi, M., Uchida, Y., Yumura, M., Yamamoto, I., Fukuda, H., Kaneda, S., Mannami, T., Kokumai, Y., and Tanaka, S. Reduction of concomintant cell-mediated immunity level in advanced cancer patients. *GANN Monogr. Cancer Res.*, **16**, 141–152 (1974).

21. Orita, K., Miwa, H., and Kaneda, S. Correlation between morphological blast formation rate and functional ^{3}H-thymidine uptake in mixed lymphocyte culture in the presence of PHA. *Acta Med. Okayama*, **28**, 253–257 (1974).

22. Orita, K., Miwa, H., Fukuda, H., Yumura, M., Uchida, Y., Mannami, T., Konaga, E., and Tanaka, S. Preoperative cell-mediated immune status of gastric cancer patients. *Cancer*, **38**, 2343–2348 (1976).

23. Orita, K., Miwa, H., Ogawa, K., Suzuki, K., Sakagami, K., Konaga, E., Kokumai, Y., and Tanaka, S. Reduction of immunological surveillance level in cancer patients. *GANN Monogr. Cancer Res.*, **16**, 53–62 (1974).

24. Orita, K., Miwa, H., Mannami, T., Konaga, E., Yumura, M., Fukuda, H., Uchida, Y., Nakahara, H., and Hayashi, S. Cancer immunotherapy with surgery. *Acta Med. Okayama*, **31**, 217–234 (1977).

25. Takasugi, M. and Klein, E. A microassay for cell-mediated immunity. *Transplantation*, **9**, 219–227 (1970).

26. Tachibana, T. and Ishikawa, M. A new micromethod for quantitation of human T- and B-lymphocytes. *Japan. J. Exp. Med.*, **43**, 227–230 (1973).

27. Yamamura, Y., Azuma, I., Taniyama, T., Ribi, E., and Zbar, B. Suppression of tumor growth and regression of established tumor with oil-attached mycobacterial fractions. *Gann*, **65**, 179–181 (1974).

FUNDAMENTAL AND PRACTICAL ASPECTS OF BCG IMMUNOTHERAPY IN PATIENTS WITH LATE STAGE OF GASTRIC CANCER

Motomichi Torisu, Tetsuro Miyahara, Toshiyuki Yamamoto, Motohiko Harada, Hiroshi Fujiwara, Yukikazu Kitamura, Masafumi Jimi, Keiichi Ohsato, Jiro Tanaka, and Mitsuyuki Fukawa

*Division of Clinical Immunology, First Department of Surgery, Kyushu University School of Medicine**

In the past 5 years, BCG immunotherapy has been carried out in various cancer patients; this paper details our practical experience. In addition, a preliminary result of BCG immunotherapy in patients with late stage gastric cancer is presented. Seventy-seven patients with incurable or inoperable gastric cancer were randomly divided into 2 groups. The first group received BCG immunotherapy, the second underwent gastrectomy or palliative operation without BCG immunotherapy. Analysis of 3-year survival in these groups showed that the BCG-treated group showed significant prolongation of a disease-free interval and survival compared with the control group.

With recent advances in diagnostic techniques including endoscopy or upper gastrointestinal series, patients with early gastric cancer have been encountered in daily medical examinations. However, it has been reported that about one-half of cancer patients had advanced disease at the time of their initial surgical explorations.

These advanced gastric cancer patients, inoperable patients or patients who undergo non-curative operation, usually face death despite the various anticancer therapies. For example, only 7.5% of stage IV gastric cancer patients in our department showed 3-year survival (6).

In the past 5 years, we have carried out BCG immunotherapy in these advanced cancer patients. In this communication, we describe the immunological parameters available for evaluating the host immunological competency and the fundamental background of BCG immunotherapy in cancer patients. In addition, we present a brief summary on the clinical study of BCG immunotherapy for patients with late stage gastric cancer.

Immunological Parameters in Patients with Advanced Cancer

Depression of cell-mediated immunological potency is generally observed in various cancer patients such as leukemia (2, 4), melanoma (1, 2, 5), breast (2), digestive organs (8), and other cancers (8). The following parameters were examined in gastric cancer

---

* Maidashi 3-1-1, Higashi-ku, Fukuoka 812, Japan (鳥巣要道, 宮原哲郎, 山本利幸, 原田素彦, 藤原 博, 北村征和, 自見雅文, 大里敬一, 田中二郎, 府川光之).

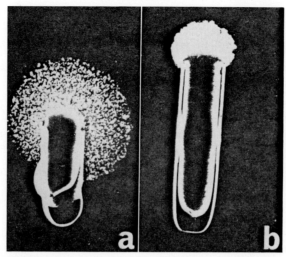

FIG. 1.   Random migration of peripheral leukocytes from a 54-year-old patient who
had gastric cancer with hepatic metastasis
   (a) Random migration activity of leukocytes on admission. His leukocytes migrated
well. (b) Three months after admission. Random migration activity was deeply suppressed.

patients for the assessment of host immunopotency: (1) Subpopulation of T and B lymphocytes in the peripheral blood (7), (2) blast forming activity of lymphocytes to phytohemagglutinin (PHA), and (3) skin tests to PHA, dinitrochlorobenzene, keyhole limpet
hemocyanin, and purified protein derivative (PPD). As previously reported (8), all
of these parameters were remarkably depressed in gastric cancer patients, and the
degree of depression correlated closely with the clinical extent of malignant disease.

   Recently, marked depression of leukocyte mobility in two different assay systems
was detected in various advanced cancer patients. One is the random migration activity and the other is the chemotactic activity of leukocytes in the peripheral blood of
these patients. The measurement of these malfunctions of the leukocyte seemed to be
a useful parameter for the assessment of host immunoreactivity. Figure 1 shows the
random migration activities of leukocytes at different stages of the disease in one patient
with advanced gastric cancer. On admission, his immunological responses were almost
normal and the vigorous random migration activity of leukocytes had been observed
(Fig. 1 a). However, despite various anticancer therapies, his symptoms progressed
and various immunological responses became depressed. In this latest stage, the random
migration activity of this patient's leukocytes was remarkably suppressed (Fig. 1b).
The leukocyte chemotactic assay is a measure of directional mobility of leukocytes
toward various chemoattractants. In this assay, similar to the random migration assay,
the leukocyte activity was impaired with the progress of the disease. These observations
suggest that cancer patients, especially in late stage, are thought to have secondary
deficiency of leukocyte mobility, which may partially explain the susceptibility to infection in these patients.

   In addition, a macrophage chemotactic inhibitor has been found in sera from
cancer patients. This inhibitor prevents guinea pig macrophages from migrating toward
chemoattractants. The appearance of this macrophage chemotactic inhibitor seems to

be correlated with the progress of the disease. As reported by Ward and Berenberg (9) chemotactic factor inactivator (CFI) is known to be present in sera from patients with Hodgkin's disease. The difference between chemotactic inhibitor in cancer patients and CFI in Hodgkin's disease is not yet clear. However, the measurement of serum macrophage chemotactic inhibitor may be a useful marker for the evaluation of host immunopotency.

Effects of BCG as an Immunotherapeutic Agent on Immunological Parameters and Clinical Prognosis in Advanced Cancer Patients

BCG is the most widely used immunostimulating agent for increasing the host defense against tumors in man and animals. In the clinical field, it was reported that the use of BCG can prolong the disease-free intervals, especially in leukemia (4) and melanoma (5).

In the past 5 years, we have carried out BCG immunotherapy in various late stage cancer patients who were inoperable or underwent non-curative operation. Figure 2

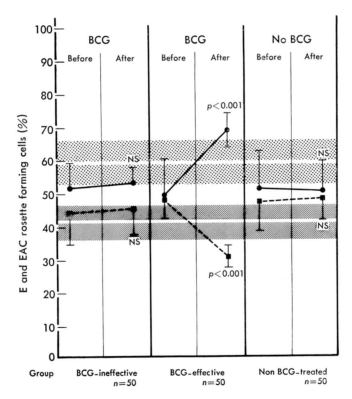

FIG. 2.   Changes of T and B cell subpopulations before, and 1 month after, BCG injection

In BCG-ineffective or control groups, T and B cell proportions did not change significantly after BCG therapy or surgery. In contrast, in BCG-effective group, significant improvement of these proportions was noted soon after BCG therapy compared with before injection. ● T cell; ■ B cell; ▒, ░ mean±SD of 37 healthy volunteers.

shows changes in lymphocyte subpopulations before and 1 month after BCG immunotherapy. One hundred and fifty patients with inoperable or incurable cancers were divided into 3 groups. The first was 50 patients who died within 1 year after ineffective BCG therapy, the second group was 50 patients who survived more than 2 years, and the remaining 50 patients without BCG immunotherapy, who succumbed within 1 year, served as a control. All 100 patients receiving BCG showed the marked depression of T cell levels and elevated B cell levels before BCG inoculation. After BCG inoculation, in the BCG-ineffective group, the T cell level remained depressed and the difference before and after BCG therapy was not significant. In contrast, in the BCG-effective group, the T cell level increased markedly to above the normal range, $69.8 \pm 5.5\%$. The difference in T cell number before and after BCG treatment was statistically significant ($p < 0.001$). Other immunological parameters also improved significantly after BCG treatment parallel to the changes of T and B cell subpopulations. These findings suggest that BCG may enhance the immunopotency of cancer patients and that there is a significant correlation between cell-mediated immunoreactivity and the clinical course of malignant disease.

Maintenance of Immunopotentiation by BCG

The most important essentials for the success of BCG immunotherapy is to maintain the high levels of immunoreactivity of cancer patients by additional injections of BCG under the continuous careful monitoring of various parameters. As described previously (8), even if the suppressed immunoreactivity of patients with advanced cancer can be successfully enhanced by a single injection of BCG, various immunological responses still decrease with time. Once host immunopotency becomes depressed after BCG inoculation, it seems irreversible and is difficult to recover by additional injections of BCG. Consequently, the host succumbs to the rapid tumor growth. Thus, the immunoreactivity enhanced by BCG in patients with cancer does not last for a long period (8). Therefore, the determination of the optimal time for a booster injection becomes practically important. Besides the various immunological parameters described above, observation of Koch's phenomenon (3) seemed to be a useful method for this purpose (8). Briefly, 1 μg of PPD was injected on the anterior aspect of the arm contralateral to BCG injection. Twenty-four hours later, the site of injection of BCG was examined, and the size of erythema was graded. If the erythema appeared and exceeded 2.5×2.5 cm in size, a booster injection was considered not yet necessary. In contrast, the appearance of a weaker reaction indicated the necessity of an additional injection of BCG. The determination of the optimal time for a booster injection is necessary in carrying out the immunotherapy and for this purpose various immunological parameters and Koch's phenomenon should be examined frequently so as not to lose the opportune moment.

BCG Immunotherapy in Patients with Late Stage Gastric Cancer

From the standpoint mentioned above, a brief summary of BCG immunotherapy for patients with gastric cancer which is the most frequently encountered malignant disease in Japan will be given.

1) Patients

Seventy-seven patients with stage IV gastric cancer were entered in the trial, 39 in the BCG-treated group and 38 in the control group, as shown in Table I. Numbers of patients and ranges of age in these 2 groups were essentially the same. In this trial 28 (72%) out of 39 BCG-treated patients and 29 (76%) out of 38 control patients underwent the non-curative gastrectomy and the remainder in both groups received the palliative operation. The degree of histological differentiation of cancers is thought to have an intimate effect on survival. In the present study, the proportions of histological types in these 2 groups was similar and no discrepancy of histological types was noted between the BCG-treated and control groups.

TABLE I. BCG Immunotherapy in Gastric Cancer (Stage IV)

Group	Age (yr.)	Operability		Histology	
		Non-curative	Inoper-able		
39 patients treated with BCG	23–79	28	11	Poorly differentiated adenocarcinoma	22
				Moderately differentiated adenocarcinoma	4
				Well-differentiated adenocarcinoma	5
				Signet ring cell carcinoma	8
38 patients (control)	25–82	29	10	Poorly differentiated adenocarcinoma	19
				Moderately differentiated adenocarcinoma	6
				Well-differentiated adenocarcinoma	3
				Signet ring cell carcinoma	11

2) Protocol for immunotherapy

BCG immunotherapy was performed according to our standard protocol previously described (*8*). In brief, 20 mg of living BCG was given intradermally on the volar aspect of the forearm as an initial dose. The time for booster injection was determined from various immunological parameters and Koch's phenomenon. If necessary, 1–5 mg of BCG was given as an additional booster dose. However, the use of a high dose of living BCG at the time of reinjection can cause various side effects. Therefore, other non-specific immunostimulants such as Levamisole, PS-K, or OK-432 were used to reduce the additional BCG dose. In addition, in patients with carcinomatosus peritonitis accompanied with a large amount of ascitic fluid, intraperitoneal injection of OK-432 or BCG cell-wall skeleton (*10*) was carried out to reduce the ascites.

3) Survival rate

The percent survival results of BCG-treated and control groups are shown in Fig. 3. In the control group, a steep decline in survival range occurred and the 3-year survival decreased to 8.2%. In contrast, patients in BCG-treated group showed a more steady decline curve which gave a higher percent survival at any time of the study compared with the control curve. Three-year survival of this group elevated to the extent of 20%.

The mean survival periods in these 2 groups are shown in Table II. In BCG-treated and control groups, mean survival periods were 15.8 and 7.9 months, respec-

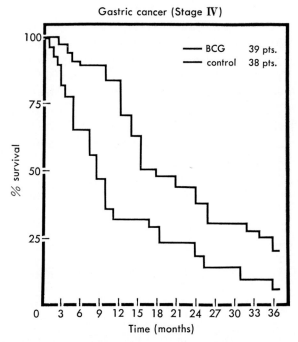

FIG. 3. Effect of BCG immunotherapy on 3-year survival of patients with stage IV gastric cancer

TABLE II. Randomized Study of Gastric Cancer (Stage IV)

Group	Range (months)	Mean survival (months)	Statistical significance
39 patients treated with BCG	2.5–36	15.8	$p < 0.001$
38 patients (control)	1.3–36	7.9	

tively. The difference in these 2 groups was statistically significant ($p < 0.001$). From these observations, it might be suggested that the enhancement of immune response by BCG prolongs the disease-free interval and survival in patients with late stage gastric cancer.

REFERENCES

1. Eilber, F. R., Nizze, J. A., and Morton, D. L. Sequential evaluation of general immune competence in cancer patients: Correlation with clinical course. *Cancer*, **35**, 660–665 (1975).
2. Gutterman, J. U., Mavligit, G. M., Burgess, M. A., Cardenas, J. D., Blumenschein, G. R., Gottlieb, J. A., McBride Ch. M., McCredie, K. B., Bodey, G. P., Rodriguez, V., Freireich, E. J., and Hersh, E. M. Immunotherapy of breast cancer, malignant melanoma, and acute leukemia with BCG: Prolongation of disease-free interval and survival. *Cancer Immunol. Immunother.*, **1**, 99–107 (1976).
3. Koch, R. I. Weitere Mittheilungen über ein Heilmittel gegen Tuberculose. *Deutsch. Med. Wochenschr.*, **13**, 1029–1032 (1890).

4. Mathé, G., Amiel, J. L., Schwartzenberg, L., Schneider, M., Catton, A. R., Schlumberger, J. R., Hayat, M., and De Vassel, F. Active immunotherapy for acute lymphoblastic leukemia. *Lancet*, **i**, 697–699 (1969).

5. Morton, D. L., Eilber, F. R., Malmgren, R. A., and Wood, W. C. Immunological factors which influence response to immunotherapy in malignant melanoma. *Surgery*, **68**, 158–164 (1970).

6. Ohsato, K., Itoh, H., and Nagata, T. Five years survival in various stages of gastric cancer in our surgical department. *Geka Chiryo (Surg. Diagn. Treat.)*, **15**, 437–441 (1972) (in Japanese).

7. Tachibana, T. and Ishikawa, M. Quantitation of T and B lymphocytes. *Japan. J. Exp. Med.*, **43**, 227–230 (1973).

8. Torisu, M., Fukawa, M., Nishimura, M., Harasaki, H., Kai, S., and Tanaka, J. Immunotherapy of cancer patients with BCG: Summary of four years experience in Japan. *Ann. N. Y. Acad. Sci.*, **277**, 160–186 (1976).

9. Ward, P. A. and Berenberg, J. L. Defective regulation of inflammatory mediators in Hodgkin's disease: Supernormal levels of chemotactic-factor inactivator. *New Engl. J. Med.*, **290**, 76–80 (1974).

10. Yamamura, Y., Azuma, I., Taniyama, T., Sugimura, K., Hirao, F., Tokuzen, R., Okabe, M., Nakahara, W., Yasumoto, K., and Ohta, M. Immunotherapy of cancer with cell-wall skeleton of *Mycobacterium bovis*-Bacillus Calmette-Guérin: Experimental and clinical results. *Ann. N. Y. Acad. Sci.*, **277**, 209–227 (1976).

CLINICAL TRIALS. III.
IMMUNOTHERAPY
OF ACUTE LEUKEMIA

CHEMOIMMUNOTHERAPY OF ACUTE
MYELOCYTIC LEUKEMIA

James F. Holland, J. George Bekesi, and Janet Cuttner

*Department of Neoplastic Diseases, Mount Sinai School of Medicine**

The prolongation of survival periods of AKR mice with spontaneous leukemia treated with combination chemotherapy plus immunization with neuraminidase-treated AKR spleen cells was observed. This and other experimental data allowed clinical trials in acute myelocytic leukemia with neuraminidase-treated allogeneic myeloblasts. The clinical results indicate that neuraminidase-treated cells constitute a highly effective immunotherapeutic adjuvant. The usefulness of methanol-extraction residue (MER) of BCG in cancer immunotherapy is also discussed.

We have demonstrated a major augmentation of cure rate in mice bearing leukemia L1210 (*1*) by using chemotherapy and immunotherapy in the form of neuraminidase-treated leukemic cells of the same strain (*2, 3*). Other neuraminidases do not work, apparently because they do not remove nearly so much sialic acid with 2–6 linkage as does the *Vibrio cholerae* neuraminidase. Upon incubation the leukemogenicity of cells is eliminated but their immunogenicity is enhanced. Major protection can be demonstrated in immunoprophylaxis experiments (*2, 3*). Treatment with the nitrosourea, methyl 1-(2-chloroethyl)-3-cyclohexy-1-nitrosourea (CCNU), led to 20% cures by chemotherapy alone. In addition to the chemotherapy, immunization with the specific tumor on day 3 or 6, or 9, 11, or 15 after transplantation, using 10^7 neuraminidase-treated L1210 leukemic cells, caused as many as 90% of animals to survive for 60 days or more. If the tumor burden is allowed to become larger, by allowing a longer time for tumor to grow before chemotherapy starts, chemotherapy is less effective and chemoimmunotherapy is also less effective, attaining a maximum of 50% survival. Cure of the L1210 leukemia in animals treated by nitrosoureas alone allowed 90% of them to withstand a challenge of 1,000 viable L1210 cells. Those cured by the chemotherapy plus immunotherapy, however, withstood a challenge of 10^4 in all animals, and 90% in two experiments withstood 10^5 or 10^6 cells—100 to 1,000 times more resistant (*4*).

Chemoimmunotherapy in AKR Mice with Spontaneous Leukemia

Leukemia L1210 is a transplanted lymphocytic tumor and the possibility of genetic drift between tumor and host, allowing for changes that would propitiate immunotherapy, prompted us to study autochthonous AKR leukemia. Immunization alone with neuraminidase-treated leukemic thymocytes from other old AKR mice, given either intraperitoneally or subcutaneously, to newly diagnosed AKR leukemic mice

---

* New York, New York 10029, U.S.A.

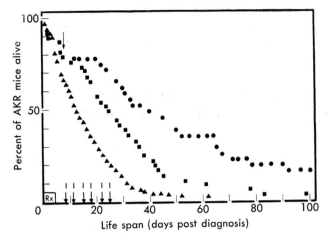

FIG. 1. Effect of chemotherapy and chemotherapy+immunization with neuraminidase-treated leukemic (AKR) spleen cells
      ▲ historical control;   ■ vincristine+dexamethasone;   ● vincristine+dexame-
thasone and immunization.

caused no augmentation of survival. Reducing the leukemic body burden by chemotherapy before giving immunotherapy, however, caused major survival extension (Fig.
1). Based upon these observations in an autochthonous tumor (*1, 5*), we initiated a study
of human acute myelocytic leukemia. This leukemia was chosen because suggestive
evidence of immunogeneity of myeloblasts existed, and because the poor results with
chemotherapy alone made it an easier disease than acute lymphocytic leukemia in
which to undertake highly experimental treatments.

Chemoimmunotherapy of Acute Myelocytic Leukemia

1. Immunization with neuraminidase-treated myeloblasts

Leukemic blasts are harvested from untreated patients with acute myelocytic
leukemia who have leukocytosis, using a Haemonetics Centrifuge. If granulocytes re-
present more than 5% of harvested cells they are removed by glass or nylon adherence.
Thereafter myeloblasts and other nonadherent cells are frozen in a programmed manner in 10% dimethyl sulfoxide. They are thawed immediately prior to use, separated
from nonviable cells by centrifugation on a human serum albumin cushion, and then
incubated with *Vibrio cholerae* neuraminidase. This enzyme, which requires calcium
to attach to the cell surface, is removed by multiple washes in ethylenediaminetetra-
acetate so that neuraminidase itself is not given to the patient, only the cells minus
their sialic acid. Each batch of cells is reserved for a particular patient in quantity for
at least a treatment period of 6 months. Each batch of cells is analysed for its sialic
acid content and is demonstrated to be immunogenic in mixed cell cultures. Those
few which are poorly immunogenic are not used. Pooled cells are not employed.

Immediately after washing following the incubation with neuraminidase, cells are
injected into patients with acute myelocytic leukemia in remission from chemotherapy.
Some 50 intradermal sites are chosen to provide stimulus to multiple lymph node areas

and to allow the largest possible exposure at the surface of interaction between immuno-gen and the host's responding cells. Multiple intradermal areas of injection are a sig-nificant feature that differentiates this from other types of cellular immunotherapy that have been given (6). In some patients we have also used injections of the methanol extract of BCG organisms (MER). Microscopically, the delayed cutaneous hypersen-sitivity lesions at the site of cell injections show inflammatory mononuclear cells and immunoblasts. The leukemic cells disappear; thousands of inoculations have been given without leukemic cellular growth or tumefaction.

2. Clinical evaluation of chemoimmunotherapy of acute myelocytic leukemia

The results of a clinical trial of patients with acute myelocytic leukemia (AML) randomly allocated to receive chemotherapy only or neuraminidase-treated cells in association with chemotherapy show important differences. The chemotherapy used is cytosine arabinoside and daunorubicin for induction, and then monthly courses of cytosine arabinoside in combination with a rotating cycle of thioguanine, cyclophos-phamide, and CCNU. Because remission in our control arm appeared short, a group of patients in the Cancer and Leukemia Group B study #7421 (CALGB) was selected who had been treated with a chemotherapeutic regimen identical to patients in this study. Since one illusory way to get a good looking treatment effect is to have a poor control, the CALGB control was also used since it represents the universe of patients treated by the same drugs. The difference between the neuraminidase-treated cells and both control subsets is significant (Fig. 2). Patients were disqualified if they were over 60, had received a slightly altered chemotherapy, had missed a marrow examination at the times set by the rigid protocol, or for similar infractions. The disqualified patients were not selectively eliminated because their results did not conform to our hypothesis (Fig. 3). The combined set of all treated patients, qualified and disqualified makes larger group sizes (Fig. 4). The graph is truncated at 36 months. Five neuraminidase-cell

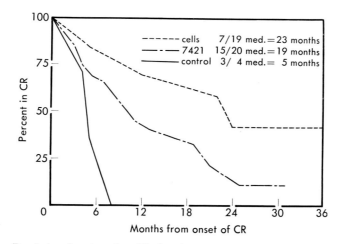

FIG. 2.   Remission duration of qualified patient
Patients with acute myelocytic leukemia treated with indicated chemotherapy (CR) based on cytosine arabinoside and daunorubicin. Control patients and patients immunized with neuraminidase-treated leukemia cells were randomly allocated. #7421 is a universe of patients treated with identical CR in CALGB.

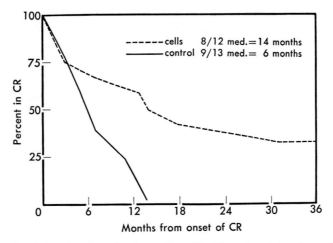

FIG. 3. Remission duration of patients disqualified for minor infractions of the protocol

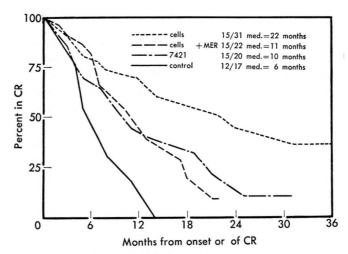

FIG. 4. Remission duration of all treated patients
See the legends for Figs. 2 and 3.

immunized patients are still in complete remission beyond 5 years. The remission times and survival are significantly different from contemporaneous controls and from the "universe" of controls of CALGB patients using the same chemotherapy.

Furthermore, a group of patients was treated with MER in addition to the neuraminidase-treated cells (Fig. 4). This additional treatment in some way interferes with the immunizing effect and returns patients to a status as if they were receiving chemotherapy alone.

3. *Immunological parameters*

We have been able to recognize *in vitro* correlates of this alteration in remission duration. The group of patients immunized by cells alone has progressively increasing blastogenesis to phytohemagglutinin (PHA) and pokeweed mitogen, and a rising number of T cells (7). The group of patients who received cells plus MER has a similarly increased number of T cells, but there is a progressive diminution in the PHA and pokeweed responses. We interpret this to be the appearance of a population of suppressor cells, evoked by MER, which alters the response of T and B cells to the mitogens. On cessation of MER administration to a few patients whose *in vitro* data suggested this phenomenon, remission has persisted and restoration of *in vitro* blastogenesis has occurred. Even though they are part of the cells-plus-MER subset, such patients appear to have longer remissions than patients continued on a full dose of MER with cells who relapse prematurely. Thus, excess immunologic stimulation appears possible with the biologic equivalent of tumor enhancement.

Chemoimmunotherapy with MER of Acute Myelocytic Leukemia

A separate investigation that has 733 patients entered is now in progress under the study chairmanship of Dr. Cuttner in the Cancer and Leukemia Group B. It is an attempt to demonstrate the value of MER used alone as an immunotherapeutic agent in acute myelocytic leukemia. The design of the study called for a standard chemotherapeutic regimen of induction, cytosine arabinoside and daunorubicin. A random segment of patients received MER on the first day of induction and monthly during maintenance. Another subset received MER during remission maintenance only. The third arm is a control receiving only chemotherapy (8). Five hundred and nine patients have been subjected to an interim analysis. There is an increase in remission frequency, 58%, associated with MER in the group of patients below the age of 60, *versus* 52% for those who did not receive MER. Adding in the 180 patients over the age of 60 for the entire group, and adjusting the two groups for equal age distribution, 48% reached M1 marrow in the MER-treated group, and 46% in those who did not receive MER. Thus MER does not make an important difference to the total population of patients who are immunized on the first day. In terms of remission induction, however, in those patients who had negative skin tests to a battery of recall antigens, MER administration on day one led to 57% remission, compared to 44% for those who had chemotherapy alone. Indeed, the changes in the group can reasonably be ascribed in port to conversion to MER reactor status of patients who were anergic to recall antigens. In such patients remission frequency was increased to the same level as for patients who were positive reactors to recall antigens.

Preliminary data on remission duration are available for two different chemotherapeutic maintenance regimens. One regimen consisted of cytosine arabinoside and thioguanine in repeated courses. For patients on this chemotherapy who received no MER, the median remission duration is 12 months; for those who received MER in maintenance only the median remission duration is 17 months; and, for uncertain reasons, those who received MER in both phases, induction and remission, have a median remission of 12 months. The other maintenance regimen called for half as much thioguanine; with their monthly courses of cytosine arabinoside, patients received vincristine and dexamethasone on alternate months. In this second subset the median remission duration of the chemotherapy-treated patients is 11 months, for those who received MER in both induction and remission, median remission was 19 months. The MER effects seem to be influenced by the chemotherapy, but since we are dealing with small sample sizes, representing only 200 patients in remission, the differences are not yet statistically significant. Other data suggest that specific doses of a particular immunostimulatory agent influence its effect (9). In addition, specific components of chemotherapeutic regimens may influence the effects of immunotherapy, just as the timing and relationship between chemotherapy and immunotherapy may.

Neuraminidase-treated cells appear for the moment to have specificity and to be a highly effective immunotherapeutic adjuvant, albeit expensive and complex. MER is relatively inexpensive, subject to further refinement, transportable, stable, safe, and noninfectious. In preliminary assessment of a large series of patients it demonstrates some efficacy in acute myelocytic leukemia.

Acknowledgment

This work was supported in part by a contract with the National Cancer Institute CB 43879; by grant from the National Cancer Institute CA 15936, CA 16118, and the T. J. Martell Memorial Foundation for Leukemia Research.

REFERENCES

1. Bekesi, J. G. and Holland, J. F. Combined chemotherapy and immunotherapy of transplantable and spontaneous murine leukemia in DBA/2 and AKR mice. *In:* "Recent Results in Cancer Research," Vol. 47, ed. by G. Mathé, Springer-Verlag, Berlin, p. 357 (1974).

2. Bekesi, J. G., St. Arneault, G., and Holland, J. F. Increase of leukemia L1210 immunogenicity by vibrio cholerae neuraminidase treatment. *Cancer Res.*, **31**, 2130 (1971).

3. Bekesi, J. G., St. Arneault, G., Walter, L., and Holland, J. F. Immunogenicity of leukemia L1210 cells after neuraminidase treatment. *J. Natl. Cancer Inst.*, **49**, 107 (1972).

4. Bekesi, J. G., Roboz, J. P., Walter, L., and Holland, J. F. Stimulation of specific immunity against cancer by neuraminidase treated tumor cells. *Behring Inst. Mitt.*, **55**, 309 (1974).

5. Bekesi, J. G., Roboz, J. P., Zimmerman, E., and Holland, J. F. Treatment of spontaneous leukemia in AKR mice with chemotherapy, immunotherapy, interferon and virazole. *Cancer Res.*, **36**, 631 (1976).

6. Holland, J. F. and Bekesi, J. G. Immunotherapy of human leukemia with neuraminidase modified cells. *Med. Clin. North Am.*, **60**, 539 (1976).

7. Bekesi, J. G., Holland, J. F., and Roboz, J. P. Specific immunotherapy with neuraminidase-modified leukemic cells. *Med. Clin. North Am.*, **61**, 1083 (1977).

8. Cuttner, J., Glidewell, O., and Holland, J. F. Advances in the treatment of acute leukemia. *In* "Recent Advances in Cancer Treatment," Raven Press, New York, pp. 13–18 (1977).

9. Perloff, M., Holland, J. F., Lumb, G. J., and Bekesi, J. G. Effects of methanol extraction residue of Bacillus Calmette-Guerin (MER) in man. *Cancer Res.*, **37**, 1191(1977).

GANN Monograph on Cancer Research 21, 1978

IMMUNOTHERAPY WITH BCG OR ITS DERIVATIVES IN ACUTE MYELOGENOUS LEUKEMIA

Susumu KISHIMOTO, Koichi ARAKI, and Taro SAITO

Second Department of Internal Medicine,
*Kumamoto University Medical School**

Current immunotherapy in acute myelogenous leukemia (AML) by the use of live BCG or its derivatives is reviewed. Immunotherapy usually consisted of administration of live BCG by scarification or multiple-puncture with or without autologous or allogeneic myeloblasts between courses of the maintenance chemotherapy after having achieved full remission. The efficacy of live BCG generally depended on the strain, viability, absence of free antigens, dose, route, and schedule of administration. Immunotherapy with live BCG alone or in combination with maintenance chemotherapy was usually effective in prolonging the median duration of remission and survival. A methanol extraction residue prepared from BCG was also effective when given alone or combined with allogeneic, irradiated, neuraminidase-treated myeloblasts. Cell-wall skeleton (CWS) identified as a "mycolic acid-arabinogalactan-mucopeptide" complex caused a significant prolongation of median survival compared with that of historical control patients, when AML patients in remission were kept on CWS intradermal injections combined with maintenance chemotherapy. Many immunological parameters, including delayed-type hypersensitivity to recall antigens, T cell counts, phytohemagglutinin responsiveness, blastogenic response, and cell-mediated cytotoxicity of peripheral lymphocytes to allogeneic blastoid cells, were enhanced in most cases while in remission. In some patients evidence for the development of immune response to autochthonous leukemic cells was obtained. This seems to indicate the rationale for immunotherapy. The toxicity due to BCG immunotherapy largely depended on the route of administration. These complications include malaise, fever, hepatic dysfunction, granulomatous hepatitis, and generalized tuberculosis. No major toxicity was observed in CWS-treated patients.

There has been currently great interest in the use of BCG vaccine in the therapy of human cancer because of promising results in prophylactic and therapeutic experiments in various animal systems and in studies in man reported recently. Immunotherapy with BCG vaccine is effective in prolonging remission duration and survival in acute leukemia. This was first reported by Mathé and his co-workers (*12*). Immunotherapy was effective in more than tripling the remission duration of acute lymphoblastic leukemia (ALL). More recently, BCG immunotherapy, with or without irradiated leukemic cells, has been applied to the treatment of acute myelogenous leukemia

---

* Honjo 1-1-1, Kumamoto 860, Japan (岸本 進, 荒木弘一, 斎藤太郎).

(AML) (*7*, *19*, *26*). This is also effective in prolonging duration of survival and/or remission compared to chemotherapy controls. In contrast, some negative results of BCG immunotherapy in ALL were reported (*10*, *20*). These negative results were criticized by Hersh *et al.* (*9*) who claimed that the failure might result from inadequate or suboptimal cytoreductive therapy before starting BCG immunotherapy in patients with advanced, relatively refractory diseases, or from the use of a relatively low dose of a relatively ineffective strain of BCG, or of a very low dose of BCG. Later, it became clear that the efficacy of BCG vaccine depends on the strain, proportion of viable organisms, absence of free soluble antigens, dose, route, and schedule of administration. Hence, it is not easy to obtain a BCG vaccine with a constant potency for clinical use.

On the other hand, BCG immunotherapy in patients with cancer may lead to serious complications (*22*). These are more frequent when given intratumorally than when given intradermally by the multiple-puncture technique. These complications include marked malaise, temperature rise, hepatic dysfunction, granulomatous hepatitis, and generalized tuberculosis. Accordingly, live BCG is not necessarily a safe immunopotentiator. It is conceivable that one of its derivative products or subfractions would be safer, invariable in potency and devoid of some of the side effects displayed by live BCG, when used as an immunopotentiator. From these considerations, varying kinds of constituents have been prepared from the BCG strain. Among these there are the methanol extraction residue (MER), cord factor, water-soluble adjuvant, mycobacterial adjuvant, and antitumor fractions (MAAF), as well as the cell-wall skeleton (CWS). All of them are effective in some types of immunopotentiation and some have been structurally identified. In this article, a review of immunotherapy with subfractions of BCG is presented and compared to that with live BCG, in acute myelogenous leukemia.

BCG and Its Derivatives

All BCG preparations are not the same in immunological and antitumor efficacy. Cell-mediated immunity is most augmented by the Pasteur, and least augmented by the Glaxo, strains, while the Phipps, Tice, and Montreal strains are intermediate (*11*). The dose of BCG given is also critical and high doses such as 6×10^8 cells per treatment are more effective immunotherapeutically than one or more log lower doses. The presence of dead organisms or free soluble antigen or both in a BCG preparation can completely or partially abrogate the efficacy of the living organisms. The standard lyophilized BCG preparations usually contain both a large amount of free soluble antigen and approximately 90% dead organisms and thus are not optimal. Fully viable preparations free of soluble antigens are better in immunotherapeutic and antitumor activity in animal systems. MER prepared from BCG is known to be effective in the immunoprophylactic and immunotherapeutic action against tumors in animals. Also, the addition of MER to chemotherapy, 1 mg intradermally, between courses of maintenance chemotherapy is reported to prolong remission duration and survival in acute myelogenous leukemia (*2*). CWS prepared from BCG is identified as "mycolic acid-arabinogalactan-mucopeptide" complex as shown in Fig. 1, and confirmed to possess a potent adjuvant activity, and capability of inducing adjuvant arthritis. When given in oil-attached droplets, it has shown immunotherapeutic efficacy in both experimental

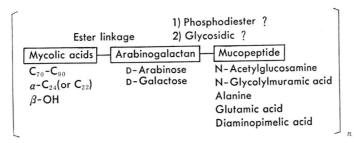

FIG. 1. Chemical structure of CWS prepared from *Mycobacterium bovis* strain BCG (*1*)

tumor systems (*1, 13*), human lung cancer (*27, 29*), and melanoma (*28*). A water-soluble adjuvant prepared by digestion of the cell wall with lysozyme is considered to consist of "arabinogalactan-mucopeptide" devoid of mycolic acid. This is also confirmed to have an adjuvant activity in animals, but has not yet been used for immunotherapy of human malignancies.

Immune Status During Immunotherapy

A therapy should not be called an immunotherapy unless the therapeutic effects are proved to be mediated by the immunological mechanisms elicited by the therapy. In view of this, the immune status has been followed using various immunological parameters in patients receiving immunotherapy. Needless to say, immunotherapy of leukemia and other human malignancies has been based on the concept that immune responsiveness, particularly cell-mediated immunity, has an important effect on tumor growth. The principal aim of immunotherapy is to boost the level of general cellular immunocompetence and to generate or increase specific reactivity to tumor-associated antigens. There have been a few studies on cell-mediated immunocompetence of leukemic patients undergoing therapy with either live BCG or its subfraction. Cell-mediated immunocompetence, as measured by various *in vivo* and *in vitro* tests is generally correlated with a good prognosis, whereas immunodepression generally has been associated with a poor prognosis.

Whether BCG immunotherapy could increase the lymphocytes was assessed by Oldham *et al.* (*15*). After having attained full remission by standard chemotherapy, 52 children with ALL were kept on immunotherapy with a Glaxo strain of BCG. All of these patients showed an increase in peripheral blood lymphocytes. Ekert *et al.* (*4*) also reported a similar result that 11 of 12 patients with ALL in full remission demonstrated a significant increase of lymphocyte counts in both the peripheral blood (PB) and bone marrow after initiation of BCG therapy. This increase in circulating lymphocytes was attributed to T lymphocytes. Figure 2 shows the changes in PB lymphocytes (PBL) in leukemic patients before and during BCG-CWS therapy in our trial. Nine of them were AML and 1 acute monocytic leukemia (AMoL) in full remission and 1 AML in partial remission when BCG-CWS was initially given. Shortly after the initiation of BCG-CWS therapy there was a significant increase of PBL ($p < 0.05$) in 7 of 11 cases. However, the leukocyte count decreased concurrently with relapse. T and B cell counts revealed that T cells, but not B cells, were responsible for the increase in PBL in these patients. The change of T cells paralleled fairly well that of

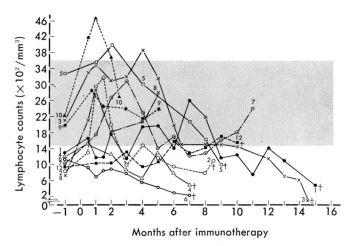

FIG. 2.   Peripheral blood lymphocytes of 9 AML, 1 AMoL and 1 smoldering AML patients before and during chemoimmunotherapy with BCG-CWS

The number in the graph corresponds to case number. + denotes death. Shadowed area indicates normal range of peripheral blood lymphocyte counts.

PBL. A similar increase in the circulating T cells was also reported in ALL patients receiving BCG therapy or AML patients receiving MER (8). Delayed-type hypersensitivity (DTH) of the skin to either specific, autologous, or allogeneic leukemic cell extracts or nonspecific antigens has been widely used as a parameter of the immune status of patients on immunotherapy. DTH to the autologous leukemic cell extracts in patients was investigated in relation to prognosis by Oren and Herberman (16) who demonstrated that survival of more than 12 months was 63.6% in the DTH positive group but only 36.3% in the DTH negative group. Moreover, Char et al. (3) showed that positive reactions to autologous blast extracts were obtained in 20 of 44 ALL and in 16 of 19 AML in remission. By contrast, positive responses were markedly diminished in relapse. By immunotherapy with BCG and allogeneic blast cells, the incidence of positive reactions did not increase to the immunizing or other allogeneic blast cells in comparison with the reactions before receiving the cells. Oldham et al. (15) stated that 10 of 23 ALL patients tested after 2–8 years of immunotherapy with BCG scarification showed positive skin test responses to extracts of allogeneic tumor-derived lymphoblastoid cell lines, whereas no positive responses were observed at 60 and 120 days of immunotherapy. The 3M KCl extracts gave a higher reactivity than crude membrane extracts. Seventy-one percent of these ALL patients tested during the first 120 days of immunotherapy responded to primary sensitization to picryl chloride compared to only 10% of normal subjects. On the other hand, apparent depression in response was observed in vivo to candidin and mumps antigen. Hyperimmunization with BCG may have blocked, transiently, the specific recall response to other antigens. In the trial of Sokal et al. (21), chronic myelogenous leukemia (CML) patients were treated with BCG and irradiated allogeneic leukemic cells and tested for DTH responses to 6 recall antigens and leukemic cell homogenates. With increasing immunization, there was an increase in frequency and intensity of positive reactivity. A similar positive conversion of skin reaction to purified protein derivative (PPD) was also ob-

TABLE I. Delayed-type Hypersensitivity Responses of 9 AML and 1 AMoL Patients
Before and During Chemoimmunotherapy with BCG-CWS

	Diameter of erythema (mm)		
	PPD	Candidin	DNCB
Before immunotherapy	9 (3–15)	15 (0–30)	− (−−+)
After immunotherapy			
in remission	33 (19–65)	28 (0–55)	╫ (+-╫)
after relapse	7 (0–16)	11 (0–39)	− (−−±)
Reactivity	Before and after / before and therapy in remission / after relapse		
Negative to positive[a]	5/0	4/0	7/0
Positive to positive	5/2	4/2	1/0
Positive to negative	0/5	0/5	0/5
Negative to positive	0/0	2/0	2/2
Number evaluable	10/7	10/7	10/7

[a] Positive: Over 10 mm erythema for PPD, over 20 mm erythema for Candidin, and definite erythema elicited by 0.1% DNCB at 48 hr.

served in 8 of 9 AML patients given BCG immunotherapy by Vogler and Chan (26). In Gutterman's trial (7), 7 of 14 patients with AML were anergic to PPD and 5 other recall antigens at the end of consolidation chemotherapy; 6 of 7 negative reactors became responsive to all antigens following BCG immunotherapy and remained in remission, whereas the remaining non-reactor relapsed shortly afterwards. As indicated in Table I, BCG-CWS therapy in our AML patients in remission enhanced reactivity to PPD, candidin and dinitrochlorobenzene (DNCB). Positive reactivity was 100% for PPD, 70% for candidin, and 80% for DNCB after 1–2 months of the immunotherapy. DTH responses seem to be well correlated to the patients' clinical status. Ekert *et al.* (4) treated 12 ALL children in remission following continuous chemotherapy for at least 12 months with intermittent courses of chemotherapy alternating with BCG inoculation during the drug-free intervals. Ten of 12 children who remained PPD-negative relapsed during this study. Few changes in skin reactivity to the other antigens such as candidin, streptokinase-streptodornase (SK-SD), and mumps were found. In addition, there was an increase in the relative response to phytohemagglutinin (PHA) in children with low initial responses. In our trial, PHA response rose in approximately 90% of cases following CWS therapy and fell down to below normal range at relapse. The PHA response was fairly well reflected by the circulating T cell counts and clinical status of the patients.

The search for antigen characteristic of leukemic cells is certainly of great importance in terms of diagnostic and therapeutic significance. The evidence for such antigens specific to human leukemic cells is based largely on observations that DNA synthesis by lymphocytes from patients in remission is stimulated by autochthonous leukemic cells (25). Taylor *et al.* (23) treated 6 AML patients in remission with live BCG and allogeneic AML blasts. Two of these patients demonstrated the blastogenic responses of remission lymphocytes to autochthonous and allogeneic AML blasts used for immunization which reached a peak at 48–72 hr of culture. This early peak response seems to be consistent with the concept of a population of lymphocytes pre-immunized to antigens carried by the blasts. In addition, the remission lymphocytes exhibited an enhanced cell-mediated cytotoxicity (CMC) not only against the allogeneic AML blasts used in immunotherapy but also to Burkitt's lymphoma cells or lymphoblastoid cells when CMC was assayed after 6-day culture with AML blasts in immunotherapy (24). A similar intensification of the reaction of remission lymphocytes to autochthonous AML or ALL blasts was also reported in patients immunized with their own leukemic blasts (5, 6, 14, 18).

Remission Duration and Survival

Remission duration and survival are most reliable parameters for evaluating the efficacy of immunotherapy. Powles et al. (19) made a prospective randomized study involving 42 patients with AML. After achieving full remission by standard chemotherapy, they were divided into two groups. One group received maintenance chemotherapy alone, the other the identical chemotherapy combined with immunotherapy consisting of irradiated allogeneic leukemic cells and BCG. Actuarial analysis predicted a median remission length for the chemotherapy group of 188 days compared with 312 days for the immunotherapy patients, and a median survival for the chemotherapy group of 303 days compared with 545 days for the group receiving chemotherapy combined with immunotherapy. Later, more encouraging data were reported by the same author (17). A study along similar lines has been made by Vogler et al. (26). AML patients achieving full remission and having consolidation chemotherapy were randomized to either 4 weeks of BCG therapy by the tine technique twice weekly followed by methotrexate (MTX), or MTX alone. The median duration of total remission in 25 patients in the BCG-MTX group was 42 weeks with 2 patients still in their first remission, whereas that in 33 patients in the MTX alone group was 32 weeks with 7 patients still in remission. The median duration of remission from the time of BCG therapy was 24.3 weeks in the BCG-MTX group and 13.4 weeks in the MTX alone group ($p < 0.05$). The median survival from diagnosis was 120 weeks in the BCG-MTX group and 75 weeks in the MTX alone group ($p < 0.05$). These data indicate that a short course of BCG therapy increases remission duration and survival in AML. Gutterman et al. (7) have demonstrated that the median duration of remission in 14 patients with AML receiving fresh, liquid, pellicle-grown Pasteur strain BCG vaccine by scarification approximately weekly between courses of remission maintenance chemotherapy was more than 72 weeks compared to that of 60 weeks in 21 patients on chemotherapy alone ($p = 0.04$).

As regards the clinical efficacy of subfractions or derivatives of BCG, Cuttner et al. (8) have shown that MER is effective in prolonging remission duration in AML patients. Besides, very encouraging data have been reported using neuraminidase-treated allogeneic myeloblasts, with or without MER, by Bekesi et al. (2). They allocated 53 patients with AML to 3 groups following successful remission induction with standard chemotherapy. All received cyclical maintenance chemotherapy, every 28 days. Neuraminidase-treated allogeneic myeloblasts or neuraminidase-treated myeloblasts plus MER were given to 2 groups. In each immunization, 10^{10} neuraminidase-treated myeloblasts were injected intradermally in approximately 48 sites. One milligram MER

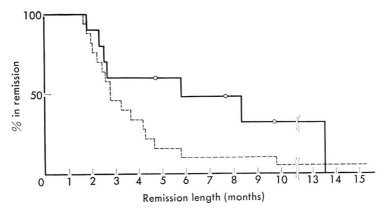

FIG. 3.   Comparison of remission length between BCG-CWS group of 9 AML and 1 AMoL patients and historical control of 17 AML patients

Solid line: BCG-CWS plus maintenance chemotherapy group. Broken line: historical control group. Open circle: still in remission.

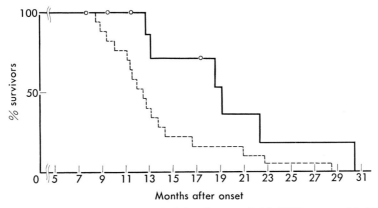

FIG. 4.   Comparison of overall survival time between BCG-CWS group of 9 AML and 1 AMoL patients and historical control group of 17 AML patients

Solid line: BCG-CWS plus maintenance chemotherapy group. Broken line: historical control group. Open circle: still in alive.

was given in 5–10 intradermal sites. The median remission duration was 20 weeks in the control group and more than 78 weeks in the groups receiving either form of immunotherapy. These differences were highly significant. Seventeen of 21 patients given chemotherapy alone died by 90 weeks compared with 5 of 32 patients on the immunochemotherapy. In our trial to evaluate the efficacy of CWS, 10 patients with AML were given 200 μg CWS intradermally at 4 divided sites, biweekly for the first 8 weeks and then monthly after having achieved complete remission by combined chemotherapy. Maintenance chemotherapy with prednisolone in cyclic 4-day courses of either 6-mercaptopurine (6MP), cytosine arabinoside, or MTX was given at intervals between injections. The median duration of remission was 23 weeks in the chemotherapy-plus-CWS group compared with 11 weeks in 17 historical control patients, as shown in Fig. 3. This difference is statistically not significant. However, Fig. 4 clearly indicates a significant difference $(p<0.05)$ in median survival between the chemoimmunotherapy group (19.2 months) and the chemotherapy group (12.5 months).

Adverse Reactions

The toxicity of BCG immunotherapy largely depends on the route of administration. As shown by Sparks *et al.* *(22)*, the intratumor injection of BCG is associated with more frequent and more severe complications than the administration of BCG by multiple-puncture tine technique or scarification. In some cases, granulomatous hepatitis was reported to develop after intratumor injections of BCG. In our 12 patients treated with CWS, erythema occurred followed by ulceration over the injected sites. This ulceration usually disappeared in 4–5 weeks. On some occasions, local lymphadenopathy was observed, with or without low-grade fever. Neither hepatotoxicity nor systemic complications were noted.

REFERENCES

1. Azuma, I., Taniyama, T., Hirano, F., and Yamamura, Y. Antitumor activity of cell-wall skeletons and peptidoglycolipids of mycobacteria and related microorganisms in mice and rabbits. *Gann*, **65**, 493–505 (1974).
2. Bekesi, J. G., Holland, J. F., Cuttner, J., Silver, R., Coleman, M., Jarowski, C., and Viceguerra, V. Immunotherapy in acute myelocytic leukemia with neuraminidasetreated allogeneic myeloblasts with or without MER. *Proc. AACR and ASCO*, 184 (1976).
3. Char, D. H., Lepourhiet, A., Leventhal, B. G., and Herberman, R. B. Cutaneous delayed hypersensitivity responses to tumor-associated and other antigens in acute leukemia. *Int. J. Cancer*, **12**, 409–419 (1973).
4. Ekert, H., Jose, D. G., Wilson, G. C., Mattews, R. N., and Lay, H. Intermittent chemotherapy and immunotherapy with BCG in remission maintenance of children with acute lymphocytic leukemia: Effects upon immunological function. *Int. J. Cancer*, **16**, 103–112 (1975).
5. Fridman, W. H. and Kourilsky, F. M. Stimulation of lymphocytes by autologous leukemic cells in acute leukemia. *Nature*, **224**, 277–279 (1969).
6. Gutterman, J. U., Mavligit, G., McCredie, K. B., Freireich, E. J., and Hersh, E. M. Autoimmunization with acute leukemia cells: Demonstration of increased lymphocyte responsiveness. *Int. J. Cancer*, **11**, 521–526 (1973).
7. Gutterman, J. U., Rodriguez, V., Mavligit, G. M., Burgess, M. A., Gejan, E., Hersh, E. M., McCredie, K. B., Reed, R., Smith, T., and Bodey, G.P.S. Chemoimmunotherapy of adult acute leukemia: Prolongation of remission in myeloblastic leukemia with BCG. *Lancet*, **ii**, 1405–1409 (1974).
8. Cuttner, J., Bekesi, J. G., and Holland, J. F. Chemoimmunotherapy of acute leukemia using MER. *Proc. AACR and ASCO*, 196 (1976).
9. Hersh, E. M., Gutterman, J. U., Mavligit, G. M., Reed, R. C., and Richman, S. P. BCG vaccine and derivatives. *J. Am. Med. Assoc.*, **235**, 646–650 (1976).
10. Leventhal, B. G., Lepourhiet, A., Halterman, R. H., Henderson, E. S., and Herberman, R. B. Immunotherapy in previously treated lymphatic leukemia. *Natl. Cancer Inst. Monogr.*, **39**, 177–187 (1973).
11. Mackaness, G. B., Auclair, D. J., and Lagrange, P. H. Immunopotentiation with BCG.

I. Immune response to different strains and preparations. *J. Natl. Cancer Inst.*, **51**, 1655–1667 (1973).

12. Mathé, G., Amiel, J. L., Schwarzenberg, L., Schneider, M., Cattan, A., Schlumberger, J. R., Hayat, M., and De Vassal, F. Active immunotherapy for acute lymphoblastic leukemia. *Lancet*, **i**, 697–699 (1969).

13. Meyer, T. J., Ribi, E. E., Azuma, I., and Zbar, B. Biologically active components from mycobacterial cell walls: Suppression and regression of strain-2 guinea pig hepatoma. *J. Natl. Cancer Inst.*, **52**, 103–111 (1974).

14. Ohno, R., Morishima, Y., Kato, Y., Sugiura, S., Takeyama, H., Wakayama, K., Ueda, R., Ezake, K., and Yamada, Y. Studies of tumor-specific antigens on leukemic cells by mixed lymphocyte-leukemic cell cultures. *Nihon Ketsueki Gakkai Zasshi* (*Acta Haematol. Japon.*), **40**, 177–182 (1977) (in Japanese).

15. Oldham, R. K., Weiner, R. S., Mathé, G., Breard, J., Simmler, M. C., Carde, P., and Herberman, R. B. Cell-mediated immune responsiveness of patients with acute lymphocytic leukemia in remission. *Int. J. Cancer*, **17**, 326–337 (1976).

16. Oren, M. E. and Herberman, R. B. Delayed cutaneous hypersensitivity reactions to membrane extracts of human tumor cells. *Clin. Exp. Immunol.*, **9**, 45–56 (1971).

17. Powles, R. Immunotherapy for acute myelogenous leukemia. *Br. J. Cancer*, **28** (Suppl. I) 262–265 (1973).

18. Powles, R. L., Balchin, L. A., Hamilton Fairley, G., and Alexander, P. Recognition of leukemia cells as foreign before and after autoimmunization. *Br. Med. J.*, **1**, 486–489 (1971).

19. Powles, R. L., Crowther, D., Bateman, C.J.T., Beard, M.E.J., McElwain, T. J., Russell, J., Lister, T. A., Whitehouse, J.M.A., Wrigley, P.F.M., Pike, M., Alexander, P., and Hamilton Fairley, G. Immunotherapy for acute myelogenous leukemia. *Br. J. Cancer*, **28**, 365–376 (1973).

20. Leukemia Committee and the Working Party on Leukemia in Childhood. Report on the treatment of acute lymphoblastic leukemia. *Br. Med. J.*, **4**, 189–194 (1974).

21. Sokal, J. E., Aungst, C. W., and Grace, J. T. Immunotherapy of chronic myelogenous leukemia. *Natl. Cancer Inst. Monogr.*, **39**, 195–198 (1973).

22. Sparks, F. C., Silverstein, M. J., Hunt, J. S., Haskell, C. M., Pilch, Y. H., and Morton, D. L. Complications of BCG immunotherapy in patients with cancer. *N. Engl. J. Med.*, **289**, 827–828 (1973).

23. Taylor, G. M., Freeman, C. B., and Harris, R. Response of remission lymphocytes to autochthonous leukemic myeloblasts. *Br. J. Cancer*, **33**, 501–511 (1976).

24. Taylor, G. M., Harris, R., and Freeman, C. B. Cell-mediated cytotoxicity as a result of immunotherapy in patients with acute myeloid leukemia. *Br. J. Cancer*, **33**, 137–143 (1976).

25. Viza, D. C., Bernard-Degani, O., Bernard, C. L., and Harris, R. Leukemia antigens. *Lancet*, **ii**, 493–494 (1969).

26. Vogler, W. R. and Chan, Y. K. Prolonging remission in myeloblastic leukemia by Tice-strain Bacillus Calmette-Guérin. *Lancet*, **ii**, 128–131 (1974).

27. Yamamura, Y., Ogura, T., Yoshimoto, T., Nishikawa, H., Sakatani, M., Itoh, M., Masuno, T., Namba, M., Yazaki, H., Hirano, F., and Azuma, I. Successful treatment of the patients with malignant pleural effusion with BCG cell-wall skeleton. *Gann*, **67**, 669–675 (1976).

28. Yamamura, Y., Yoshizaki, K., Azuma, I., Yagura, T., and Watanabe, T. Immunotherapy of human malignant melanoma with oil-attached BCG cell-wall skeleton. *Gann*, **66**, 355–363 (1975).

29. Yasumoto, K., Manabe, H., Ueno, M., Ohta, M., Ueda, H., Iida, A., Nomoto, K., Azuma, I., and Yamamura, Y. Immunotherapy of human lung cancer with BCG cell-wall skeleton. *Gann*, **67**, 787–795 (1976).

CHEMOIMMUNOTHERAPY OF ACUTE MYELOGENOUS LEUKEMIA IN ADULTS WITH BCG CELL-WALL SKELETON

Kazumasa YAMADA, Kohei KAWASHIMA, Yasuo MORISHIMA,
Koji ESAKI, Yoshihisa KODERA, and Ryuzo OHNO

*First Department of Internal Medicine,
Nagoya University School of Medicine**

The present clinical trial was designed to evaluate toxicity, immuno-logical response, and possible therapeutic benefits of immunotherapy with cell-wall skeleton of BCG (BCG-CWS) in adult patients with acute non-lymphocytic leukemia. After remission was induced and con-solidated with a quadruple combination chemotherapy (daunorubicin/ cytosine arabinoside/6-mercaptopurine riboside/prednisolone; DCMP), BCG-CWS was added to the bimonthly schedule of maintenance DCMP chemotherapy. Immunotherapy with 200 μg of oil-attached BCG-CWS mixed with 10^7 autochthonous leukemia cells was administered intra-dermally at either the upper or lower extremities every week until relapse. No serious systemic side effect attributable to BCG-CWS was noted. The most important side effect was a local skin reaction. Indurated papules developed in all patients, resulting in draining ulcerations. A substantial increase in immunological reactivity of the patients receiving BCG-CWS was noted. The skin test response to purified protein deriva-tive (PPD), Varidase, and *Candida* extract showed a definite increase. *In vitro* lymphocyte blastogenic response to PPD, concanavallin A (Con A), and pokeweed mitogen (PWM) also revealed a significant increase. The therapeutic effectiveness of BCG-CWS was evaluated in 16 adult patients with acute, non-lymphocytic leukemia receiving immunotherapy and compared to that for a historical control group of 40 consecutive patients given chemotherapy alone. The 16 BCG-CWS treated patients had a significantly longer survival time than the control group, yet there was no difference in the duration of the first remission between the two groups. Factors attributable for the improved survival in the BCG-CWS treated group are discussed.

There have been an increasing number of clinical trials in patients with a variety of neoplastic diseases which demonstrated that immunotherapy using living cells of *Mycobacterium bovis* strain BCG can favorably improve prognosis, at least temporarily, and tilt the balance in favor of the patient. The difficulties inherent in the use of living bacteria, in terms of safety, stability, and reproducibility, however, have stimulated interest in non-viable materials.

---
* Tsurumai-cho 65, Showa-ku, Nagoya 466, Japan (山田一正, 川島康平, 森島泰雄, 江崎幸治, 小寺良尚, 大野竜三).

The cell-wall skeleton of BCG (BCG-CWS) was developed by Yamamura and Azuma (*1, 2, 14*) and its chemical structure, adjuvant activities, and antitumor activities have been extensively investigated. This paper reports our clinical trial of BCG-CWS in chemoimmunotherapy of acute leukemia. The main purpose of this study was to evaluate the local and systemic toxicity of BCG-CWS, to assess its immunostimulatory effect, and to examine whether BCG-CWS prolongs remission duration and survival period of acute leukemia patients.

Remission Induction

Remissions for acute non-lymphocytic leukemia (ANLL) had been induced by 4-day courses of quadruple (DCMP) combination chemotherapy, namely, cytosine arabinoside 120 mg/m², daunorubicin 25 mg/m², 6-mercaptopurine riboside 300 mg/m², all given intravenously, and prednisolone 60 mg/m², orally. Remissions of acute lymphocytic leukemia (ALL) had been induced by DVP chemotherapy combination: Daunorubicin 25 mg/m² intravenously, on day 1–5, vincristine 2 mg intravenously, on day 1, and prednisolone 60 mg/m² daily, days 1–4, orally. Cycles were repeated every 14–21 days.

Chemoimmunotherapy (Fig. 1)

After remission was induced and consolidated by 2 cycles of regimens used for induction therapy, BCG-CWS was added to the maintenance chemotherapy regimen at the time of discharge from the hospital. During maintenance therapy, multiple combination chemotherapy was given as described above for remission induction, except that 4-day courses were repeated every 2 months. In between the maintenance chemotherapy over a period of 2 months, BCG-CWS was given weekly until the patient relapsed.

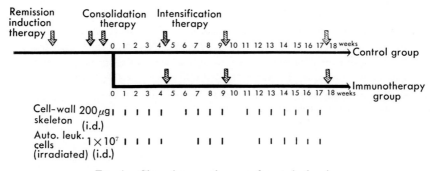

FIG. 1.   Chemoimmunotherapy of acute leukemia

Preparation of Oil-attached BCG-CWS

A uniform suspension of small oil droplets associated with BCG-CWS was obtained by grinding BCG-CWS with light mineral oil (Drakeol 6VR, Pennsylvania

Refining Co., Buttler, Pa.). Oil-attached BCG-CWS was sterilized by heating at 60° for 30 min.

Preparation of Autologous Leukemia Cells

Autologous leukemia cells were collected either from the peripheral blood or the bone marrow of the patients in the study before any treatment. These leukemia cells were washed with phosphate-buffered saline (PBS), and suspended in tissue culture medium RPMI 1640 with 1% dimethyl sulfoxide (DMSO) and 10% fetal calf serum at a concentration of $5\text{--}20 \times 10^6$ cells/ml. This suspension was frozen in multiple sterile ampules. These ampules were stored in liquid nitrogen and when required, rapidly thawed at 37°, and washed three times in PBS(−).

Method of Administration of BCG-CWS

A 0.1 ml portion of the mixture containing 200 μg of BCG-CWS and 1×10^7 autologous leukemia cells (5,000 rad irradiated) was injected intradermally at two sites, either on the upper arms or thighs.

Immunological Evaluation

1) Skin test for delayed hypersensitivity

Cutaneous hypersensitivity was evaluated by the delayed skin reaction against purified protein derivative (PPD) (Japan BCG Laboratory, Tokyo), *Candida* (Hollister-Stier Laboratories, Los Angeles, Calif.). Streptokinase-streptodornase (Varidase; Lederle Laboratories, Pearl River, N.Y.). Recall antigens were applied on day 1 of each treatment cycle to the volar forearm by inoculation in a volume of 0.1 ml through a 25-gauge needle. Delayed hypersensitivity response to these antigens was read after 48 hr.

2) In vitro lymphocyte blastogenic response to PPD, concanavalin A (Con A), and pokeweed mitogen (PWM)

Peripheral blood lymphocytes (1.5×10^5) suspended in 1 ml of RPMI 1640 medium enriched with 20% human AB serum were cultured with 1 μg PPD, 50 μg Con A, or 30 μg PWM using the microtest plate 3034 (Falcon, Oxnard, Calif.), in a CO_2 incubator (5% CO_2 and 95% air) for 5 days. Seven hours before the end of culture, 1 μCi of ³H-thymidine (³H-TdR) was added and the cells were harvested by the multiple Automated Sample Harvestor II (Microbiological Associates, Bethesda, Md.). DNA synthesis was measured by the amount of radioactivity incorporated using a liquid scintillation spectrophotometer.

3) In vitro lymphocyte blastogenic response to autologous leukemia cells

Stimulation of lymphocytes in the autologous mixed leukemia cell cultures was estimated by incubation with ³H-TdR, and DNA synthesis by determining the amount of incorporated radioactivity. DNA synthesis in the stimulated cells (in this case leukemia cells) was inhibited by prior treatment with either 25 μg/ml of mitomycin C or

4,000 rad irradiation. The mixed cell culture was performed as described above for *in vitro* lymphocyte blastogenesis to PPD, *etc.*, except that intact or irradiated leukemia cells were added to the reacting remission lymphocytes at a ratio of 1: 1 or 1: 2.

4) Serum immunoglobulin levels

The concentration of IgG, IgA, and IgM was measured by the single radial diffusion method before and during chemoimmunotherapy.

Result of Immunology with BCG-CWS

Twenty-nine patients in complete remission were entered in the study. They consisted of 21 adults (13 acute myelogenous leukemia (AML), 3 acute monocytic leukemia (AMoL), and 5 ALL) and 8 children (3 AML and 5 ALL).

1) Toxicity (Table I)

All 29 patients developed erythema and induration at the sites of injection mostly after the first vaccination. Ulceration developed in 27 patients which was generally apparent after 3 to 4 vaccinations. The ulcer discharged a serosanguinous material, which was consistently negative for significant pathogens when tested by gram stain and culture. Lesions healed slowly by granulation tissue, leaving a flat scar within 2 to 4 weeks.

Frequently, lesions from previous injections of BCG-CWS became reactive with subsequent injections at near or remote sites. In some of the patients, the dose of BCG-CWS was reduced because of these local skin reactions, to 20 µg at one site, and the interval of administration was prolonged to every 2 weeks. In this manner, the cutaneous reactions were tolerated and accepted by all patients.

No patient developed hepatomegaly or splenomegaly during the course of treatment. Eight patients developed lymphadenopathy in a lymph node draining BCG-CWS lesions. Systemic toxicity commonly consisted of malaise and fever on the day of BCG-CWS administration and for a short while thereafter. Two patients reported fever above 38.5° on the day of immunotherapy. The frequency of febrile responses did not increase with the duration of treatment. In 6 patients, hepatic dysfunctions were observed, manifested by a mild degree of elevated transaminase and alkaline phosphatase. These

TABLE I. Complications of Chemoimmunotherapy with CWS-BCG (29 Cases)

Skin reaction	
Induration	29 (100%)
Ulcer	27 (93)
Adenopathy	8 (30)
Fever	
$<38.0°$	6 (22)
$\geqq 38.0°$	2 (7)
Eruption	1 (4)
Hepatic dysfunction	6 (22)

were temporary and reversible in spite of continuation of BCG-CWS therapy. In one patient, an acne-like generalized skin eruption developed.

2) *Immunological response*

The skin test response to PPD showed that substantial stimulation of cellular immune reactivity was achieved with BCG-CWS immunotherapy (Fig. 2). Before BCG-CWS injection, 27% of patients showed a positive skin test to PPD (more than 10 mm in diameter) and after 8 vaccinations 82% became positive. To *Candida* and Varidase, the number of patients with a positive skin test also increased but less striking than in PPD. Figure 3 shows *in vitro* lymphocyte blastogenesis induced by 1 μg/ml PPD. All but one patient, who had a weak response (less than 10^4 cpm) before BCG-CWS therapy, showed an increased response during immunotherapy. Lymphocytes from most of the patients responded to Con A and PWM in the normal range before

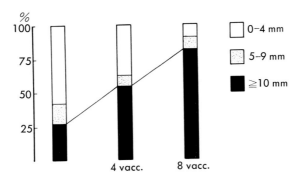

FIG. 2.   Skin test response to PPD

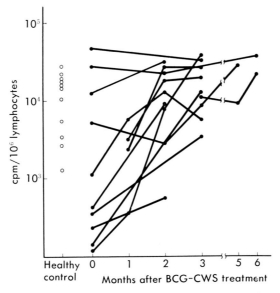

FIG. 3.   Lymphocyte blastogenic response to PPD

BCG-CWS vaccination. Lymphocytes from patients which showed a subnormal response to these mitogens, however, increased significantly to the normal range after BCG-CWS immunotherapy. Immunoglobulin levels did not show a significant change during immunotherapy.

The *in vitro* lymphocyte blastogenic response to autologous leukemia cells collected at the time of diagnosis was measured in 25 patients before immunotherapy and in some patients at the follow-up examination. Table II shows the results of one patient with AML in complete remission. A significant blastogenic response to irradiated autologous leukemia cells was noted, indicating that the lymphocytes recognized their own leukemia cells as not-self. As shown in Table III, 8 of 10 AML patients and 4 of 5 AMoL patients had a significant response to their own leukemia cells before immunotherapy. However, only 2 of 10 ALL patients showed a positive blastogenic response. Within the limited number of patients so far studied, there appeared to be no positive correlation between intensity of response and prognosis.

TABLE II. Lymphocyte Blastogenic Response to Autochthonous
Leukemia Cells (T. K., AML, 27 yr. M)

	^{3}H-TdR incorporation	
	Nov. 28, 1975	Dec. 24, 1975
	cpm$\pm$SD^a (SI)	cpm$\pm$SD^a (SI)
Lymph. $\times$ Lymph.	809$\pm$ 43 (1)	1,351$\pm$ 164 (1)
Lymph. $\times$ Blast	899$\pm$ 246	22,465$\pm$1,796 (16.6)*
Lymph. $\times$2$\times$ Blast	487$\pm$ 62	20,982$\pm$ 178 (15.5)*
Lymph. $\times$ Blast	12,185$\pm$2,505 (5.4)**	21,610$\pm$ 428 (11.3)*
Lymph. $\times$2$\times$ Blast	13,969$\pm$1,448 (7.6)**	19,228$\pm$2,358 (7.0)*
Lymph. $\times$ Blast	7,796$\pm$ 556	6,398$\pm$2,057
Blast $\times$ Blast	3,707$\pm$ 213	7,883$\pm$1,375
Lymph. $\times$ Blast	—	310$\pm$ 22
Lymph. · PHA	5,466$\pm$1,143	9,210$\pm$1,580
Lymph. · PWM	9,167$\pm$1,330	17,528$\pm$1,923

^{a} cpm/10^6 lymphocytes/hr.
* $p<0.01$; ** $p<0.05$.
☐ : irradiated.

TABLE III. Blastogenic Response of Remission Lymphocytes against
Autochthonous Leukemia Cells

Type	No. of cases	Blastogenic response		% positive
		Positive	Negative	
AML	10	8 (2)	2	80
AMoL	5	4	1	80
ALL	10	2 (2)	8	20
Total	25	14 (4)	11	56

( ) positive only against non-irradiated leukemia cells.

3) Remission length and survival time

Sixteen adult patients (13 AML and 3 AMoL) receiving chemoimmunotherapy were compared to a group of 40 consecutive patients who were consolidated and maintained with intermittent use of DCMP combination chemotherapy and cyclic maintenance chemotherapy, consisting of 100 mg 6-mercaptopurine orally q.d., 100 mg cyclophosphamide orally q.d., and 80 mg cytosine arabinoside per m² b.i.w., each alternating every 4 weeks in a cyclic fashion. Two groups were analysed for those factors known to affect the prognosis of adult leukemia. As shown in Table IV, the two groups of patients were comparable with regard to histological diagnosis and age distribution.

Figure 4 shows the duration of remission and time of relapse for the two groups of patients. The median duration of remission for the group on chemotherapy alone was 8 months but 7.8 months for the group on chemoimmunotherapy.

TABLE IV. Distribution of Diagnosis and Age for Chemotherapy
and Chemotherapy+BCG-CWS Groups

Patient characteristics	Chemotherapy (40)		Chemotherapy+CWS (16)	
Diagnosis	(%)		(%)	
AML	34 (85)		13 (81)	
AMoL	6 (15)		3 (18)	
Age (yr.)				
30	26 (65)		8 (50)	
30–40	9 (22)	28	4 (25)	30
55	5 (12)	(Med.)	2 (12)	(Med.)

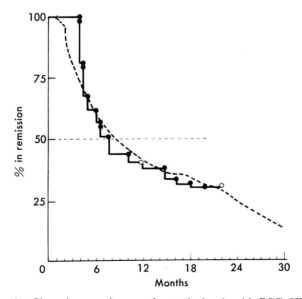

FIG. 4. Chemoimmunotherapy of acute leukemia with BCG-CWS
Remission length for AML in adults

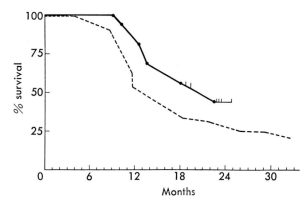

F<small>IG</small>. 5.   Chemoimmunotherapy of acute leukemia with BCG-CWS
Survival time for AML in adults
——— chemotherapy+BCG-CWS; - - - - chemotherapy.

Figure 5 shows the survival time for the two groups of patients. In contrast to the lack of beneficial effect BCG-CWS had in prolonging the first remission length, significant improvement of the survival time was noted for the immunochemotherapy group. The median survival period for the patient group on chemotherapy alone was 13 months, whereas for group with BCG-CWS as well, it was 20.5 months. Six out of 16 patients receiving immunotherapy have survived from 19 to 25 months.

Comments

Until recently, living BCG has attracted preferential attention as an immuno-therapeutic agent for neoplastic disease. When living BCG is used, however, there are several practical disadvantages. Serious side effects, including disseminated BCG infection and granulomatous hepatitis, have been reported when a high dose of live BCG was administered (*10*). Among BCG preparations there are apparently strain differences in virulence and in immunological and antitumor efficacy (*7*). The presence of dead organisms or freely soluble antigens in a BCG vaccine preparation is said to abrogate the efficacy of living organisms (*5*). Thus, standardization and preservation of living BCG seem to be difficult.

BCG-CWS, which is purified from the cells of *M. bovis* strain BCG, is a polymer of the mycolic acid-arabinogalactan-mucopeptide complex. In experimental animals BCG-CWS was shown to possess a potent adjuvant activity in humoral and cell-mediated immune responses and to augment the functions of both helper and cytotoxic T cells (*11*). Its antitumor activity was exhibited in transplantable tumor systems in syngeneic mice (*13*) and in guinea pigs (*8*). The tumor growth of mastocytoma P815-X2, melanoma B16, EL4 leukemia, and Line 10 hepatoma was suppressed when these tumor cells were inoculated with oil-attached BCG-CWS. Systemic and specific tumor immunity was induced in the animals in which tumor growth was suppressed (*1*). A successful clinical trial of BCG-CWS was reported for a case of malignant melanoma (*15*). The primary tumor which was treated intralesionally with oil-attached BCG-CWS regressed together with metastatic inguinal lymph nodes without any significant complications.

In the present study, no serious side effect attributable to BCG-CWS was noted. The temperature elevation was mild and transient. The local skin reactions, however, often became severe with draining ulcers. It usually required 2 to 4 weeks for the lesions to heal. The initial starting dose, 100 μg at two sites, was often reduced and the interval of administration was prolonged because of remaining ulcerative skin lesions. Although these reactions were acceptable and tolerable to most of the patients, the appropriate administration dosage and schedule seem to be 100 μg at two sites weekly until ulcerative local reactions appear, and 50 to 20 μg, depending upon the intensity of the reaction, every 2 weeks at an alternating site of the extremities. The local skin reactions observed during BCG-CWS administration seemed to resemble the reported skin lesions during immunotherapy with the methanol extraction residue of BCG (9). The intensity and the duration of the lesions, however, seem to be less in the case of BCG-CWS.

The rationale for nonspecific immunotherapy is supported by data correlating the relationship between immunocompetence and prognosis of acute leukemia patients. By repeated BCG-CWS administration there was a substantial and consistent increase in the immunological status of the patients. Skin test response to PPD showed a definite increase after several BCG-CWS administrations. Before BCG-CWS only 27% of the patients showed a positive skin reaction to PPD, and after the immunotherapy 82% became positive. Since Japanese adults show about 80 to 85% positive skin test to PPD, BCG-CWS apparently increased the responsiveness to PPD of the leukemia patients to the normal level. In our previous study, only about 45% of adult acute leukemia patients were positive to repeated PPD skin tests during their remission period. Positive skin reactions to *Candida* and Varidase changed from 32 and 57% to 46 and 80%, respectively, after several BCG-CWS administrations. *In vitro* lymphocyte blastogenic response to PPD also showed a definite increase after immunotherapy. In 5 out of 6 patients whose lymphocytes showed subnormal responses to PPD before BCG-CWS immunotherapy, the blastogenic response reached the healthy adult range after several BCG-CWS administrations. Lymphocytes of most of the patients responded to Con A and PWM at the normal level even before BCG-CWS therapy, although lymphocytes which showed a subnormal response to both mitogens responded at the normal level after immunotherapy.

Tumor-specific antigens appear to exist on leukemia blast cells. Several investigators have shown by a variety of *in vitro* and *in vivo* techniques that the leukemic patient can mount a humoral and/or cell-mediated immune response to their own leukemia cells or to tumor antigen extracted from the leukemia cells (3, 4, 6). Twelve of 15 patients with ANLL showed evidence suggesting tumor-specific immunity as measured by lymphocyte blastogenic response to autologous leukemia cells. In contrast, only 2 of 10 patients with ALL had positive response. The results indicate a rationale for the use of nonspecific as well as specific immunotherapy in ANLL, but probably not in ALL. Tumor-specific immunity as measured by lymphocyte blastogenic response to autologous leukemia cells could be correlated with subsequent prognosis (6), yet such evidence was not observed in the present study.

In evaluating the clinical effect of immunotherapy compared to that of historical controls, the present study demonstrated that the 16 BCG-CWS treated adult ANLL patients had a significantly longer survival period than 40 patients maintained on chemotherapy alone and there was no difference in the duration of the first remission between the two groups. The increase in survival length produced is principally made up of two components; prolongation of the first remission and length of survival after the first relapse. The first component, prolongation of the first remission, could not be obtained in this study. It is imperative to emphasize that minimal leukemia cell load is a prerequisite for evoking host ability to kill leukemia cells immunologically. In this sense, our protocol of a maintenance chemotherapy adjunct to immunotherapy is thought not to be intense enough to induce a minimum leukemia cell residue, particularly in terms of the interval of maintenance chemotherapy.

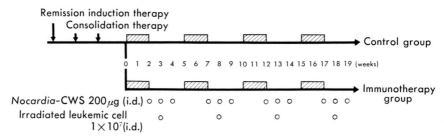

FIG. 6.   Randomized trial of chemoimmunotherapy for actue myelogenous leukemia
///// intensification with quadruple combination chemotherapy.

The prolongation of survival period, after the first relapse, produced by immunotherapy can be provided by two factors: (1) The ease with which patients enter a second and third remission. This is the case which accounts for our data on the therapeutic efficacy of BCG-CWS in terms of prolongation of survival period, *i.e.*, 50% of patients on immunotherapy achieved a second remission. Whittaker and Slater (*12*) presented similar data in their study on immunotherapy of AML using intravenous BCG. Thirty-seven patients were randomised to maintenance treatment with daunorubicin/cytosine arabinoside or to identical chemotherapy and intravenous BCG. The 18 BCG-treated patients had a significantly longer survival time than the 19 patients maintained on chemotherapy alone. There was no difference in the duration of first remission between the two groups and they concluded that improved survival in the BCG group appeared to be due entirely to the high rate of remission at the second and third re-induction therapy. (2) By heightening resistance to microbial infection, and by protecting immunologically reactive tissue from the insults of chemotherapy, BCG-CWS may protect leukemia patients at critical times in the course of the disease against secondary infection, and they make possible more intensive chemotherapy even at a late stage with reduced risk. This interpretation is supported, in part, by demonstration of a substantial increase in immune responses following BCG-CWS therapy.

There have been increasing criticisms on the validity and justification for using a historical control assessment system for the therapeutic benefit of immunotherapy. Reflecting on all the matters discussed above, we have set up a new protocol of chemoimmunotherapy of acute leukemia as shown in Fig. 6. The main aspects of this protocol are as follows: 1) A randomized trial has been employed, 2) *Nocardia rubra*-CWS (*11*) has been used instead of BCG-CWS, and 3) maintenance chemotherapy has been intensified, given monthly instead of every 2 months. This new protocol is under investigation.

REFERENCES

1. Azuma, I., Ribi, E., Meyer, T. J., and Zbar, B. Biologically active components from mycobacterial cell walls. I. Isolation and composition of cell-wall skeleton and component P_3. *J. Natl. Cancer Inst.*, **52**, 95–101 (1974).
2. Azuma, I., Taniyama, T., Hirano, F., and Yamamura, Y. Antitumor activity of cell-wall skeleton and peptidoglycolipids of *Mycobacteria* and related microorganisms in mice and rabbits. *Gann*, **65**, 493–505 (1974).
3. Fridman, W. H. and Kourilsky, F. M. Stimulation of lymphocytes by autologous leukemia cells in acute leukemia. *Nature*, **224**, 277–279 (1969).
4. Gutterman, J. U., Hersh, E. M., McCredie, K. B., Bodey, G. P., Rodriguez, V., and Freireich, E. J. Lymphocyte blastogenesis to human leukemia cells and their relationship to serum factors, immunocompetence, and prognosis. *Cancer Res.*, **32**, 2524–2529 (1972).
5. Hersh, E. M., Gutterman, J. U., Mavligit, G. M., Reed, R. C., and Richman, S. P. BCG vaccine and its derivatives. Potential, practical considerations and precautions in human cancer immunotherapy. *N. Engl. J. Med.* **235**, 646–650 (1976).
6. Leventhal, B. G., Halterman, R. H., and Rosenberg, E. B. Immune reactivity of leukemia patients to autologous blast cells. *Cancer Res.*, **32**, 1820–1825 (1972).
7. Mackaness, G. B., Auzlair, D. J., and Lagrange, P. H. Immunopotentiation with BCG. I. Immune response to different strains and preparation. *J. Natl. Cancer Inst.*, **51**, 1655–1667 (1973).
8. Meyer, T. J., Ribi, E. E., Azuma, I., and Zbar, B. Biologically active components from mycobacterial cell walls. II. Suppression and regression of strain-2 guinea pig hepatoma. *J. Natl. Cancer Inst.*, **52**, 103–111 (1974).
9. Moertel, C. G., Ritts, R. E., Jr., Schutt, A. J., and Hahn, R. G. Clinical studies of methanol extraction residue fraction of Bacillus Calmette-Guérin as an immunostimulant in a patient with advanced cancer. *Cancer Res.*, **35**, 3075–3083 (1975).
10. Sparks, F. C. Hazards and complications of BCG immunotherapy. *Med. Clin. North Am.*, **60**, 499–509 (1976).
11. Taniyama, T., Watanabe, I., Azuma, I., and Yamamura, Y. Adjuvant activity of mycobacterial fractions. *In vitro* adjuvant activity of cell walls of mycobacteria, nocardia, and corynebacteria. *Japan. J. Microbiol.*, **18**, 415–426 (1974).
12. Whittaker, J. A. and Slater, A. J. The immunotherapy of acute myelogenous leukemia using intravenous BCG. Abstracts of "Immunotherapy of Cancer—Present Status of Trials in Man," October 27–29, Bethesda, Md., p. 33 (1976).
13. Yamamura, Y., Azuma, I., Taniyama, T., Ribi, E. E., and Zbar, B. Suppression of tumor growth and regression of established tumor with oil-attached mycobacterial fractions. *Gann*, **65**, 179–181 (1974).
14. Yamamura, Y., Azuma, I., Taniyama, T., Sugimura, K., Hirao, F., Tokuzen, R., Okabe, M., Nakahara, W., Yasumoto, K., and Ohta, M. Immunotherapy of cancer with cell-wall skeleton of *Mycobacterium bovis*-Bacillus Calmette-Guérin: Experimental and clinical results. *Ann. N.Y. Acad. Sci.*, **276**, 209–227 (1976).
15. Yamamura, Y., Yoshizaki, K., Azuma, I., Yagura, T., and Watanabe, T. Immunotherapy of human malignant melanoma with oil-attached BCG cell-wall skeleton. *Gann*, **66**, 355–363 (1975).

GANN Monograph on Cancer Research 21, 1978

SPECIFIC ACTIVE IMMUNOTHERAPY OF ACUTE LEUKEMIA IN CHILDREN AND HOST IMMUNE RESPONSES AGAINST LEUKEMIC ANTIGENS

Tadasu Izawa, Tamotsu Yoshizumi, and Minoru Sakurai

*Department of Pediatrics, Mie University School of Medicine**

Previous evidence from our own and other laboratories indicated that leukemic cells carried a specific and common antigen. Children with acute leukemia were immunotolerant to this antigen on admission or relapse, but had recovered immunologically several months after remission induction. In order to cope with residual leukemic cells during remission, a monthly specific active immunotherapy with BCG and adjuvant was given to 17 children with acute blastic leukemia, combined with maintenance chemotherapy.

One to 4×10^8 8,000 rad irradiated leukemic cells in 2 ml of suspension was injected intracutaneously within the area of 5×5 cm, and BCG was given in the same area of the skin by the multiple-puncture method.

Of the 17 children, two developed hematological relapse within 8 months and one developed central nervous system leukemia after 2 years. The remaining 14 children continued their first remission from 8 to 36 months (median remission duration 17.1 months). Although the clinical course so far has been satisfactory, the effect of chemoimmunotherapy cannot be evaluated, since the time of observation is too short and the patients were not randomized. As immunological parameters, delayed-type skin reaction, *in vitro* lymphocyte cytotoxicity assay, and blastogenic response were performed. These results correlated well with the clinical status of the patients.

It is generally agreed that leukemic cells differ antigenically from normal hematopoietic cells. Our previous evidence also indicates the presence of a specific leukemic antigen, common to leukemic cells among children with acute leukemia (*3*). Untreated children with acute leukemia were immunologically deficient both specifically and nonspecifically. Nonspecific cellular and primary humoral immune responses were generally involved in these children, and delayed-type skin reaction and circulating antibodies against autologous and allogeneic leukemic cell extracts were invariably negative (*4, 5*). Despite the initial immune deficiency, children can recover from it as complete remission continues along with maintenance chemoimmunotherapy. The rational support for specific active immunotherapy lies in experimental leukemic mice (*9*). Up to 53% leukemic mice that had been partially treated by chemotherapy, were cured only by specific immunotherapy combined with various adjuvants. The spleen lym-

---

* Edobashi 2-174, Tsu, Mie 514, Japan (井沢 道, 吉住 完, 桜井 実).

211

phocytes of immunologically cured mice were proved, under cinematographic microscopy, to attack and destroy target leukemic cells.

When leukemic cells were retransplanted to the cured mice, they could not tolerate
more than 1×10^6 cells. This indicated that the immunological eradication of tumor
cells might be limited, and that for successful immunotherapy, the tumor load should
be minimized to a certain threshold by chemotherapy.

Chemoimmunotherapy of Acute Leukemia in Children

Active immunotherapy was started for children with acute leukemia at our institute
in May 1973. By December 1974, 9 children had been on immunotherapy with monthly
subcutaneous injection of $2-4 \times 10^7$ irradiated leukemic cells with BCG as adjuvant.
The clinical results were unsatisfactory (6). Among 9 children, 4 died and 3 relapsed.
In January 1975, the method of chemoimmunotherapy was revised, as in Protocol 7501
(Fig. 1). Autologous and allogeneic irradiated leukemic cells, $1-4 \times 10^8$, were injected
monthly intracutaneously in an area of 2×2 cm, and BCG was given at the same site
of injection by a multiple-puncture method (about 60 needle punctures).

Maintenance chemotherapy consisted of daily, oral 6-mercaptopurine and weekly,
intravenous methotrexate (MTX). Vincristine and steroids, and intrathecal MTX
were given once every 3 months for reinforcement. Maintenance chemotherapy was
suspended one week before and after monthly immunotherapy, when a complete remission continued over 6 months. Eighteen children with acute blastic leukemia were
registered on this protocol and 17 had entered complete remission to receive chemoimmunotherapy. Of the 17 children, 3 relapsed. Two of them had developed hematological relapse within 8 months and the remaining one developed central nervous sys-

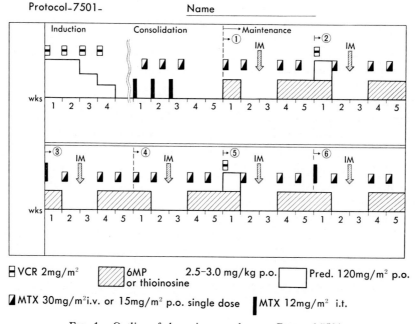

FIG. 1.   Outline of chemoimmunotherapy, Protocol 7501

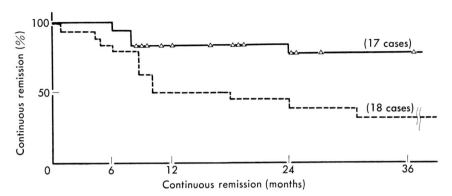

FIG. 2.   Duration of continuous complete remission after initial induction in children with ALL on chemotherapy and chemoimmunotherapy

Chemoimmunotherapy (Protocol 7501); chemotherapy (Total Therapy Protocol VIII).

tem (CNS) leukemia after 2 years. Fourteen children are now in continuous remission for 8 to 36 months, with a median duration of 17.1 months. The evaluation of this chemoimmunotherapy will be carried out in 2 years (Fig. 2).

Mathé *et al.* (7) reported their cumulative survivals of 100 patients with acute lymphoblastic leukemia (ALL), and 23 patients were in continuous remission for over 5 years. He stressed the superiority of active immunotherapy over conventional intensive chemotherapy, pointing out several advantages, including no late relapse and absence of the severe side effects of chemotherapeutics.

Certain groups of American hematologists were rather skeptical of immunotherapy in ALL. They felt that their chemotherapeutic regimen would exceed Mathé's results, and that Mathé's original claim for the benefit of active immunotherapy could not be proved by subsequent studies (1).

Host Immune Responses to the Leukemic Antigens

For the immunologic evaluation of chemoimmunotherapy, children were tested by delayed-type skin reaction, *in vitro* lymphocyte cytotoxicity, and blastogenic response (4).

Table I shows the results of skin tests. Autologous and allogeneic leukemic cell extracts were used as antigen. None of the children showed a positive reaction on admission to either autologous or allogeneic cell extracts, but the rate of positive reaction increased as the remission duration lengthened. The skin reaction turned positive in 6 of 9 children between 6th and 12th month of remission. It appeared that skin reaction correlated well with the clinical status of the patients. The reaction turned negative or weakened when relapse occurred, and it never became positive among those children whose relapse had occurred during early course of therapy.

For the lymphocyte cytotoxicity assay, ^{51}Cr-labeled leukemic cells were cultured with lymphocytes for 8 hr and then the chromium released in the culture medium was counted by a γ-scintillation counter. Figure 3 shows the results. When percent lysis values were plotted according to the skin reaction or the clinical status of children at the time of testing, there was some correlation among them but this is not statistically

TABLE I. Skin Reaction to Autologous and Allogeneic Leukemic Cell Extracts

Clinical status	Admission		Remission duration						Relapse	
			1–6 months		6–12 months		Over 12 months			
Leukemic antigen	Auto.	Allo.	Auto.	Allo.	Auto.	Allo.	Auto.	Allo.	Auto.	Allo.
Positive reaction/ No. tested	0/13	0/58	3/13	42/91	6/9	57/81	3/4	46/65	1/5	6/25
(Positive reaction in %)	(0)	(0)	(23.1)	(46.2)	(66.7)	(70.4)	(75)	(70.8)	(20)	(24)

Auto., autologous leukemic cell extracts; allo., allogeneic leukemic cell extracts.

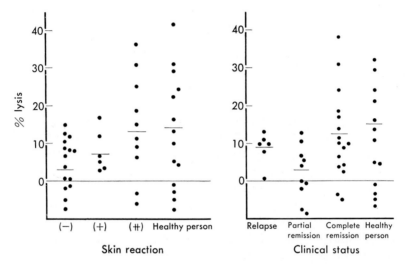

FIG. 3. Lymphocyte cytotoxicity assay against human leukemic cells, and its relation to skin reaction and clinical status of the patients with acute leukemia

significant. Significantly higher values of percent lysis were obtained during remission, but they may still be low at this time.

From our experience with this assay, values of percent lysis varied on each testing so that they could not be compared with each other during the immunotherapy courses.

For the assay of blastogenic response mitomycin C-treated leukemic cells were cultured with lymphocytes for 96 hr and the stimulation index (SI) was obtained by counting ^{3}H-TdR incorporated into the insoluble DNA of lymphocytes. The mean values of SI were higher during complete remission than in early remission or bone marrow relapse. In our survey, SI was not higher than that of acute myelocytic leukemia reported by Powles (8) or by Gutterman (2).

Figure 4 illustrates the plotted SI with patients of different clinical status. In the first two columns, the SI for children with bone marrow relapse is shown, and in the next two columns, with CNS relapse. In the remaining 7 columns SI values for children in complete remission were plotted. The SI was evidently higher among children in remission and interestingly, SI was also higher in children with CNS relapse.

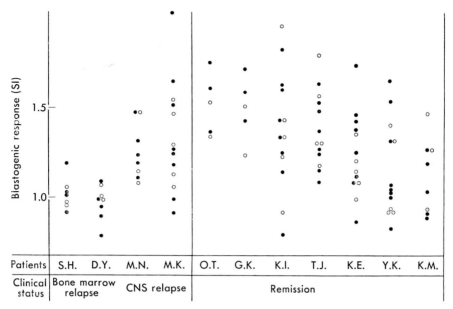

FIG. 4. Lymphocyte blastogenic response to various leukemic cells used as stimulator cells

○ leukemic cells used as antigen for immunotherapy; ● leukemic cells not used as antigen for immunotherapy.

CONCLUSION

Although some hematologists are skeptical of Mathé's initial claim, a rational basis is still in favor of specific active immunotherapy of acute lymphoblastic leukemia, and its clinical effects and methodology should be re-evaluated. Since the immunological eradication of residual leukemic cells is considered to be limited, basic chemotherapy might be essential for successful immunotherapy, thus there is a place for chemo-immunotherapy for maintenance.

REFERENCES

1. Bernstein, I. D. and Wright, P. W. Immunology and immunotherapy of childhood neoplasia. *Pediat. Clin. North Am.*, **23**, 93–109 (1976).
2. Gutterman, J. U., Hersh, E. M., Mavlight, G., and Freireich, E. J. Cell-mediated and humoral immune response to acute leukemia cell and soluble leukemia antigen. *In* "Recent Results in Cancer Research," Vol. 47, ed. by G. Mathé and R. Weiner, Springer-Verlag, Berlin/Heidelberg/New York, pp. 97–112 (1974).
3. Izawa, T., Sakurai, M., Atsuta, Y., and Yoshizumi, T. Antigenicity of leukemia and antiserum therapy. *Shōnika Kiyō* (*Japan. J. Pediat.*), **12**, 346–362 (1966) (in Japanese).
4. Izawa, T. and Sakurai, M. Immune status of children with acute leukemia. *Shōnika Rinshō* (*Japan. J. Pediat.*), **30**, 1007–1012 (1977) (in Japanese).
5. Izawa, T., Sakurai, M., Kamiya, H., and Taki, M. Immunological studies on leukemia, with special references to the circulating antibodies against leukemic antigen. *Int. Congr. Pediat.*, **9-39**, 201–205 (1971).

6. Izawa, T. and Sakurai, M. Active immunotherapy of acute leukemia in children. *Rinshō Men'eki* (*Japan. J. Clin. Immunol.*), **8**, 1099–1104 (1976) (in Japanese).
7. Mathé, G. Cancer active immunotherapy. *In* "Recent Result in Cancer Research," Vol. 55, ed. by G. Mathé, Springer-Verlag, Berlin/Heidelberg/New York, pp. 96–121 (1976).
8. Powles, R. L., Balchin, L. A., Fairley, G. H., and Alexander, P. Recognition of leukemic cells as foreign before and after autoimmunization. *Br. Med. J.*, **1971-1**, 486–489 (1971).
9. Sakurai, M., Uchida, Y., and Izawa, T. Immunotherapy of acute leukemia in children and its fundamental studies. *Gan to Kagaku Ryōhō* (*Cancer Chemother.*), **3**, 439–448 (1976) (in Japanese).

ANTITUMOR EFFECT OF BCG CELL-WALL SKELETON IN ACUTE LEUKEMIA

Hiroyuki Nakamura,[*1] Katsuhiko Miyoshi,[*1] Hirotoshi Shibata,[*1]
Akira Hayashi,[*2] Toru Masaoka,[*1] and Junsuke Yoshitake[*1]

*Center for Adult Diseases, Osaka,[*1] and Third Department of
Internal Medicine, Osaka University Medical School[*2]*

Although demonstrated in murine leukemia, the antitumor activity of BCG has not yet been reported in human leukemia. Two cases of acute leukemia have recently been successfully treated with BCG cell-wall skeleton (BCG-CWS). One patient had acute promyelocytic leukemia, the other had acute myelogenous leukemia, and they relapsed after chemotherapy-induced complete remission. The relapse was detected early by the routine study of blood cells by the leucoconcentration and 5,000 differential methods. Both patients have successfully achieved remissions by the administration of BCG-CWS and they are still in complete remission in the absence of any maintenance chemotherapy. The duration of remission is more than 3 years for the case of acute promyelocytic leukemia and more than 1 year and 8 months for the case of acute myelogenous leukemia.

Recent multi-agent induction chemotherapy produced complete remission in 70 to 80% of adult acute leukemia (*1, 2, 5*). Unfortunately, in most patients the complete remissions are invariably followed by a relapse. This relapse is generally thought to be due to proliferation of the leukemic cells that have persisted and whose presence has not been detected in routine examination (*10*). We have shown that examinations of the cells in the blood of patients in remission are indispensable for early detection of relapse. The leucoconcentration technique is useful for this purpose (*4, 6*). Immunotherapy with BCG has been reported to be effective in prolonging chemotherapy-induced remissions (*3 9, 12, 14, 15*). However, it remains unclear whether BCG has an antitumor effect on the leukemic cells or if it merely prolongs remissions by as yet unknown mechanisms. We have recently observed in two cases of patients with acute leukemia that BCG cell-wall skeleton (BCG-CWS) treatment resulted in the induction of remission, indicating an antitumor effect of this agent on leukemic cells.

Antitumor Effect of BCG in Murine Leukemia

Effective immunotherapy of established murine leukemia has been observed after the administration of BCG alone or in combination with irradiated leukemia cells (*7, 8, 11*). Mathé *et al.* showed that immunotherapy with BCG alone or in combina-

---

[*1] Nakamichi 1-3-3, Higashinari-ku, Osaka 537, Japan (中村博行, 三好勝彦, 柴田弘俊, 正岡徹, 吉武淳介).

[*2] Fukushima 1-1-50, Fukushima-ku, Osaka 553, Japan (林 昭).

tion with irradiated leukemia cells could not only prolong the survival of leukemic mice but also cure murine L1210 leukemia if the number of leukemic cells did not exceed 10^5 per whole body (8). A similar effect of BCG was observed in an isogeneic, transplantable, murine lymphoid leukemia (AKR) growing as an ascites tumor (11). Furthermore, among several cytotoxicity assays tested, only the antibody-dependent lymphocyte-mediated cytotoxicity correlated well with the growth of ascites tumor cells, suggesting that this cytotoxicity may play a major role in the BCG-induced tumor reduction (11).

BCG Immunotherapy of Acute Leukemia

With the development of highly effective regimens for remission induction, leukemic relapse rather than induction failure has now become the major obstacle to successful therapy of acute leukemia. Masaoka *et al.* estimated that 10^{10} to 10^{11} leukemic cells were usually present in the blood when acute leukemia was first diagnosed (6). Although recent combination chemotherapy can reduce the number of leukemic cells to the range of 10^5 to 10^7 (6), it usually fails to eradicate an entire tumor cell population. Mathé concluded that this failure of chemotherapy was inevitable (7), citing the finding of Skipper *et al.* (13) that a given dose of any kind of chemotherapeutic drug killed a constant fraction of cells regardless of the total number of leukemic cells present in the animal. In practice, toxicity of chemotherapeutic agents also limits their use. Consequently, leukemic cells may well remain in the tissues of patients who are considered to be in complete remission (10). Mathé *et al.* showed that immunotherapy could cure an experimental murine leukemia if the number of leukemic cells did not exceed 10^5 (8) and that it might offer a relatively safe method for eradicating residual leukemic cells. There has been an increasing interest in BCG immunotherapy for maintenance treatment of acute leukemia. In fact, BCG given alone or in combination with irradiated leukemic cells has significantly prolonged remissions (3, 9, 12, 14, 15). However, the antitumor activity of BCG has not been reported in acute leukemia.

Antitumor Effect of BCG-CWS in Acute Leukemia

Recently we observed the antitumor effect of BCG-CWS in two cases of patients with acute leukemia.

1) Case histories

Case 1. F. N., a 35-year-old woman was admitted to the Center for Adult Diseases, Osaka, in August 1974, because of fever and vaginal bleeding. A gynecologist found pancytopenia and referred her to this hospital. Physical examination was unremarkable except for the presence of pallor and fever. The hematocrit was 19%, the white cell count was 400/mm³ with 0.8% abnormal promyelocytes (peroxidase-positive; Auer rods present), 22% neutrophils, 75% lymphocytes, 0.4% monocytes, and 1.4% myelocytes. The platelet count was 58,000/mm³. A bone marrow aspiration revealed normal cellularity with 64% of abnormal promyelocytes. The diagnosis of acute promyelocytic leukemia was made and the patient received a 4-day course of daunorubicin and 2 courses of combination chemotherapy (daunorubicin, cytosine arabinoside, 6-mercaptopurine riboside, and betamethasone) which led to complete remission of the disease. 6-Mercaptopurine and methotrexate were administered as maintenance chemotherapy and the patient was discharged in September, 1974.

Case 2. N. K., a 27-year-old woman was admitted to the Center for Adult Diseases, in October 1975, with complaints of fever and petechiae in the breast and bilateral upper arms. An abnormal blood count was found one month before the admission. Physical examination disclosed no abnormalities except for the presence of petechiae in the breast. The hematocrit was 28%; the white cell count was 6,300/mm³ with 40% leukemic myeloblasts, 25% neutrophils, and 21% lymphocytes. The platelet count was 33,000/mm³. A bone marrow aspiration revealed hypercellularity with 51% leukemic myeloblasts. A diagnosis of acute myelogenous leukemia was made and the patient received 2 courses of combination chemotherapy (daunorubicin, cytosine arabinoside, 6-mercaptopurine, and betamethasone) which led to complete remission of the disease. As maintenance chemotherapy 6-mercaptopurine was administered, and the patient was discharged in December 1975.

Both patients showed a similar course after the induction of complete remission (Figs. 1 and 2). Since acute hepatitis developed 3 months (case 1) and 2 months (case 2) after discharge, the maintenance chemotherapy was discontinued and immunotherapy with BCG-CWS and PS-K (a polysaccharide isolated from *Coriolus versicolor* of the Polyporaceae family of Basidiomycetes) was instituted. In March 1976 (case 1) and in February 1976 (case 2), leukemic cells (2 to 7 per 5,000 leukocytes) were found consistently for several weeks in the peripheral blood by 5,000 differential. Auer rods were noted occasionally in the leukemic cells of case 1 (Fig. 3). Accordingly, BCG-CWS

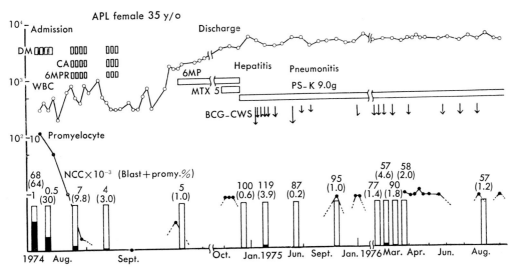

FIG. 1. Clinical course of case 1 (F.N.)

WBC, the white cell count; promyelocyte, the number of leukemic promyelocytes per mm³; DM, daunorubicin; CA, cytosine arabinoside, 6MPR, 6-mercaptopurine riboside; NCC, nucleated marrow cell count; 6MP, 6-mercaptopurine; MTX, methotrexate. Numbers show nucleated marrow cell counts. Numbers in parentheses indicate the percentage of myeloblasts and promyelocytes in marrow aspirates (shown as shaded areas in the bar graph).

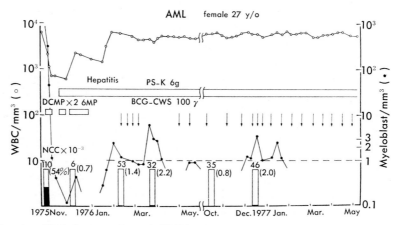

Fig. 2. Clinical course of case 2 (N.K.)
  DCMP: combination chemotherapy (daunorubicin, cytosine arabinoside, 6-mercap-
topurine, and betamethasone).

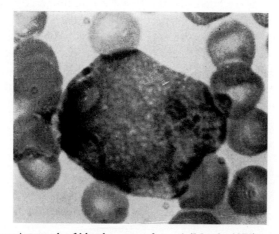

Fig. 3. Photomicrograph of blood smears of case 1 (March, 1976)
  Cells were collected by means of the leucoconcentration technique. Note the Auer
rod. May-Grünwald-Giemsa stain. ×1,000.

was administered to both cases once a week for a period of 3 weeks. In both cases, the
number of leukemic cells decreased gradually from the blood. In December 1976,
however, a peripheral blood sample taken from case 2 showed a re-appearance of
leukemic cells (Fig. 2). BCG-CWS was again given once a week for a period of 3 weeks.
After several weeks, leukemic cells disappeared from the blood. Until December 1977,
they were treated every 2 or 3 weeks with an intradermal injection of BCG-CWS.
Up until the present, both patients are still in complete remission without any maintenance chemotherapy. In both patients, bone marrow aspiration revealed normal cellularity with less than 5% blast cells and the number of leukemic cells in the blood is
less than 1 per 5,000 leukocytes.
  In these two cases, the repeated injections of BCG-CWS resulted in disappearance
of leukemic cells from the blood. When the relapse was detected in its early stage by

means of the leucoconcentration technique, the number of leukemic cells present in the blood was roughly estimated to be in the range of 10^6 to 10^7 (Figs. 1 and 2). This result suggests that a short, intensive course of immunotherapy with BCG-CWS has an antitumor effect, at least when the number of leukemic cells is less than 10^7. With the development of immunopotentiating agents, immunotherapy will offer a relatively safe method for eradicating the residual leukemic cells.

ADDENDUM

Leucoconcentration Technique

We have shown that examinations of the cells in the blood of patients in remission by means of the leucoconcentration technique and 5,000 differential are very useful for early detection of relapse of the disease (5, 6). This technique was previously described in detail (4, 6). Briefly, peripheral blood (5 ml) was mixed with one-half volume of Haemacel (Hoechst) containing 10 units of heparin per milliliter. The mixture was allowed to stand at an angle of $45°$ at room temperature for approximately 20 min until almost all red blood cells had sedimented. The supernatant plasma containing leukocytes was collected and centrifuged at $80 \times g$ for 10 min. The packed cells are smeared on a glass slide and stained with May-Grünwald-Giemsa. The differential count of 5,000 cells in this smear is essentially the same as a routine differential count on the basis of 100 leukocytes.

Acknowledgment

We would like to thank Drs. Y. Yamamura and I. Azuma for supplying BCG-CWS.

REFERENCES

1. Gale, R. P. and Cline, M. J. High remission-induction rate in acute myeloid leukemia. *Lancet*, **i**, 497–499 (1977).
2. Glucksberg, H., Buckner, C. D., Fefer, A., DeMarsh, Q., Coleman, D., Dobrow, R. B., Huff, J., Kjobech, C., Hill, A. S., Dittman, W., Neiman, P. E., Cheever, M. A., Einstein, A. B., Jr., and Thomas, E. D. Combination chemotherapy for acute nonlymphoblastic leukemia in adults. *Cancer Chemother. Rep.*, **59**, 1131–1137 (1975).
3. Gutterman, J. U., Rodriguez, V., Mavligit, G., Burgess, M. A., Gehan, E., Hersh, E. M., McCredie, K. B., Reed, R., Smith, T., Bodey, G. P., and Freireich, E. J. Chemo-immunotherapy of adult acute leukemia. Prolongation of remission in myeloblastic leukemia with BCG. *Lancet*, **ii**, 1405–1409 (1974).
4. Hiura, M., Nose, T., Fukuda, H., and Yoshitake, J. Leucoconcentration technique. *Seijin Byo (Adult Diseases)*, **16**, 58–69 (1976) (in Japanese).
5. Masaoka, T. Supportive therapy of acute leukemia. *In* "Ketsueki Sikkan no Sinpo (Recent Advances in Hematology)," ed. by F. Takaku, Kanehara Shuppan, Tokyo, pp. 228–234 (1978) (in Japanese).
6. Masaoka, T., Hasegawa, Y., Tatsumi, N., Yoshitake, J., Ueda, T., Takubo, T., Shibata, H., Nakamura, H., and Senda, N. On the analysis of decrease curve of leukemic cells during treatment of acute leukemia. *Acta Haematol. Japon.*, **39**, 1–10 (1976)
7. Mathé, G. Active immunotherapy. *Adv. Cancer Res.*, **14**, 1–36 (1971).
8. Mathé, G., Pouillart, P., and Lapeyraque, F. Active immunotherapy of L1210 leukemia applied after the graft of tumor cells. *Br. J. Cancer*, **23**, 814–824 (1969).

9. Mathé, G., Schwarzenberg, L., Delgado, M., and De Vassal, F. Active immunotherapy trials on acute lymphoid leukemia, lymphosarcoma and acute myeloid leukemia. *Eur. J. Cancer*, **13**, 445–455 (1977).

10. Mathé, G., Schwarzenberg, L., Mery, A. M., Cattan, A., Schneider, M., Amiel, J. L., Schlumberger, J. R., Poisson, L., and Wajcner, G. Extensive histological and cytological survey of patients with acute leukemia in "complete remission." *Br. Med. J.*, **1**, 640–642 (1966).

11. Olsson, L., Florentin, I., Kiger, N., and Mathé, G. Cellular and humoral immunity to leukemia cells in BCG-induced growth control of a murine leukemia. *J. Natl. Cancer Inst.*, **59**, 1297–1306 (1977).

12. Powles, R. L., Russell, J., Lister, T. A., Oliver, T., Whitehouse, J.M.A., Malpas, J., Chapuis, B., Crowther, D., and Alexander, P. Immunotherapy for acute myelogenous leukemia: A controlled clinical study 2 1/2 years after entry of the last patient. *Br. J. Cancer*, **35**, 265–272 (1977).

13. Skipper, H. E., Schabel, F. M., Jr., and Wilcox, W. S. Experimental evaluation of potential anticancer agents. XIII. On the criteria and kinetics associated with the "curability" of experimental leukemia. *Cancer Chemother. Rep.*, **35**, 1–111 (1964).

14. Vogler, W. R. and Chan, Y. K. Prolonging remission in myeloblastic leukemia by Tice-strain Bacillus Calmette-Guérin. *Lancet*, **ii**, 128–131 (1974).

15. Whiteside, M. G., Cauchi, M. N., Paton, C., and Stone, J. Chemoimmunotherapy for maintenance in acute myeloblastic leukemia. *Cancer*, **38**, 1581–1586 (1976).

CLINICAL TRIALS. IV. IMMUNOTHERAPY OF MALIGNANT MELANOMA

GANN Monograph on Cancer Research 21, 1978

IMMUNOCHEMOTHERAPY OF MALIGNANT MELANOMA WITH BCG CELL-WALL SKELETON

Masao Oguro,*1 Toshiyuki Takagi,*1 Hisashi Majima,*1 and Kimiko Ishiguro*2

*Division of Hematology and Chemotherapy, Chiba Cancer Center Hospital,*1 *and Division of Chemotherapy, Chiba Cancer Center Research Institute*2

Eight patients with malignant melanoma were treated by immuno-chemotherapy (chemotherapy with BCG cell-wall skeleton (BCG-CWS)) and followed up for 46 months. Two out of 8 cases with malignant melanoma received intralesional BCG-CWS injection with complete regression of the injected sites and showed regression of distal metastasis in one. One case received cryosurgery which suggested immunological response and revealed partial regression.

The indication and limitation of immunotherapy, and relationship between various immunological parameters and prognosis of malignant melanoma are discussed.

Since the report of Foley (2) in 1953, tumor immunology has developed rapidly. By the progress of these experimental studies, the possibility of human tumor immunotherapy was strongly considered. Hence, various trials of human immunotherapy have been performed in many types of human neoplasm. Among these neoplasms, malignant melanoma was indicated as the most suitable tumor for the subject of immunotherapy for the following reasons: (1) Malignant melanoma showed spontaneous regression which was a higher rate when compared with those of other malignant tumors (5), (2) antimelanoma antibodies were observed in sera from patients with malignant melanoma, (6) and (3) melanoma-specific antibody titers were closely related to extension of the disease (7). These three factors led us to the conclusion that theoretically potentiation of tumor-specific antibodies probably causes suppression of the tumor growth as a final cure by means of immunotherapy.

In general, there are two types of immunotherapy, active and passive. BCG is widely used as an active immunotherapeutic agent. However, BCG itself has variable potency and gives side effects (8) such as fever, allergic reaction, and liver damage. Therefore, Azuma et al. (3) produced BCG cell-wall skeleton (BCG-CWS) which had some of the potency of BCG as an immunotherapeutic agent (9), yet had less side effects. We used BCG-CWS for immunopotentiation therapy.

Antitumor Effects of BCG-CWS

Yamamura et al. (10) showed that BCG-CWS is an antitumor immunopotentiator against malignant melanoma. We treated 8 cases of malignant melanoma (Table I).

---

*1, *2 Nitona-cho 666-2, Chiba 280, Japan (小黒昌夫, 高木敏之, 馬島 尚, 石黒公子).

TABLE I. Clinical Data and Treatment of Patients with Malignant Melanoma

Name	Age (yr.) sex	Primary location	Stage	Spread of disease before BCG-CWS (after BCG-CWS)	Previous treatment (with BCG-CWS)	BCG-CWS method / total dose / dose (μg) / (μg)	Effect survived months (death)
T. M.	63 M	L-gum	III	L-neck nodes Liver · lung ↓ (Brain)	Radiation 5-FU (DTIC)	i.c. 400 / 1,200	None (10)
K. T.	65 F	R-foot	III	Generalized ↓ (No change)	Surgery (ACNU)	i.c. 200 / 1,000	None (11)
G. E.	48 M	Back	III	R-supraclavicular L-femur ↓ (Generalized)	Surgery (Bleo)	i.c. 200 / 3,600	None (20)
N. O.	34 M	Lip	II	L-neck L-submandibular ↓ (Disappear)	Surgery VCR·Bleo· CCNU·DTIC (None)	i.t. 300–500 / 9,600 i.c. 200	Effective 46
S. S.	63 M	L-axilla	I	None ↓ (None)	Surgery (None)	i.c. 200 / 1,800	Disease-free 11
H. H.	64 M	R-thigh	I	None ↓ (None)	Surgery (None)	i.c. 200 / 2,000	Disease-free 10
M. T.	32 M	R-foot	II	R-inguinal nodes ↓ (No change)	None (ACNU·VCR) Cryosurgery	i.t. 600 / 2,200 i.c. 200	Effective 7
E. I.	54 M	R-axilla	I	None ↓ (None)	DTIC·ACNU· VCR Radiation (None)	i.c. 200 / 3,200	Local recurrence 11

5-FU, 5-fluorouracil; Bleo, bleomycin; i.c., intracutaneous injection; i.t., intratumor injection.

Two cases (cases N.O. and M.T.) who had received intralesional injections (300 μg) revealed regression of the tumor. Especially in case N.O., metastatic lesions of non-injected areas also revealed complete regression. Three ineffective cases belonged to a late stage III. Two other cases (S.S. and H.H.) belonged to stage I, had resection of the primary lesion, and received intracutaneously 200 μg BCG-CWS per 1–2 weeks for more than 10 months with disappearance of disease. The histological findings of tumors after intralesional injection of BCG-CWS revealed massive necrosis in the injected area surrounded by tubercle-like lesions.

By electron microscopic examination (Fig. 1), destruction of tumor cell membrane, changes of nuclear membrane, and swelling of mitochondria were observed, which suggested destruction of cells. The above findings suggested that immunotherapy with BCG-CWS was effective in early stages (stages I–II), but not in advanced stages.

Effect of BCG-CWS Therapy on Immunological Parameters

Morton et al. (7) reported usefulness of skin tests with purified protein derivative (PPD) and 1-chloro-2, 4-dinitrobenzene (DCNB) as immunological parameters in ef-

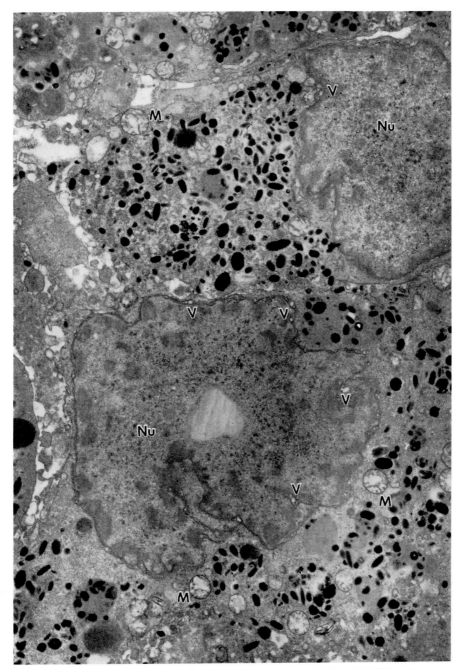

FIG. 1. Electron microscopic findings of melanoma cell in BCG-CWS injected melanoma nodule
  Nu, nucleus with low electron density; M, swelling mitochondria; V, tiny vacuoles in surrounding nuclear membrane.

TABLE II. Changes of Immunological Parameters in BCG-CWS Treatment

Name	PPD (+)	PPD (−)	DNCB (+)	DNCB (−)	Lymphocyte count	T cell	Blast formation (PHA)	Ig. G A M	Clinical course survived months (death)
T.M.	(+)			(−)	↘	↘	ND	↓ → →	Progressive (10)
K.T.	↘	↓	∧↘	↗	↘		↗↓ → →		Progressive (11)
G.E.	⇄			↘	↘	↗	↗	→ → →	Temporally arrested (20)
N.O.	↘	↓		↗	↘	↘		↓ → →	Arrested 46
S.S.	↓	↓		↗	↗	→		→ → →	Disease-free 11
H.H.	↘	↘		↗	↗	↘		→ → →	Disease-free 10
M.T.	↓	↓		↗	→	↘		→ → →	Arrested 7
E.I.	↓	↓		↗	↘	↗		↓ → ↑	Local recurrence 11

ND : not done.

fective cases. Theoretically, lymphocyte blast formation, T and B cell as cellular immunoparameters, should be evaluated in patients with immune reactions to the therapy. In our study, however, no clear correlation was observed (Table II). Even in patients who responded to BCG-CWS, these parameters revealed dissociation. Only in the case of absolute number of lymphocytes and a positive change of PPD skin test showed correlation in responding patients. These results may indicate that the so-called immunological parameters had no correlation with response of the patient.

BCG-CWS Therapy and Other Related Therapy

Since the ideal therapy of malignant melanoma is the combination of surgical removal of the primary lesion with wide resection of regional lymph nodes, immunotherapy may play an important role for eradication of any remaining minor metastasis. Cryosurgery has effects not only by freezing death of a local tumor, but also the immune response systemically is suggested (1). We tried cryosurgery on case M.T. This patient is under observation and the final result is not known at this time. As a chemotherapy of malignant melanoma, 5-(3, 3-dimethyl-1-triazeno) imidazole-4-carboxamide (DTIC), vincristine (VCR), and 1, 3-bis (2-chloroethyl)-1-nitrosourea (BCNU) combination was thought to be most effective (4). We treated case E.I. with 1-(4-amino-2-methyl-5-pyrimidinyl) methyl-3-(2-chloroethyl)-3-nitrosourea hydrochloride (ACNU), DTIC, and VCR, and this patient showed tumor regression. This patient was given maintenance therapy with BCG-CWS but the primary lesion relapsed 3 months later. However, no metastasis was noticed.

Another case (N.O.) had been treated with DTIC, VCR, and 1-(2-chloroethyl)-3-cyclohexyl-1-nitrosourea (CCNU), etc. (Fig. 2) and had a one-year remission. After

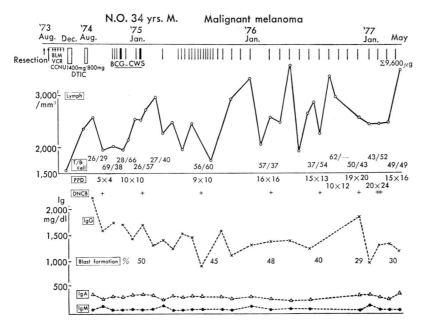

FIG. 2. Clinical course of a patient with malignant melanoma

relapse one year later, DTIC therapy had no response. Then, the patient had an intralesional injection of BCG-CWS with shrinkage or disappearance of metastatic lesions. The patient had over 46 months of survival with normal daily life. Based on these results, we concluded that BCG-CWS had a major role as an adjuvant therapy.

Side Effects of BCG-CWS

In the case of intracutaneous injection, ulceration of the local site and occasional fever (37–38°) were noted. In the case of intralesional injection, fever was observed for 2–3 days. No other side effects were noticed, except for occasional positive C-reactive protein (CRP) in laboratory examination. As a result of these observations, the side effects of BCG-CWS were considered to be mild and tolerable.

CONCLUSION

It is too early to evaluate the present status of immunotherapy because of short experience and shortage of appropriate parameters. Immunotherapy has more limited applications compared with those of other modalities, because it is only effective on a small number of tumor cells. For these reasons, immunotherapy has to be used only in appropriate periods.

The incidence of malignant melanoma is low in Japan and our experience is also limited. Thus we cannot draw conclusions on the effect of immunotherapy. Even so, BCG-CWS is one of the anticancer immunopotentiators and further accumulation of clinical experience is necessary.

REFERENCES

1. Albin, R. J. Immunological aspects of cryosurgery. Consideration of recent experimental and clinical developments. Their implication and indications for further study. *Low Temp. Med.*, **2**, 61–73 (1976).
2. Foley, E. J. Antigenic properties of methylcholanthrene induced tumors in mice of the strain of origin. *Cancer Res.*, **13**, 835–837 (1953).
3. Azuma, I., Taniyama, T., Hirao, F., and Yamamura, Y. Antitumor activity of cell-wall skeletons and peptidoglycolipids of mycobacteria and related microorganisms in mice and rabbits. *Gann*, **65**, 493–505 (1974).
4. Luce, J. K. Chemotherapy of melanoma. *Semin. Oncol.*, **2**, 179–185 (1975).
5. McGovern, V. J. Spontaneous regression of melanoma. *Pathology*, **7**, 91–99 (1975).
6. Morton, D. L., Malmgren, R. A., Homes, E. C., and Ketcham, A. S. Demonstration of antibodies against human malignant melanoma by immunofluorescence. *Surgery*, **64**, 233–240 (1968).
7. Morton, D. L., Eilber, F. R., Malmgren, R. A., and Wood, W. C. Immunological factors which influence response to immunotherapy in malignant melanoma. *Surgery*, **68**, 158–164 (1970).
8. Sparks, F. C., Silverstein, M. J., Hunt, J. S., Haskell, C. M., Pilch, Y. H., and Morton, D. L. Complications of BCG immunotherapy in patients with cancer, *N. Engl. J. Med.*, **289**, 827–830 (1973).
9. Yamamura, Y., Azuma, I., Taniyama, T., Ribi, E., and Zber, B. Suppression of tumor growth and regression of established tumor with oil-attached mycobacterial fractions. *Gann*, **65**, 179–181 (1974).
10. Yamamura, Y., Yoshizaki, K., Azuma, I., Yagura, T., and Watanabe, T. Immunotherapy of human malignant melanoma with oil-attached BCG cell-wall skeleton. *Gann*, **66**, 355–363 (1975).

IMMUNOTHERAPY OF MALIGNANT MELANOMA

Kazuyuki Ishihara and Ken-ichi Hayasaka

Department of Dermatology, National Cancer Center Hospital*

In continuation of studies on immunotherapy of human malignant melanoma using living BCG, BCG cell-wall skeleton (BCG-CWS), Picibanil (a streptococcal preparation), and a transfer factor, treatment using living BCG is described.

The treatment was given to 37 cases of malignant melanoma, by oral administration in 19 cases, intratumor injection in 10 cases, and intradermal injection in 8 cases. For oral administration, 80–160 mg was administered once a week; this was effective in 19 cases and slightly effective in 4 cases. Intratumor injection was effective in 7 out of 10 cases. Intradermal injection was effective in 2, and slightly effective in 1, out of 8 cases. Side effects were not observed after oral administration, but fever, anorexia, and/or an influenza-like syndrome were observed in many cases after intratumor or intradermal administration. Lymph node swelling and liver hypofunction were sometimes observed.

Cellular immunity (protein antigen of tubercle bacilli, dinitrochloro-benzene, lymphocyte blast transformation test, lymphocyte cytotoxicity test, *etc.*) during BCG therapy is also described.

Maligant melanoma is known to give an extremely unfavorable prognosis, especially in stages II and III. Radiotherapy or chemotherapy is so ineffective that only a fatal prognosis can be expected. On the other hand, maligant melanoma is one of the tumors having an immunity (*2*), and many reports have been published on its immunotherapy (*1, 3, 4*).

We have tried the use of living BCG, BCG cell-wall skeleton (BCG-CWS), PSK (a polysaccharide preparation), Picibanil (a streptococcal preparation), and Levamisole as immunotherapy of human malignant melanoma; 37 cases treated with living BCG are herein reported.

Mode of Administration

1) Oral administration

Ampules containing 40 or 80 mg of living BCG (Japan BCG Laboratory, Tokyo) (its 0.5 mg being equivalent to 2.0×10^7 cells) were used. The content of each ampule was dissolved in physiological saline or a suitable fluid and diluted to an appropriate volume with a beverage, such as fruit juice. The initial dosage was 40–80 mg, and a maximum, 160 mg. The administration was made once a week or once a fortnight according to the results of cell-mediated immunity testing.

---

* Tsukiji 5-1-1, Chuo-ku, Tokyo 104, Japan (石原和之, 早坂健一).

2) Intratumor injection

An ampule containing 5 mg of living BCG was used. The contents were dissolved in physiological saline to make the volume 1 ml and this volume was injected once a week or once a fortnight. The initial dosage was 0.5 mg and the maximum, 3 mg. After the tumor regressed, BCG was given by intracutaneous injection or orally.

3) Intracutaneous injection

Administration was made with the same materials as for intratumor injection. The initial dosage of 0.2–0.5 mg was injected intracutaneously in the inner part of the forearm. The dosage was augmented according to the intensity of response, to a maximum of 5 mg. For the first 3 months, the administration was made once every 2 or 3 weeks, and then once every 4 weeks thereafter.

Indicated Stage for BCG Immunotherapy

BCG immunotherapy was carried out for cases in stage II (regional lymph node involvement of primary basin only) and in stage III (disseminated spread) of malignant melanoma. Patients in stage II were mostly postoperative cases and those in stage III were all cases including postoperative cases.

Immunological Examination

In addition to the general clinical examinations, tests for cell-mediated immunity such as the skin test (2, 4-dinitrochlorobenzene (DNCB), protein antigen of tubercle bacilli (PPD)), lymphocyte blast transformation (LBT) test, lymphocyte cytotoxicity test (LCT), and T and B lymphocyte population test were carried out.

Criteria for Judgement

Results were compared with those of the control group which did not receive the BCG therapy. For cases in stage II, the therapy was considered as slightly effective when neither recurrence nor metastasis occurred 1 or 1.5 years after wide resection of the regional lymph node, and as effective if neither recurrence nor metastasis occurred for more than 1.5 years. For cases in stage III, the therapy was considered as effective when there was a complete or marked regression of the tumor, or when a patient has survived more than 1.5 years, and as slightly effective if a patient survives just 1.5 years.

Clinical Effect

1) Oral administration

The total of 19 cases treated with BCG therapy included 6 patients in stage II and 13 in stage III. The therapy was effective in 1 case, slightly effective in 2 cases, and ineffective in 3 cases in stage II. In 3 patients in whom the therapy was effective, a positive response and/or elevation in the response to both DNCB and PPD due to BCG therapy was observed.

For patients in stage III, the therapy was effective in 6 cases, slightly effective in 2 cases, and ineffective in 6 cases. Response to DNCB and PPD tests in this group was similar to the effective cases in stage II. Among 16 cases which showed a positive response and/or rise in the response to DNCB and PPD, an effective result was observed in 10 cases. The therapy had no effect in all the patients who showed a negative response.

2) Intratumor injection

This mode of administration was carried out on cases in stage III with skin metastasis. Among the 10 cases given this therapy it proved effective in 7 cases. The response to DNCB and PPD was elevated in 8 of 10 cases, while it remained negative in all ineffective cases, even after the treatment. A rise in LBT was observed in 3 cases, but the presence of such a function is important and a value above the standard would be no problem.

3) Intracutaneous injection

This mode of treatment was carried out on cases in stages II and III in which intratumor injection was impossible or the tumor was not observed clinically. Among 3 cases in stage II, the therapy was effective in 2 cases and ineffective in 1 case. Among 5 cases in stage III, the therapy was slightly effective in only 1 case, being ineffective in the remaining 4 cases.

Side Effects

A fever of 37–38° was observed in almost all the cases given intracutaneous or intratumor injection, but the fever subsided in 1 or 2 days. Some cases showed anorexia or an influenza-like syndrome. One case each of lymph node swelling and liver hypofunction were observed among 18 cases given intracutaneous or intratumor injection, but the symptoms became normal 3 weeks after discontinuation of BCG administration. In some cases, oral administration of 400 mg of isoniazid and intramuscular injection of streptomycin were given. Practically no side effects were observed after oral administration.

Relationship between Immune Response and Therapeutic Effect (Table I)

Changes in cell-mediated immunity play an important part in immunotherapy; one cannot expect a favorable effect for cases without immune responses, although this does not hold for cases which show positive results from the beginning. Among the total of 37 cases given BCG therapy, 14 cases showed positive responses to both DNCB and PPD before the treatment and 11 of these cases showed some effect from this treatment. For 8 cases which showed a positive reaction to either DNCB or PPD and which became positive to both tests after BCG therapy, the treatment was effective in 6 cases. The treatment was also effective in 2 of 4 cases in which the response was negative to both PPD and DNCB before the treatment, but became positive after the treatment. In contrast, the treatment was ineffective in 7 cases with a negative response to both PPD and DNCB even after treatment.

TABLE I. Relationship between Immune Responses and Therapeutic Effect

Admin. route	No. of cases	Before treatment		After treatment		PHA		Effect			
		PPD	DNCB	PPD	DNCB	Ele-vate	No change	+	±	−	Un-known
Oral (19 cases)	4	+	+	++	++	2	2	1	2	1	
	3	+	+	+	+	1	2	1	1	1	
	3	−	+	+	+	2	1	2		1	
	2	−	+	−	+	1	1	1		1	
	2	−	−	+	+	0	2	1		1	
	2	−	−	−	+	0	1		1	1	
	3	−	−	−	−	0	3			3	
Intra-tumor (10 cases)	4	+	+	++	++	2	2	4			
	2	−	+	+	+	1	1	2			
	2	−	−	+	+	0	2	1		1	
	2	−	−	−	−	0	2			2	
Intra-cutaneous (8 cases)	3	+	+	+	+	0	3		1	1	1
	3	−	+	+	+	1	2	1		1	1
	2	−	−	−	−	0	2			2	

PHA: phytohemagglutinin.

These facts seem to suggest that it is important to raise the cell-mediated immunity and to maintain it in the treatment of malignant melanoma. In addition, since all the cases of malignant melanoma treated by living BCG reported here had been proved insensitive to various treatment trials, a more effective immunotherapy should be developed with improvement in therapeutic procedures.

CONCLUSION

Although judgement of the effect of immunotherapy is rather difficult, the present series of treatments with living BCG has shown that the treatment can be evaluated by examining the host's cell-mediated immunity. A therapeutic effect cannot be expected in cases which do not respond by a rise in immune response. Combined use of chemotherapy naturally should be considered, but it would have to be assessed individually.

Acknowledgment

We thank Prof. Yuichi Yamamura of Osaka University for kindly supplying us with BCG-CWS.

REFERENCES

1. Gutterman, J. V., Mavligit, G., McBride, C., Frei, E., III, Freireich, E. J., and Hersh, E. M. Active immunotherapy with B.C.G. for recurrent malignant melanoma. *Lancet*, i, 1208–1212 (1973).
2. Ishihara, K. Cell-mediated immunity of malignant melanoma. *Japan. J. Dermatol., Ser. B*, **74**, 696–698 (1975).

3. Ishihara, K. Immunity of malignant melanoma. *In* "Human Cancer and Immunity," ed. by G. Fujii *et al.*, Life Science, Tokyo, pp. 346–349 (1976) (in Japanese).

4. Tanaka, T. Immunotherapy of cancer with living BCG. *In* "Human Cancer and Immunity," ed. by G. Fujii *et al.*, Life Science, Tokyo, pp. 238–252 (1976) (in Japanese).

SUMMARY REMARKS

PRESENT STATUS AND FUTURE DIRECTIONS FOR CANCER IMMUNOTHERAPY

William D. Terry

Immunology Branch, Division of Cancer Biology and Diagnosis,
*National Cancer Institute**

In the past decade, the possible application of immunologic techniques and manipulations to the diagnosis and treatment of cancer has received a great deal of attention from physicians, patients with cancer, and the public press. Claims for new vaccines or other immunotherapies are announced in the newspaper almost as frequently as the *shinkansen* (bullet train) departs from Osaka to Tokyo. The difference is that the *shinkansen* almost always gets there, and on time, while the new immunotherapies seem to run into trouble as soon as they leave the station and frequently disappear before they reach the next one.

It is reasonable for anyone viewing the great excitement about immunology and cancer to assume that this is a newly discovered relationship. To put this in perspective, we must consider this quotation: "The chief objective of all studies upon immunity against cancer is, naturally, the finding of some means by which this fearful disease in human beings may be successfully combatted" (2). This quote is brought to your attention not because it is particularly informative but because it comes from an article published by Drs. Coca and Gilman in *Phillip. J. Sci.* in 1909. Tumor immunology, and specifically, immunotherapy was being pursued by physicians in Germany in the 1880's, so this is certainly a field with a significant history. In order to consider the present status and future directions of immunotherapy, it is useful to consider some of its historical origins.

Brief History of Immunotherapy

In 1891, William Coley published a paper concerning a patient with recurrent sarcoma who developed erysipelas right on the surface of the tumor (3). Not only did the patient survive this severe and frequently fatal streptococcal infection, but, in addition, his tumor became necrotic and regressed completely. Coley discovered several similar cases in the literature and reasoned that if "naturally" occurring streptococcal infections of tumors could lead to regression, perhaps intentional infections would cause the same effect. He therefore began injecting streptococci into tumors and indeed found that a few of these tumors responded with remarkable regressions. For various reasons, Coley concluded that the effective agent was probably not the streptococcus, but rather some bacterial product and he began to use bacteria-free filtrates, at first derived only from streptococci, subsequently from mixtures of bacteria. These became known as Coley's mixed bacterial toxins or Coley's toxins, and they were used by Coley and others for a number of years before they became unfashionable.

---

* Bethesda, Maryland 20014, U.S.A.

Some 50 years later, another clinical observation led to renewed interest in immunotherapy. Edmund Klein was treating skin cancers with topical chemotherapy. He noted that those patients who became allergic to the chemotherapy and gave delayed hypersensitivity reactions in the areas of treatment had much more tumor regression than did patients who were not allergic. Klein began to intentionally sensitize patients to chemicals, such as dinitrochlorobenzene, and then applied the chemical on their skin cancers. With a number of skin cancers, Klein showed that delayed hypersensitivity reactions could make tumors regress (8).

At about the same time, Mathé began some trials of immunotherapy in children with leukemia (11), Morton began to inject BCG into melanoma lesions (12), and the modern era of immunotherapy had been launched.

Evaluation of Current Immunotherapy

In the past 15 years, a number of agents have been studied for effectiveness against a variety of human tumors. I will briefly review those studies that have already provided statistically evaluable results that give some promise of leading to useful treatments. A general framework in which to consider immunotherapy is shown in Table I. Active immunotherapy implies that the patient is being stimulated and his own immune elements are expected to respond. In adoptive or passive immunotherapy, the patient is supplied with immune elements he appears to lack, or that are functionally depressed. The term "nonspecific" is meant to imply that the agent is stimulating immune activity not only against the tumor but also against anything immunogenic. Specific implies that the agent or treatment has immunologic specificity for the tumor.

TABLE I.   General Framework of Immunotherapy

I. Active immunotherapy
    A. Nonspecific stimulation
       1. BCG, BCG extracts (*e.g.*, MER), and BCG fractions (*e.g.*, cell-wall skeleton)
       2. *Corynebacterium parvum (C. parvum)*
       3. Other bacterial and viral vaccines
       4. Chemical immunostimulants
    B. Specific immunization
       1. Native autologous or allogeneic tumor cells or cell membrane extracts
       2. Chemically or enzymically modified tumor cells or cell membrane extracts
II. Adoptive or passive immunotherapy
    A. Nonspecific
       1. Thymosin
    B. Specific
       1. Transfer factor
       2. Immune RNA
       3. Antibodies

1) BCG
a) Intralesional BCG in malignant melanoma metastatic to skin
Numbers of studies have shown that the injection of living BCG organisms into

melanoma skin metastases leads to eradication of the injected tumor deposits. This work is, in a sense, a direct extension of the experiments of Coley and Klein. Occasionally an uninjected skin lesion will regress and very rarely a visceral metastasis will regress. The usual finding, however, is that this is local treatment having an effect only on injected nodules, and that systemic disease progresses while local disease is controlled or cured. It is alleged that patients with disease limited to the skin survive longer as a result of intralesional therapy, but there has not yet been a study to critically test this clinical impression. Until such a study is performed, intralesional therapy must be considered local therapy not known to be superior to surgery or other local forms of treatment in terms of patient survival.

b) Intrapleural BCG in lung cancer

McKneally and colleagues have explored the effect of placing living BCG organisms into the pleural space following surgery for bronchogenic carcinoma (*10*). In a prospective study, patients have been randomized to receive BCG postoperatively, followed after 2 weeks with a 3-month course of isoniazid, or to receive postoperative isoniazid alone. Patients with stage I disease have shown significant prolongation of remission and survival apparently as a result of the intrapleural BCG. Although this has been a well-planned, randomized trial, only a relatively small number of patients has been treated. A large scale, multi-institutional study will be carried out to determine whether this result can again be obtained and an answer should be available within the next 1.5–2 years.

It should also be noted that related preliminary trials using fractions of the BCG organism intrapleurally have been carried out in Japan (*21*) and that a randomized, controlled trial of these fractions in lung cancer has now been initiated. It will be most interesting in the future to compare the results obtained with BCG to those obtained with BCG fractions.

c) Systemic BCG in adult acute myelogenous leukemia (AML)

Multiple studies have suggested that the systemic use of BCG in conjunction with chemotherapy in AML leads to prolongation of survival (*6, 16, 19*). Results of those studies utilizing contemporaneous controls lead to the conclusion that although survival was somewhat prolonged, remission duration did not change, suggesting that the use of BCG prolonged survival after relapse.

All other trials using BCG fall into one of three categories: i) Trials have been completed and they are negative, ii) trials are in progress and therefore cannot yet be evaluated, and iii) trials are either complete or in progress, but have such faulty design that they will never be interpretable. Unfortunately, far too many trials of immunotherapy fall into this category.

2) Agents related to BCG

A number of BCG fractions, such as cell walls, cell-wall skeletons, and cord factor, as well as BCG extracts, such as the methanol-extracted residue (MER) are being assessed for clinical efficacy. There is preliminary evidence that the addition of MER to chemotherapy may increase the number of patients achieving complete remission in adult AML (*4*). All other trials of MER or BCG fractions are as yet inevaluable.

3) *Corynebacterium parvum*

a) *Systemic C. parvum in advanced breast cancer*

In this trial, patients with advanced breast cancer are randomly assigned to treatment with chemotherapy (cytoxan, adriamycin, methotrexate, and 5-fluorouracil) or the same chemotherapy plus weekly subcutaneous injections of *C. parvum* (15). There is no difference between the two groups in response rate, duration of response, or survival. If, however, only those patients who do respond with tumor regression are compared to those patients who respond to chemotherapy plus *C. parvum*, the responders to immunochemotherapy survive significantly longer than do those responding to chemotherapy alone. The numbers of patients in this study are quite small and it will be important to repeat this trial.

Intravenous administration of *C. parvum* is being investigated, but these studies, as well as others using subcutaneous *C. parvum*, are not evaluable at present.

4) *Other bacterial and viral vaccines*

Other bacteria, such as *Pseudomonas* and *Mycobacterium tuberculosis*, and viruses such as smallpox, are being used as attempted treatments for human cancer but as yet, none of these investigations are evaluable.

5) *Chemical immunostimulants*

The antihelminthic, levamisole, apparently has some immunostimulatory effect and has been assessed for usefulness in cancer patients.

a) *Levamisole in advanced breast cancer*

Patients with unresectable breast cancer were treated with radiotherapy alone or radiotherapy plus levamisole (17). Survival has been significantly prolonged in those patients receiving levamisole. Again, this conclusion is based on the treatment of relatively few patients, and a more extensive study of this combined treatment would be desirable.

b) *Levamisole in lung cancer*

Patients with resectable lung cancer are randomly assigned to receive levamisole for 3 days before surgery and then every 2 weeks for 2 years after surgery, or to receive a placebo (1). Analysis of this study shows no difference between treatment and control groups. However, if only those patients weighing less than 70 kg are considered, there is significant prolongation of disease-free survival in those receiving levamisole. Since all patients received the same total dose of levamisole, it is postulated that there may be a dose effect and that only patients under 70 kg received an adequate quantity of levamisole.

Many other studies are in progress, but they are not evaluable at this time.

6) *Specific immunization*

Numerous trials of specific immunization with unmodified (13) or modified (7) tumor cells are in progress, but data are not yet evaluable.

7) *Adoptive or passive immunotherapy*

Clinical trials utilizing transfer factor (9), immune RNA (14), and antibodies (20) are in progress but data are not yet evaluable. The use of hormone or hormones derived from the thymus and referred to as thymosin or thymopoetin is beginning to be evaluated in cancer patients (5).

The Future of Immunotherapy

While the results of the first 15 years of modern immunotherapy may appear to be meager, they are quite significant and point the way to our future efforts.

In the first place, it must be clear that clinical immunotherapy has thus far taken advantage of only a small part of the potential of the immune system to interact with tumors. Considerable additional basic research into such areas as the role of suppressor cells, the nature of tumor antigens, the possibility of making tumor cells more immunogenic and dozens of other problems that appear to control the host response to tumors must be pursued. This will require continued fundamental investigations into the immune system itself and the nature of regulation and control of immune responses in the general sense, until we fully comprehend the complexities and interactions of this system.

At the same time we must study the ways in which tumors interact with and influence the function of the immune system. With this information in hand, we will be able to design more sophisticated immunotherapies, first in the preclinical, and then in the clinical setting. As a major portion of this task, we will have to discover or create animal tumors that are biologically analogous to human tumors and that will be predictive of the effects seen when immunologic manipulations are tried in man.

Once we have such models and we have some effective immunotherapies, we must find laboratory tests the results of which correlate well with the results of treatment. We do not have sensitive indicators of whether or not our treatment is having the desired effect; and in preclinical and clinical trials, we have only the crude indicators of tumor recurrence or death. The development of appropriate laboratory tests will almost surely require more knowledge of the biology of tumors, the effect of immunotherapeutic agents on the immune system and the mechanism whereby this is converted into effective antitumor activity.

In the clinic, we have a fairly clear agenda. We must carry out large-scale, well-designed trials in an attempt to reproduce positive effects seen in preliminary trials. Once we have convinced ourselves that the results are real, we must attempt to understand the mechanisms by which the results have been obtained. For example, it appears that BCG really does cause a slight prolongation of survival in AML. Unfortunately, however, we are in the position of the man drinking from the Sake bottle. He knows that as the Sake bottle gets lighter, his legs get heavier, but he is not sure why. We must understand what is happening, so that we can build on these observations and make them more significant and more broadly applicable. The comments about the need for predictive laboratory tests bear repeating. Progress in the clinic will be painfully slow until we have laboratory tests useful for monitoring treatment.

We will have to use immunotherapy earlier in the course of treatment and earlier in the course of the disease. Almost all animal experiments indicate that an immunotherapeutic manipulation that is curative "early" in the disease is useless "late" in the disease. One attempt to use "early" immunotherapy is the trial being conducted by Rosenberg (18) in primary melanoma patients with no clinical evidence of dissemination (clinical stage I). Primary lesions are hemisected and half of the lesion used to determine the diagnosis and the level of invasion. Patients are then randomized to have conventional treatment (wide surgical excision) or immunotherapy with intralesional BCG, followed 2 weeks later by conventional surgery. There are no evaluable results from this treatment yet, but this illustrates a way in which immunotherapy can be tested for effect early in cancer treatment.

We must identify the active components in such organisms as BCG and learn how to use these components in place of the organisms. The work being done in Osaka by Professor Yamamura and Dr. Azuma in analyzing the chemical nature of active components is of critical importance in providing the next generation of immuno-therapeutic agents. We must keep abreast of advances in basic immunology and seek ways to apply in the clinic newly available information about the immune system.

Finally, we must be sure that what we do in the clinic produces significant information. General medicine is filled with examples of treatments based not on fact, but on clinical impressions. Many of these treatments are worthless. In cancer medicine, we need look no further than the surgical treatment of breast cancer where for decades the treatment of choice was based on the clinical impression that more radical surgery was beneficial to the patient. Careful study of this matter does not appear to support this time-honored clinical impression.

The lesson as far as immunotherapy is concerned is that we must not uncritically accept "exciting preliminary results" or studies showing "no significant difference but with strong trends," or studies that are poorly controlled, or not controlled at all. There are examples of "positive" immunotherapy trials that become "negative" immunotherapy trials when repeated with a randomized control group. The use of randomization can create many difficulties in dealing with patients, and it takes much longer to acquire enough patients to achieve an evaluable result. But when that trial is completed, we know with reasonable certainty whether the test treatment was better than the control treatment. It is only by acquiring this type of information that the field of immunotherapy will be able to create a firm foundation and then build a series of effective treatments.

In conclusion, my assessment is that all of current immunotherapy is experimental, and that there is no example of an immunotherapeutic treatment that can be recommended as the treatment of choice for any cancer. There are numerous interesting observations and, 2 years from now, we will know whether some of these observations can be converted into routine treatments. The real future of immunotherapy is impossible to predict. It is my speculation that in 5 to 10 years some forms of immunotherapy will play a significant role in the treatment of some cancers, either alone or in combination with other forms of cancer therapy. Converting that speculation into reality will take considerable intelligence, hard work, and a certain amount of good luck.

REFERENCES

1. Amery, W. K. A placebo-controlled levamisole study in resectable lung cancer. *In* "Immunotherapy of Cancer: Present Status of Trials in Man," ed. by W. D. Terry and D. B. Windhorst, Raven Press, New York, pp. 191–201 (1978).

2. Coca, A. F. and Gilman, P. K. The specific treatment of carcinoma. *Phillip. J. Sci.* (*Med. Sci.*), **4**, 391–402 (1909).

3. Coley, W. B. Contributions to the knowledge of sarcoma. *Ann. Surg.*, **14**, 199–220 (1891).

4. Cuttner, J., Glidewell, O., and Holland, J. F. Chemoimmunotherapy of acute myelocytic leukemia with MER. *In* "Immunotherapy of Cancer: Present Status of Trials in Man," ed. by W. D. Terry and D. B. Windhorst, Raven Press, New York, pp. 405–413 (1978).

5. Goldstein, A. L., Cohen, G. H., Rossio, J. L., Thurman, G. B., Brown, C. N., and Ulrich, J. T. Use of thymosin in the treatment of primary immunodeficiency diseases and cancer. *Med. Clin. North Am.*, **60**, 591–606 (1976).

6. Gutterman, J. U., Hersh, E. M., Rodriguez, V., McCredie, K. B., Mavligit, G., Reed, R., Burgess, M. G., Smith, T., Gehan, E., Bodey, G. P., Sr., and Frierich, E. J. Chemoimmunotherapy of adult acute leukemia: Prolongation of remission in myeloblastic leukemia with BCG. *Lancet*, **ii**, 1405–1409 (1974).

7. Holland, J. F. and Bekesi, J. G. Immunotherapy of human leukemia with neuraminidase-modified cells. *Med. Clin. North Am.*, **60**, 539–549 (1976).

8. Klein, E., Holtermann, O., Milgrom, H. G., Case, R. W., Klein, D., Rosner, D., and Djerassi, I. Immunotherapy for accessible tumors utilizing delayed hypersensitivity reactions and separated components of the immune system. *Med. Clin. North Am.*, **60**, 389–418 (1976).

9. LoBuglio, A. F. and Neidhart, J. A. Transfer factor—A potential agent for cancer therapy. *Med. Clin. North Am.*, **60**, 585–590 (1976).

10. McKneally, M. G., Maver, C., and Kausel, H. W. Regional immunotherapy of lung cancer with intrapleural BCG. *Lancet*, **i**, 377–379 (1976).

11. Mathé, G., Schwarzenberg, L., De Vassal, G., Delgado, M., Pena-Angulo, J., Belpomme, E., Pouillart, P., Machover, D., Misset, J. L., Pico, J. L., Jasmin, C., Hayat, M., Schneider, M., Cattan, A., Amiel, J. L., Musset, M., and Rosenfeld, C. Chemotherapy followed by active immunotherapy (A.I.) in the treatment of acute lymphoid leukemias (A.L.L.) for patients of all ages. *In* "Immunotherapy of Cancer: Present Status of Trials in Man," ed. by W. D. Terry and D. B. Windhorst, Raven Press, New York, pp. 451–469 (1978).

12. Morton, D. K., Eilber, F. R., Holmes, E. C., Sparks, F. C., and Ramming, K. BCG immunotherapy as a systemic adjunct to surgery in malignant melanoma. *Med. Clin. North Am.*, **60**, 431–439 (1976).

13. Morton, D. L., Holmes, E. C., Eilber, F. R., Sparks, F. C., and Ramming, K. P. Adjuvant immunotherapy of malignant melanoma: Preliminary results of a randomized trial in patients with lymph node metastases. *In* "Immunotherapy of Cancer: Present Status of Trials in Man," ed. by W. D. Terry and D. B. Windhorst, Raven Press, New York, pp. 57–64 (1978).

14. Pilch, Y. H., Ramming, K. P., and deKernion, J. B. Clinical trials of immune RNA in the immunotherapy of cancer. *In* "Immunotherapy of Cancer: Present Status of Trials in Man," ed. by W. D. Terry and D. B. Windhorst, Raven Press, New York, pp. 539–556 (1978).

15. Pinsky, C. M., DeJager, R. L., Wittes, R. E., Wong, P. P., Kaufman, R. J., Mike, V., Hansen, J. A., Oettgen, H. F., and Krakoff, I. H. *Corynebacterium parvum* as adjuvant to combination chemotherapy in patients with advanced breast cancer. *In* "Immunotherapy of Cancer: Present Status of Trials in Man," ed. by W. D. Terry and D. B. Windhorst, Raven Press, New York, pp. 647–654 (1978).

16. Powles, R. L., Russell, J., Lister, T. A., Oliver, T., Whitehouse, J.M.A., Malpas, J.,

Chapuis, B., Crowther, D., and Alexander, P. Immunotherapy for acute myelogenous leukaemia: Analysis of a controlled clinical study 2-1/2 years after entry of the last patient. *In* "Immunotherapy of Cancer: Present Status of Trials in Man," ed. by W. D. Terry and D. B. Windhorst, Raven Press, New York, pp. 315–327 (1978).

17. Rojas, A. F., Feierstein, J. N., Glait, H. M., and Olivari, A. J. Levamisole action in breast cancer stage III. *In* "Immunotherapy of Cancer: Present Status of Trials in Man," ed. by W. D. Terry and D. B. Windhorst, Raven Press, New York, pp. 635–645 (1978).

18. Rosenberg, S. A. and Rapp, H. J. Intralesional immunotherapy of melanoma with BCG. *Med. Clin. North Am.*, **60**, 419–430 (1976).

19. Vogler, W. R., Bartolucci, A. A., Omura, G. A., Miller, D., Smalley, R. V., Knospe, W. H., and Goldsmith, A. S. A randomized clinical trial of BCG in myeloblastic leukemia conducted by the Southeastern Cancer Study Group. *In* "Immunotherapy of Cancer: Present Status of Trials in Man," ed. by W. D. Terry and D. B. Windhorst, Raven Press, New York, pp. 365–373 (1978).

20. Wright, P. W., Hellstrom, K. E., Hellstrom, I., Warner, G., Prentice, R., and Jones, R. F. Serotherapy of malignant melanoma. *In* "Immunotherapy of Cancer: Present Status of Trials in Man," ed. by W. D. Terry and D. B. Windhorst, Raven Press, New York, pp. 135–148 (1978).

21. Yamamura, Y. Immunotherapy of lung cancer with oil-attached cell-wall skeleton of BCG. *In* "Immunotherapy of Cancer: Present Status of Trials in Man," ed. by W. D. Terry and D. B. Windhorst, Raven Press, New York, pp. 173–179 (1978).

SUBJECT INDEX